# Asian Perspectives on Public Health

This book series aims to foster the multiple perspectives and dimensions of Public Health and welcomes a diversity of theories, interpretations, and experiences by academics and practitioners from various disciplinary backgrounds. It encompasses public health topics that promote and protect the safety and improvement of the health of communities through education, policymaking, and research for disease and injury prevention. The series engages with an increasingly interdisciplinary field drawing extensively on the natural and social sciences and the humanities. It welcomes and explores new methods that offer new insights into how systems and infrastructure influence population health, such as network analysis and practice-based research networks. Another new engagement area will be social epidemiology, including life course epidemiology. The series welcomes contributions from psychologists, sociologists, demographers, anthropologists, and biologists in this realm. It also welcomes monographs and edited volumes on a wide field of health impacts of human-caused disruptions of Earth's natural systems, including Planetary Health, One Health, Eco-Health, and Conservation Medicine.

Pradip Chouhan · Kailash Chandra Das ·
Avijit Roy · Nanigopal Kapasia ·
Margubur Rahaman · Jayanta Das
Editors

# Women's Health Dynamics in South Asia

## Perspectives, Challenges, and Innovations

Springer

*Editors*
Pradip Chouhan
Department of Geography
University of Gour Banga
Malda, West Bengal, India

Avijit Roy
Department of Geography
Malda College
Malda, West Bengal, India

Margubur Rahaman
Department of Migration and Urban Studies
International Institute for Population Sciences (IIPS)
Mumbai, Maharashtra, India

Kailash Chandra Das
Department of Migration and Urban Studies
International Institute for Population Sciences (IIPS)
Mumbai, Maharashtra, India

Nanigopal Kapasia
Department of Geography
Malda College
Malda, West Bengal, India

Jayanta Das
Department of Geography
Rampurhat College
Rampurhat, West Bengal, India

ISSN 2731-7242 ISSN 2731-7250 (electronic)
Asian Perspectives on Public Health
ISBN 978-981-95-2320-7 ISBN 978-981-95-2321-4 (eBook)
https://doi.org/10.1007/978-981-95-2321-4



This Springer imprint is published by the registered company Springer Nature Singapore Pte Ltd.
The registered company address is: 152 Beach Road, #21-01/04 Gateway East, Singapore 189721, Singapore

# Foreword

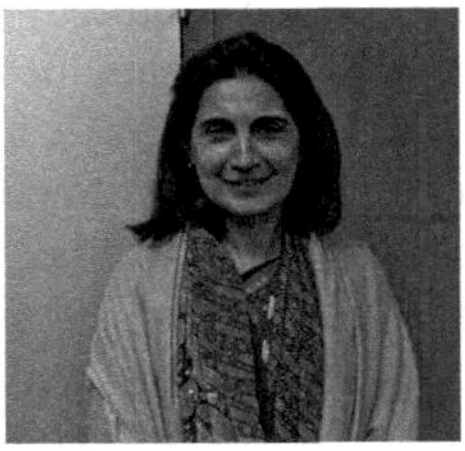

The World Health Organization (WHO) defines health as "a state of complete physical, mental and social well-being and not merely the absence of disease or infirmity." The health of women and girls falls particularly short of attaining good health, because in many societies, particularly those that are patriarchal, women and girls are uniquely disadvantaged in terms of the limited priority accorded their health, their limited ability to exercise their right to seek health care, and the overall imbalance in gender roles that exacerbate their risks of ill-health.

In the authoritarian patriarchal setting that characterizes most of South Asia, gender relations are typically unbalanced, and many women and girls have limited agency to make choices affecting their own lives and health. While access to schools, workplaces, and new opportunities has begun to erode the power wielded by fathers and husbands, not enough is known about whether and how these changes have affected the health and agency of women and girls in the region.

This volume, *Women's Health Dynamics in South Asia: Perspectives, Challenges and Innovations*, provides a view of the contemporary situation in the countries of the region. For example, its chapters delve into the adverse physical, reproductive, and mental health consequences experienced by disadvantaged groups of women. These authors focus on sexual and reproductive health matters, ranging from pregnancy-related care and abortion, to pregnancy-related care and outcomes, and the extent to which women in the region exercise their right to make reproductive health-related choices. Others have focused on mental health of specific groups of disadvantaged women, including poor pregnant women, indigenous women, those experiencing life-threatening disease, and so on. Other chapters have honed in on the health outcomes of hard to reach sub-groups, for example, women those trafficked, homeless, and tribal, forcibly displaced or affected by humanitarian crises. Insights, moreover, come from a variety of methodologies. Several authors have further analysed data from the Demographic and Health surveys (NFHS in India), while others present findings from small and more dedicated surveys, and a large number have drawn insights from qualitative studies. Despite the range of thematic areas and the variety of methodologies employed, several have pointed to similarities and differences spanning more than one setting of the region, and almost all have highlighted the importance of a range of social determinants that underlie health outcomes in every setting.

This volume should serve as a springboard for further research and syntheses of evidence from the region. Currently, its chapters shed light, in-depth, on poorly addressed issues and sub-populations—for example, poor and voiceless women in a single or a few settings. What is needed is more in-depth comparative analyses of physical, reproductive, and/or mental health outcomes among disadvantaged women, including those experiencing trafficking, those affected by climate change, or those affected by political unrest and forced displacement, across various South Asian settings. Such a probing analysis would enable a better understanding of challenges facing a particular outcome in each setting, as well as promising practices that have enabled improvements in outcomes. Chapters open a slew of questions for deeper analysis, for example, What are the factors underlying deviations from the region-level norm in certain settings? What are the factors—programmatic and other—that account for poor outcomes among last mile sub-groups? What has worked to reverse disadvantages and can promising initiatives be generalized across the region? In short, findings invite a host of further research to both highlight poorly explored issues and delve into explaining factors underlying these inconsistencies in various geographies.

Shireen J. Jejeebhoy
Director, Aksha Centre for Equity
and Wellbeing, Distinguished Visiting
Faculty, International Institute for
Population Sciences, Mumbai, India
President, International Union for
the Scientific Study of Population,
2022–2025

# Preface

The health of women in South Asia is intricately woven into the region's social, cultural, economic, and political fabric. Understanding this complex interplay of women's health will make roadmap of achieving sustainable development. Recognizing the critical importance of these issues, this volume, *"Women's Health Dynamics in South Asia: Perspectives, Challenges, and Innovations,"* brings together a diverse range of research studies that explore various aspects of women's health across the South Asian region.

This book is organized into four thematic sections, each addressing a critical dimension of women's health Part I Introduction discusses the overview of women's health in Global South. Part II Gender, Displacement, and Health Vulnerabilities explore the impact of environmental, socio-political transition and women's health. This sub-section includes trafficking, natural disasters, and women's health. Part III Sexual, Reproductive, and Maternal Health delve into the reproductive health dynamics, including judicial perspectives of abortion, caesarean deliveries, and maternal health care. Part IV Mental Health, Social Support, and Well-being focuses on the often-overlooked area of women's mental health. This sub-section examines the women's mental health challenges.

The authors bring together a wealth of knowledge and expertise, offering insights that are both deeply rooted in the local context and broadly relevant to global health discussions. Therefore, this volume is not just a collection of research findings, but also policy attentions and further research prospects. It is our hope that this book will serve as a catalyst for change, inspiring new research, informing policy, and ultimately improving the health and well-being of women in South Asia. We also acknowledge the resilience and strength of the women whose lives are the focus of this work. We hope it will serve as a valuable resource for those engaged in the study and practice of women's health, and that it will contribute to the ongoing efforts to improve health outcomes for women in South Asia and around the world.

Malda, West Bengal, India — Prof. Pradip Chouhan
Mumbai, India — Prof. Kailash Chandra Das
Malda, West Bengal, India — Dr. Avijit Roy
Malda, West Bengal, India — Dr. Nanigopal Kapasia
Mumbai, India — Dr. Margubur Rahaman
Rampurhat, West Bengal, India — Dr. Jayanta Das

# Acknowledgements

The creation of this volume, *"Women's Health Dynamics in South Asia: Perspectives, Challenges, and Innovations,"* has been a collaborative effort that would not have been possible without the invaluable contributions of numerous individuals and institutions.

Firstly, we express our deepest gratitude to the contributing authors. Your dedication to research and your commitment to addressing the complex issues surrounding women's health in South Asia have been the driving force behind this work. Your insights and expertise have greatly enriched this volume. We extend our sincere thanks to the reviewers whose critical evaluations and thoughtful suggestions have significantly enhanced the quality of this book. Your expertise and attention to detail ensured that each chapter meets the highest academic standards. We are also deeply grateful to the institutions and organizations that provided financial support, resources, and an environment conducive to research. Your support was vital in bringing this project to fruition.

Our heartfelt thanks go to the editorial team, Satvinder Kaur, our editor in Humanities and Social Sciences (India, Southwest Asia, Middle East) at Springer Nature Singapore, along with Silky Abhay Sinha, our Production Editor for their relentless efforts in managing and coordinating the various aspects of this publication. Your professionalism, dedication, and meticulous attention to detail have been essential in shaping this book. We would like to acknowledge the participants in the studies presented in this volume. Your voices and experiences are at the core of this work, and we are committed to ensuring that this book reflects the realities of your lives. Lastly, we are thankful to our families and friends for their unwavering support and encouragement throughout this journey. Your patience and understanding have been a constant source of strength.

It is our sincere hope that this book will serve as a valuable resource for researchers, policymakers, and advocates working to improve the women's health and well-being in South Asia. We dedicate this work to the resilience, strength, and courage of the women in this region, whose stories of struggle and triumph continue to inspire us.

Malda, West Bengal, India — Prof. Pradip Chouhan
Mumbai, India — Prof. Kailash Chandra Das
Malda, West Bengal, India — Dr. Avijit Roy
Malda, West Bengal, India — Dr. Nanigopal Kapasia
Mumbai, India — Dr. Margubur Rahaman
Rampurhat, West Bengal, India — Dr. Jayanta Das

# About This Book

The volume offers a comprehensive view to understanding the complex and multi-faceted world of women's health in South Asia, aligning closely with Sustainable Development Goals-3 (SDGs-3) on "good health and well-being." It examines the critical aspects, such as maternal and newborn health, healthcare choice, and utilization. It includes perspectives on environmental, socio-cultural, and individual-level behavioural aspects of women's health outcomes. Furthermore, it highlights present-day women's health issues with the light of COVID-19 pandemics, refugee-hood, and mind-psychiatric epidemics. It contextualizes the women's health rights and development landscape with evaluating existing policies, programs, and potential gaps affecting women's health and well-being. Employing advanced geospatial techniques, including spatial modelling and quantitative approaches, the volume offers multidimensional insights into women's health, shaping dialogue around health programs and policies. It is a rich source for academics, researchers, graduate students, and health professionals in the fields of women's health development.

## Key Features

Highlights contemporary issues related to complex web of women's health in South Asia.

Deals with the issue of women's health rights, maltreatment and evidence-based policy attentions.

Offers mixed method approaches in the social sciences and GIS modelling to advance women's health research.

# About This Book

# Contents

# Editors and Contributors

## About the Editors

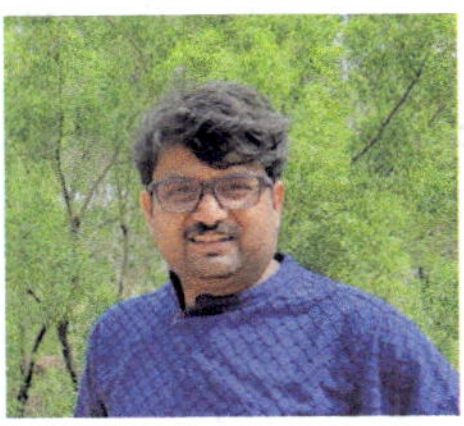

**Dr. Pradip Chouhan** is a Professor at the Department of Geography, University of Gour Banga, Malda, West Bengal, India. Earlier he was an Assistant Professor at the Department of Geography, Jadavpur University, Kolkata. His areas of research interest are fertility behaviour, public health, maternal health and child health. Actively engaged in teaching and research in Population Geography for nearly two decades, Prof. Chouhan has published more than 50 research papers in Scopus and Web of Science-indexed journals, edited 3 books and authored 1 book. He is an academic editor of PLOS One and Scientific Reports Journal and a reviewer of Scopus and Web of Science-indexed journals. He has completed a major research project funded by the Indian Council of Social Science Research, Ministry of Human Resource, Govt. of India. Dr. Chouhan has also completed one minor research project funded by the University Grants Commission. He has successfully supervised 7 Ph.D. and 8 M.Phil scholars. Recently, Dr. Chouhan has published two edited books entitled 'Sexual and Reproductive Health of Women Dimensions and Perspectives' and 'Climate Crisis, Social Responses and Sustainability Socio-ecological Study on Global' from Springer Nature.

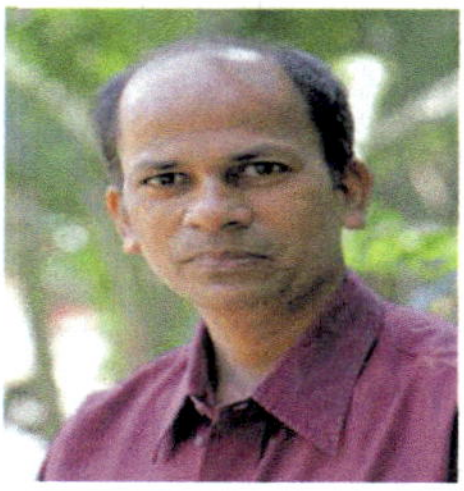

**Dr. Kailash Chandra Das** is a demographer and social geographer by training. He has completed his Ph.D. in Population Study from International Institute for Population Sciences (IIPS), Mumbai, India. Currently he is working as professor and head in the department of migration and urban studies at IIPS, Mumbai. He has more than 26 years of teaching and research experience, has completed more than 30 research projects either alone or in collaboration with other researchers. He has also guided 40 Ph.D. and M. Phil research scholars in writing their dissertations. The author has published more than 60 research papers in peer reviewed national and international journals and has written four books. He is also the convener of the South Asian Centre for Labour Mobility and Migrants (SALAM), a knowledge hub which is a joint collaboration of three UN organisations (ILO, IOM, and UN Women), five South Asian institutions (one from Bangladesh, Nepal, Pakistan, Sri Lanka, and India), University of California, Berkeley (USA) and United Nation University (UNU-MERIT, Maastricht, Netherland). He has visited more than 25 countries for conference, seminar, meeting, and other academic assignments.

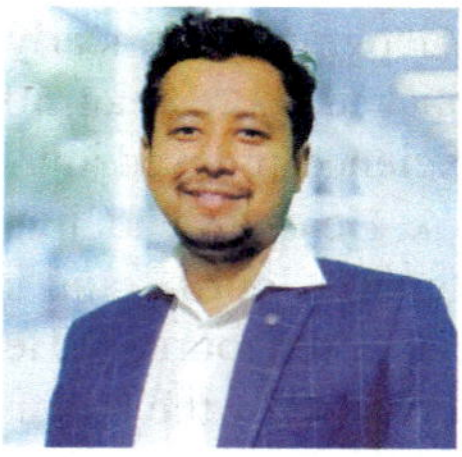

**Dr. Avijit Roy** is a State Aided College Teacher in the Department of Geography at Malda College in Malda, West Bengal, India. He teaches courses related to Population Geography, Gender Studies, Regional Planning, Urban Geography, Social, and Cultural Geography. Dr. Roy completed his Ph.D. in Geography from University of Gour Banga. He conducts research in a range of settings across the globe. His current research interests lie in women's sexual and reproductive health, maternal morbidity and mortality, maternal and newborn health, geriatrics, healthcare services, child marriage, violence against women and spatial analysis. He has published more than 35 research papers in reputed Scopus- and Web of Science–indexed journals. Recently, he has coedited three scholarly volumes—Sexual and Reproductive Health of Women: Dimensions and Perspectives, Environment and Public Health: Insights Towards Theory, Evidences and Sustainable Solutions, and Sustainable Women's Health: Perspectives from South Asia—published by Springer Nature. Dr. Roy serves as an academic editor for PLOS ONE, BMC Public Health, Frontiers in Reproductive Health and Scientific Reports

(Nature Portfolio). He is also the guest editor of the Scientific Reports Collection titled "Understanding the Determinants and Consequences of Violence." His work reflects a multidisciplinary approach that integrates geography, public health, and social policy to address critical health and gender-related issues in South Asia and beyond.

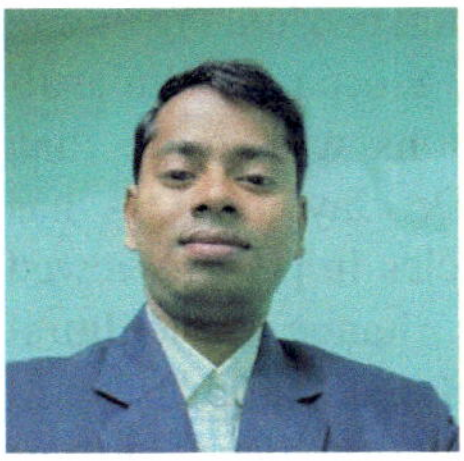

**Dr. Nanigopal Kapasia** is an Assistant Professor in the Department of Geography at Malda College, Malda, West Bengal, India. He has completed his PhD degrees from the Department of Geography and Applied Geography, University of North Bengal, India. His interested research field is social and cultural geography especially on Public Health, Maternity Care Services and Emerging Challenges related to women's health. Dr. Kapasia has published more than 20 research articles in reputed national and international journals.

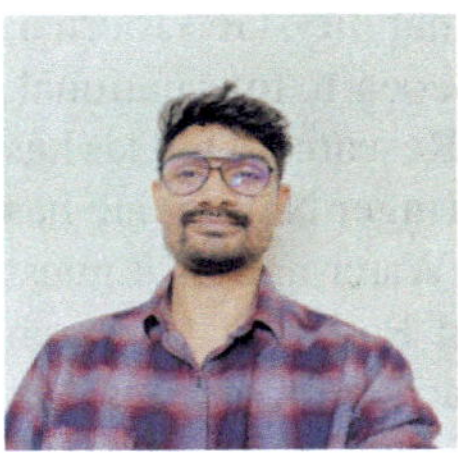

**Dr. Margubur Rahaman** is a health geographer with over six years of research experience, currently serving as a Senior Research Fellow at the Department of Migration and Urban Studies, IIPS, Mumbai. He holds an MPhil in Population Studies and dual Master's degrees in Geography and Population Studies. Recently, he completed his doctoral work on maternal health among homeless women in Kolkata, exploring the complex interplay between environment, homelessness, and reproductive health. Currently, he is working as Project Research Scientist II, Department of Community and Family Medicine, AIIMS Gorakhpur, India. Specializing in sexual and reproductive health, migration, and environment and public health, he has published several research articles and book chapters. Dr. Rahaman also serves as an editorial board member of BMC Public Health and PLOS One journals, with his research spanning diverse fields, including environment, health, and healthcare management.

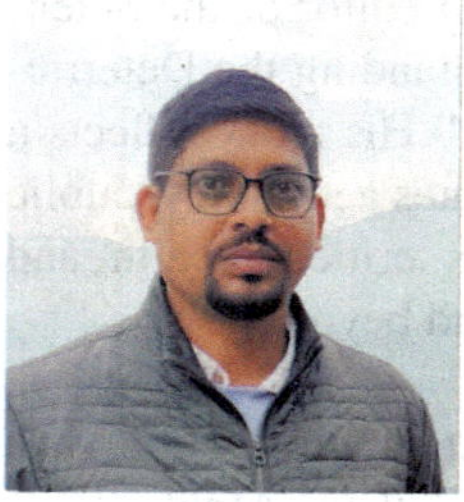

**Dr. Jayanta Das** is an Assistant Professor at the Department of Geography in Rampurhat College, University of Burdwan, West Bengal, India. He has completed his Post Graduate and PhD degrees from the Department of Geography and Applied Geography, University of North Bengal, India. His research interest includes agricultural modelling and sustainable management studies, groundwater, flood, drought analysis, climate change, watershed management, hydrological modelling, water quality, geospatial data analysis, data mining, and GIS applications with more than 15 academic years of experience. Dr. Jayanta Das has published more than 50 scholarly articles in peer-reviewed journals, focusing mainly on climate change, agricultural suitability analysis, natural and man-made hazards analysis, risk management, and spatial data analysis. He has been reviewing many journals such as Advances in Space Research, Natural Hazard, Arabian journal of geosciences, Archives of agronomy and soil science, Climatic Change, Environment, Development and Sustainability, Geo Journal, Sustainability, SN Applied Sciences, Geocarto International, Environmental Science, and Pollution Research. Dr. Das has also published 3 edited books with Springer Nature. He has served as an editor for the Journal of Water and as a guest editor for Environmental Science and Pollution Research (ESPR), published by Springer. His academic endeavours are further highlighted by his leadership in organizing international seminars and receiving prestigious awards for his research contributions.

## Contributors

**Kumudika Adikaram Boyagoda** Department of Demography, Faculty of Arts, University of Colombo, Colombo, Sri Lanka

**Jam Bilal Ahmad** Taxila Institute of Asian Studies, Quaid-I-Azam University Islamabad, Islamabad, Pakistan

**Farooq Ahmed** Department of Anthropology, The Islamia University of Bahawalpur, Bahawalpur, Punjab, Pakistan

**K. Arun** MTech Geoinformatics Student, Department of Geography, Bharathidasan University, Tiruchirappalli, India

**M. A. Arya** Research Scholar (UGC - SRF), Department of Geography, Bharathidasan University, Tiruchirappalli, India

**Mohsin Atta** Department of Psychology, University of Sargodha, Sargodha, Punjab, Pakistan

**Bontha V. Babu** Socio-Behavioural, Health Systems and Implementation Research Division, Indian Council of Medical Research, New Delhi, India

**Dhananjay W. Bansod** Department of Public Health and Mortality Studies, International Institute for Population Sciences, Mumbai, India

**Bishwajeet Besra** Department of Migration and Urban Studies, International Institute for Population Sciences, Mumbai, Maharashtra, India

**Kapil Bhati** Research Scholar, Bennett University Greater Noida, Greater Noida, India

**Adam Dubin** Faculty of Law, Universidad Pontificia Comillas, Madrid, Spain

**Jannatul Ferdous** Department of Public Administration, Comilla University, Cumilla, Bangladesh

**Manisha Gore** Faculty of Medical Health Sciences, Symbiosis Community Outreach Programme Extension, Symbiosis International Deemed University, Lavale, India

**Haritha Guduru** Icfai Business School (IBS), IFHE, Hyderabad, India

**Rahul Jain** Research Scholar, Bennett University Greater Noida, Greater Noida, India

**R. Jegankumar** Professor and Head, Department of Geography, Bharathidasan University, Tiruchirappalli, India

**Rushikesh Premdas Khadse** Department of Public Health and Mortlity Studies, International Institute for Population Sciences, Mumbai, India

**Amartya Krishnaditya** MIT School of Bioengineering Sciences and Research, Rajbaug Campus, Loni Kalbhor, Maharashtra, India

**Mukesh Kumar** Department of Migration and Urban Studies, International Institute for Population Sciences, Mumbai, Maharashtra, India

**R. S. Libina** Research Scholar, Department of Geography, Bharathidasan University, Tiruchirappalli, India

**Najma Iqbal Malik** Department of Psychology, University of Sargodha, Sargodha, Punjab, Pakistan

**Dhananjay D. Mankar** School of Health Systems Studies, Tata Institute of Social Sciences, Mumbai, India

**Ravi Kant Maurya** Department of Statistics, Mahatma Gandhi Kashi Vidyapith, Varanasi, India

**Suchismita Mishra** Department of Economics, Bangalore University, Bangalore, Karnataka, India

**Julia Morgan** Department of Human Sciences, Public Health and Wellbeing, University of Greenwich, London, UK

**Nethra Senadhi Pathirana** Department of Demography, Faculty of Arts, University of Colombo, Colombo, Sri Lanka

**T. Rajendra Prasad** Department of Economics, Bangalore University, Bangalore, Karnataka, India

**Quratulain** Department of Psychology, University of Sargodha, Sargodha, Punjab, Pakistan

**Menka Rai** Amity Law School, Amity University, Noida, Uttar Pradesh, India

**Prashna Samaddar** Xavier Law School, St. Xavier's University, Kolkata, West Bengal, India

**Anuj Singh** Department of Mathematics (Sciences), Indian Institute of Information Technology Ranchi, Ranchi, India

**Aradhya Singh** School of Law, UPES, Dehradun, Uttarakhand, India

**Neha Singh** Jaipuria Institute of Management, Jaipur, India

**Nirupama Singh** Content Manager - Historian, Tagbin Services Pvt. Ltd., Gurgaon, Haryana, India

**Shreya Srivastava** Institute of Law, Nirma University, Ahmedabad, India

**S. Syama** MTech Geoinformatics Student, Department of Geography, Bharathidasan University, Tiruchirappalli, India

**Aman Kr Tiwari** Krantisinh Nana Patil College of Veterinary Science, MAFSU, Shirwal, Maharashtra, India

**Ravita Yadav** Department of Migration and Urban Studies, International Institute for Population Sciences, Mumbai, Maharashtra, India

**Ambar Zahra** Counseling Centre, University of Sargodha, Sargodha, Punjab, Pakistan

# Abbreviations

| | |
|---|---|
| ALP | Abortion Later in Pregnancy |
| ANC | Antenatal Care |
| ANM | Auxiliary Nurse and Midwife |
| ANOVA | Analysis of Variance |
| AOR | Adjusted Odds Ratio |
| APA | American Psychopathological Association |
| ASHA | Accredited Social Health Activists |
| CA | Cognitive Anxiety |
| CHWs | Community Health Workers |
| CI | Confidence Interval |
| COVID-19 | Corona Virus-19 |
| CS | Caesarean Section |
| DHS | Demographic and Health Survey |
| FGD | Focused Group Discussion |
| GBV | Gender-Based Violence |
| HSWG | Health Sector Working Groups |
| ICMR | Indian Council of Medical Research |
| IFGO | International Federation of Gynaecology and Obstetrics |
| IIPS | International Institute for Population Sciences |
| ILO | International Labour Organization |
| IOM | International Organization for Migration |
| IRHIS | Integrated Refugee Health Information System |
| ISCG | Inter-Sector Coordination Group |
| LHV | Lady Health Visitor |
| MHME | Ministry of Health and Medical Education |
| MHPSS | Mental Health and Psychosocial Support |
| MTP | Medical Termination of Pregnancy |
| NFHS | National Family Health Survey |
| NGOs | Non-governmental Organization |
| NIH | National Institute of Health |
| NIMH | National Institute of Mental Health |

| | |
|---|---|
| NLM | National Library of Medicine |
| NPC | National Planning Commission |
| OBCs | Other Backward Caste |
| PD | Psychological Distress |
| PHY ABS | Physical Abuse |
| PNC | Postnatal Care |
| PSUs | Primary Sampling Units |
| PSY ABS | Psychological Abuse |
| QLACS | Quality of Life in Adult Cancer Survivors |
| QoL | Quality of Life |
| RRRC | Refugee Relief and Repatriation Commissioner |
| SA | Somatic Anxiety |
| SBA | Skilled Birth Attendant |
| SDGs | Sustainable Development Goals |
| SDH | Social Determinants of Health |
| SENS | Standardized Expanded Nutrition Surveys |
| SEX ABS | Sexual Abuse |
| SGBV | Sexual and Gender-Based Violence |
| SHR | Sexual Health Rights |
| SMMHCS | Scale for Measuring Maternal Health Care Services |
| SRHR | Sexual and Reproductive Health and Rights |
| STICSA | State-Trait Inventory for Cognitive and Somatic Anxiety |
| UL | Upper Limit |
| UN | United Nation |
| UNFP | United Nations Population Fund |
| UNHCR | United Nations High Commission for Refugees |
| WHO | World Health Organisation |

# Part I
# Introduction

# Chapter 1
# Women's Health in South Asia: An Introduction

**Avijit Roy and Margubur Rahaman**

**Abstract** South Asia is home to nearly half a billion women, where systemic gender disparities in education, employment, and healthcare persist. The region faces critical women's health challenges, including high maternal mortality rates, widespread anemia, and mental health issues exacerbated by gender-based violence and migration-related stressors. Adolescent girls are particularly vulnerable, with high rates of child marriage, teenage pregnancies, and limited access to sexual and reproductive health services. Migration presents both opportunities and risks for women's health. While remittances can improve healthcare access and autonomy, female migrants often face socio-economic exploitation, mental health struggles, and barriers to access the services. Gender-sensitive policies, such as pre-departure training of the migrants, counselling of the migrant's left behinds and health insurance schemes, are essential to mitigate these risks. Addressing these issues this chapter, therefore, explores the quires of refugeehood and health vulnerabilities, enforcing laws against reproductive health matters, and psychological health among women in Global South. Prioritizing women's health is not only an ethical imperative but also a cornerstone for sustainable development in South Asia. Future efforts must focus on scalable interventions and robust data systems to track progress and ensure equitable outcomes.

**Keywords** South Asia · Migration · Reproductive health · Women's health

A. Roy
Department of Geography, Malda College, Malda, West Bengal, India

M. Rahaman (✉)
Department of Migration & Urban Studies, International Institute for Population Science, Mumbai, India
e-mail: margubur48@gmail.com

All India Institute Of Medical Sciences (AIIMS), Gorakhpur, India


P. Chouhan et al. (eds.), *Women's Health Dynamics in South Asia*, Asian Perspectives on Public Health, https://doi.org/10.1007/978-981-95-2321-4_1

## 1.1 Background

South Asia is home to around 953 million women, representing 48% of the region's population (World Bank, 2023). Despite their significant stock, persistent gender-based systemic disparities in education, economic participation, and healthcare access exist in the region. For instance, the female literacy rate is still low in the area (UNESCO, 2025). Regarding female workforce participation, the participation rate in South Asia (28.8%) is lower than the global average (World Bank, 2024). Along with educational and employment lagging, strong patriarchal norms substantially affect women's health and well-being in South Asia. Regarding Critical Health Challenges, South Asia accounts for 17% of global maternal deaths, with Afghanistan and Pakistan having the highest mortality ratios (World Health Organization, 2025). About 50.1% of women suffer from anemia in South Asian countries (Keya, 2023). Depression rates among women are also prevalent in the region, particularly among gender-based violence victims (Kanougiya & Shrivastava, 2024). Sustainable health research is vital to address South Asia's intersecting crises of gender inequality, poor healthcare access, and climate threats. Prioritizing women's health is not just an ethical imperative—it's an economic and social necessity for the region's future.

## 1.2 Migration and Women's Health

Although, south Asia is known as hotspot of both internal and cross-border migration, the nexus between migration and women's health is one of the neglected research topics in south Asia. Migration, whether internal or international, has profound implications for women's health. The region, characterized by high levels of labor migration (both male and female), sees complex interactions between migration, remittances, and health outcomes (Jones, 2020). While migration can empower women economically and socially, it also exposes them to vulnerabilities that negatively impact their well-being. Observing the existing findings, migration often leads directly to household economic growth through remittances, which open window to invest on girls' education, nutrition and women's healthcare (Ullah et al., 2019). For instance, studies from Pakistan show that remittances contribute to better maternal health services, including antenatal and postnatal care (Mahmood et al., 2022). Similarly, female migrant workers' remittances found to be linked with improved dietary diversity among them in Sri Lanka (Dharmadasa & Karunarathna, 2022). In Bangladesh, women in remittance-receiving households report higher contraceptive use, suggesting improved reproductive health autonomy (Anwar & Mughal, 2016). Along with positive role of remittance of women's health, the women who migrate for work often advance financial and healthcare autonomy. Female migrants have higher agency in seeking reproductive healthcare compared to non-migrant women (Georgiadis, 2008). Cross-border labor migration or rural-urban internal migration opens the opportunity to get better health care facility which shapes the women's health. International migrants, sometimes receive employer-provided health insurance, enhancing their healthcare access. Internal migrants moving to urban areas in Pakistan and India often gain access to superior healthcare facilities compared to rural regions (Rahaman & Das, 2024).

Just opposite side of positive migration outcome invites several challenges and obstacle which negatively affects women's health For instance, many South Asian women working abroad, especially in domestic sectors, face exploitative conditions, long working hours, and abuse, leading to stress, depression, and physical injuries (Ahmad et al., 2005). In particular, a recent study highlights that Nepalese female migrants in the Middle East experience high rates of sexual harassment, contributing to PTSD and other mental health disorders (Adhikary et al., 2011). Research in Pakistan shows that left-behind wives of male migrants report higher anxiety and depression (Mughal & Aldrich, 2020). In Sri Lanka, female migrants often delay marriage and childbirth, which can lead to complications due to advanced maternal age. Irregular migrants in India often avoid healthcare due to fear of deportation, leading to untreated chronic illnesses (Rahaman & Das, 2024). Internal slum or pavement dwellers female migrants face barriers like high costs and discrimination in accessing public health services (Rahaman et al., 2025).

To mitigate risks and enhance benefits, South Asian nations should adopt gender-sensitive migration policies. It is essential to organize gender exclusive pre-departure training on legal literacy and rights, health insurance provisions, health check-ups and mental health counselling program. Nepal introduced such program under Foreign Employment Act. Furthermore, bilateral agreements with host countries to ensure safe working conditions. Health insurance schemes for migrants could also improve the healthcare access, particularly for female migrants. For instance, the Awaz Health Insurance scheme which was launched by the Kerala Government in 2017 to cover the accidents and medical expenses of state migrant workers. Community health programs targeting wives of male migrants to address mental health issues. Mobile health clinics in high low wage female labor migration clusters could also be step to reach affordable and quality health services. To implement such initiatives, call for gender-disaggregated migration and health data.

## 1.3 Mental Health of Adolescent Girls

Adolescent girls in South Asia face growing mental health crises, exacerbated by gender discrimination, digital harms, and weak support systems. About one-third of South Asian adolescent girls report depressive symptoms, linked to academic pressure, early marriage, and gender-based violence (Murshid, 2017). In India, girls aged 15–19 have higher the suicide rate of boys (Philip et al., 2022), driven by social restrictions and lack of autonomy. A substantial number of girls face cyberbullying, sexual extortion (sextortion), and non-consensual image sharing in South Asia (Dakua et al., 2024). Lack of awareness about cyber laws and cyber literacy increases such risk among girls in South Asia. School-based mental health programs need to be strength. Digital literacy and laws campaigns to combat misinformation and exploitation.

## 1.4 Sexual and Reproductive Health Among Women

South Asia bears a disproportionate burden of adolescent reproductive and maternal health challenges, driven by socio-cultural, economic, and systemic healthcare barriers. With nearly 50 million adolescent girls at risk of early marriage and pregnancy, the region faces persistent public health crises that demand urgent intervention. South Asia accounts for 45% of global child marriages, with 30% of girls married before 18 (UNICEF, 2023). In Bangladesh, 59% of women aged 20–24 was married before 18, while Nepal and Afghanistan report rates exceeding 40% (UNICEF, 2023). Early marriage leads to teenage pregnancies, contributing to one-fifth of total births in the region (Poudel et al., 2022).

As a consequence of teen age child bearing, teen mothers face twice the risk of maternal mortality compared to mature women. Obstructed labor, eclampsia, and postpartum hemorrhage are leading causes of death among teen mothers (UNICEF, 2023). Anemia also prevalent among adolescent girls in South Asia. Chronic undernutrition exacerbates pregnancy complications. Low BMI (<18.5) in 25% of adolescent mothers increases risks of low birth weight (WHO, 2025). Regarding the menstrual hygiene, 27% of adolescent girls do not use improved sanitary napkins in India (Karjee et al., 2023). A substantial number of girls report missing school during menstruation due to stigma and lack of facilities. In the areas of sexual and reproductive infection, infections like UTIs and reproductive tract infections (RTIs) are prevalent due to unhygienic practices.

Regarding the drivers of adolescent health vulnerability, socio-cultural Factors plays significant role. For instance, South Asian patriarchal norms permit and promote early marriage which limits their educational opportunity and increase the risk of sexual and reproductive health vulnerability. In addition, stigma around adolescent sexuality prevents access to sexual and reproductive health (SRH) services. Regarding healthcare settings, lack of adolescent-friendly clinics in rural areas another significant concern to access the health service. Although, almost all south Asian countries enacted law against child marriage and introduced cash intensive for marriage after legal age of marriage, still the issue is prevalent in South Asia may be due to intergenerational social cultural acceptance of such practices. Therefore, there is need more awareness on child marriage and pregnancy risk factors, adolescent girl schooling enrolment and dropout audits regularly, school health program to prevent such practice.

## 1.5 Conclusion

The evidence presented highlights the critical yet under-addressed nexus between gender, health, and development in South Asia, where systemic inequities continue to constrain the potential of nearly 1 billion women and girls. Despite constituting half of the population, women face disproportionate burdens. Health indicators reveal alarming disparities, particularly regarding maternal mortality, anemia, and undernutrition. These challenges are exacerbated by climate change impacts and inadequate health systems. Sustainable progress demands urgent, multisectoral action: (1) implementing gender-responsive healthcare policies with adolescent-friendly services; (2) enforcing legal protections against child marriage and cybercrime while expanding economic opportunities; and (3) investing in intersectional research to address caste, class, and geographic disparities. The demographic dividend of South Asia's youth population cannot be realized without prioritizing women's health as foundational to development. Addressing these gaps through evidence-based policies and strengthened health systems is not merely an ethical imperative but an economic necessity to unlock the region's full potential and achieve equitable, resilient growth. Future efforts must translate research into scalable interventions while monitoring progress through gender-disaggregated data systems.

## References


Adhikary, P., Keen, S., & van Teijlingen, E. (2011). Health issues among nepalese migrant workers in the Middle East. *Health Science Journal, 5*(3), 169–175.

Ahmad, F., Shik, A., Vanza, R., Cheung, A. M., George, U., & Stewart, D. E. (2005). Voices of South Asian women: Immigration and mental health. *Women & Health, 40*(4), 113–130.

Anwar, A. I., & Mughal, M. Y. (2016). Migrant remittances and fertility. *Applied Economics, 48*(36), 3399–3415.

Dakua, T., Rahaman, M., & Das, K. C. (2024). An analysis of the spatial and temporal variations of human trafficking in India. *Cogent Social Sciences, 10*(1), 2293315.

Dharmadasa, R. A. P. I. S., &Karunarathna, G. K. S. S. (2022). Migration, remittances and household welfare: evidence from Sri Lanka. *Sri Lanka Journal of Economic Research, 10*(1).

Georgiadis, K. (2008). Migration and reproductive health: a review of the literature. *Work. Pap*, (01). https://uis.unesco.org/bdds

Jones, G. W. (2020). New patterns of female migration in South Asia. *Asian Population Studies, 16*(1), 1–4.

Kanougiya, S., & Shrivastava, S. (2024). Intimate partner violence and mental health outcomes in South Asia. *Handbook on Sex, Gender and Health: Perspectives from South Asia*, 1–41.

Karjee, S., Rahaman, M., & Biswas, P. C. (2023). Contextualizing the socio-economic and spatial patterns of using menstrual hygienic methods among young women (15–24 years) in India: A cross-sectional study using the nationally representative survey. *Clinical Epidemiology and Global Health, 20*, Article 101253.

Keya, T. A. (2023). Prevalence and predictors of anaemia among women of reproductive age in South and Southeast Asia. *Cureus, 15*(12).

Mahmood, T., Kumar, R., Rehman, A. U., & Pongpanich, S. (2022). International remittances and women's reproductive health care: Evidence from Pakistan. *Health Systems & Reform, 8*(1), Article e2064792.

Murshid, N. S. (2017). Parents, friends, and depression: A multi-country study of adolescents in South Asia. *Children and Youth Services Review, 79*, 160–165.

Philip, S., Issac, T. G., Sharda, A., & Shekhar, A. (2022). Suicide prevention strategy in India. *The Lancet Psychiatry, 9*(3), 192.

Poudel, S., Razee, H., Dobbins, T., & Akombi-Inyang, B. (2022). Adolescent pregnancy in south Asia: A systematic review of observational studies. *International Journal of Environmental Research and Public Health, 19*(22), 15004.

Rahaman, M., & Das, K. C. (2024). Differentials in self-reported health status and healthcare utilization among homeless women during the antenatal period in urban settings: Does migration status matter? *Journal of Migration and Health, 10*, Article 100246.

Rahaman, M., Gajbhiyeand, K. S., & Das, K. C. (2025). Homeless women's multifaceted vulnerabilities in India: A research roadmap delineation. In *Sexual and reproductive health of women: Dimensions and Perspectives* (pp. 17–33). Springer Nature Singapore.

Ullah, S., Majeed, M. T., &Kiani, A. K. (2019). The Influence of Remittances on Education and Health Outcomes: An Analy-sis for South Asian Countries. *Jinnah Business Review*, 71.

UNESCO. (2025). Adult literacy in South Asia is lower among women than among men (2023)

UNICEF. (2023). Child marriage. https://www.unicef.org/rosa/what-we-do/child-protection/child-marriage

World Bank. (2023). Labor force, female (% of total labor force) - South Asia. https://data.worldbank.org/indicator/SP.POP.TOTL.FE.ZS?locations=8S

World Bank. (2024). Labor force, female (% of total labor force) - South Asia. https://data.worldbank.org/indicator/SL.TLF.TOTL.FE.ZS?locations=8S

World Health Organization. (2025). Maternal mortality. https://www.who.int/publications/i/item/9789240108462

# Part II
# Gender, Displacement, and Health Vulnerabilities

# Chapter 2
# Impact of Trafficking on Women's Health: Evidence from Sri Lanka

**Nethra Senadhi Pathirana and Kumudika Adikaram Boyagoda**

**Abstract** Health is a major, but less documented area of trafficking. When focused, it is dominated by women's sexual and reproductive health. Yet trafficked women face other health issues created by working environments, living conditions, poor sanitation, inadequate nutrition, limited health care access, etc. A comprehensive analysis of trafficked women's health is therefore warranted to gauge the full impact of trafficking on health, which is the aim of this study. Sri Lanka is a hub for trafficking, and the need is essential. Primary data from 94 family members who lodged complaints about a trafficked female family member at the Repatriation Section of the Ministry of Foreign Employment, Sri Lanka provides the data for the study. The respondents were selected by applying purposive sampling method, and the analysis was based on the triangulation of quantitative (survey) and qualitative (in-depth interviews) data. The majority (97%) of the women have migrated as labour migrants and ended up being trafficked. 'Very bad or bad' health was reported by 92%, due to physical illnesses (57%—mainly blood pressure, skin diseases, breathing difficulties/asthma, heart diseases), mental issues (93%—mainly sleeplessness, anxiety, declining self-aggrandizement), or disabilities (19%—mainly leg and hand). Physical (76%) and mental (69%) harassment at work and harassment from recruitment agency personnel (13%) were the main reasons for health conditions. Health risks are cumulative, and could even lead to death. While strict state regulation on illegal migration is needed, since most of the trafficked are legal labour migrants, policy should target the well-being of migrant workers at destinations.

**Keywords** Trafficked women · Physical health · Mental health · Sexual exploitation · Sri Lanka

N. S. Pathirana (✉) · K. Adikaram Boyagoda
Department of Demography, Faculty of Arts, University of Colombo, Colombo, Sri Lanka
e-mail: nethra@demo.cmb.ac.lk

K. Adikaram Boyagoda
e-mail: kumudikaboyagoda@demo.cmb.ac.lk

 
P. Chouhan et al. (eds.), *Women's Health Dynamics in South Asia*, Asian Perspectives on Public Health, https://doi.org/10.1007/978-981-95-2321-4_2

## 2.1 Introduction

Trafficking of humans is a grave and organized criminal offence that frequently spans across international borders and jurisdictions. Individuals, irrespective of sex and age are trafficked for a multitude of exploitative objectives such as forced labour, sexual exploitation, domestic servitude, and removal of organs. The International Labour Organization—ILO (2020) reports that traffickers exploit 25 million people each year, with the victims generating substantial profits for their captors. The industry is estimated to bring in US$150 billion annually and continues to expand (DHT, 2024).

Women are particularly affected by human trafficking. Data indicates that for every ten victims identified globally in 2018, approximately five were adult females and two were young girls. Gender inequality and the widespread violation of women's human rights are significant factors driving the high number of women caught in the trafficking cycle. Violation of women's human rights together with gender inequality are notable components that drive the high number of women caught in the cycle of trafficking. Feminization of poverty exacerbates this issue (United Nations Office on Drugs & Crime, 2020). The distribution of detected trafficking victims globally by age and sex is depicted in Fig. 2.1.

It is evident from Fig. 2.1 based on data from 162 countries for the year 2018 that a noticeable 65% of the trafficked are females, either women or girls. Multifaceted determinants make women more vulnerable to exploitation and susceptible to traffickers. The fact that women represent a significant proportion of trafficking victims globally, highlights the urgent need for targeted interventions to address the unique challenges they face in this context. UNODC (2023) reported that women victims were exploited in three main ways (Fig. 2.2).

Statistics from the UNODC (2023) indicate that gender inequality and widespread human rights abuses against women are primary factors driving women into the trafficking cycle, and this is exacerbated by the feminization of poverty (Zimmerman

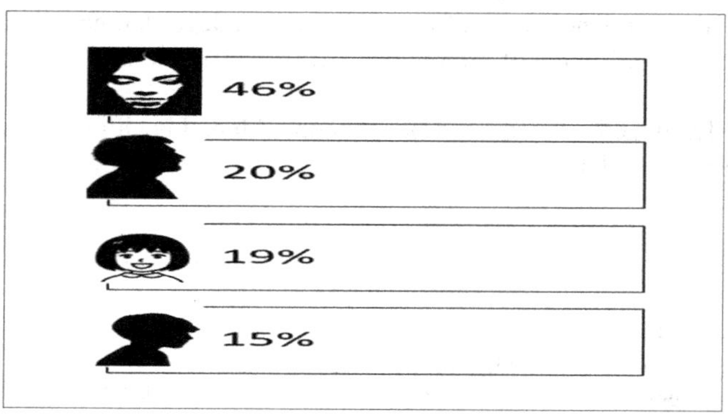


**Fig. 2.1** Distribution of trafficking victims globally by age and sex (2018). *Source* United Nations Office on Drugs and Crime (UNODC), (2023)

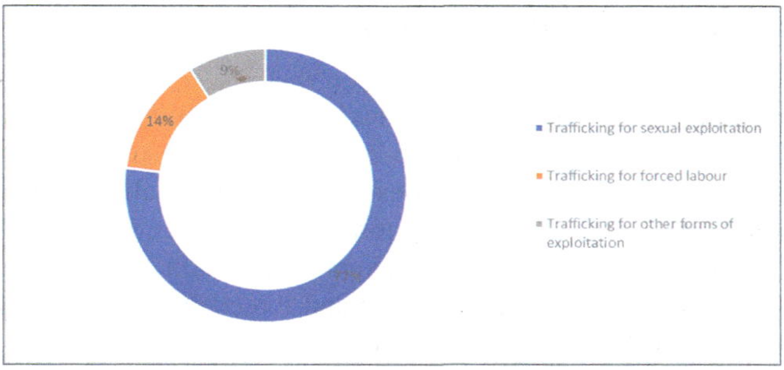


**Fig. 2.2** Forms of exploitation faced by trafficked women victims (2018). *Note* Other forms of human trafficking are the removal of organs, forced begging, etc. *Source* UNODC (2023)

et al., 2011). Figure 2.2 shows, that sexual exploitation, forced labour, removal of organs, and forced begging (among other factors) make women more vulnerable than men. According to UNODC data (2023), regional variations in trafficking patterns reveal a prevalence of male forced labour in Europe, Central Asia, and the Americas. Conversely, South Asia, East Asia, the Pacific, Africa, and the Middle East report higher incidences of trafficking among females and girls.

Studies highlight that the health impacts of female trafficking are significant issues in Asian countries, warranting attention as a major concern. Most trafficked individuals come from vulnerable situations characterized by poverty, low education, abuse, and malnutrition, which persist through travel, transportation, and recruitment stages of trafficking (Zimmerman et al., 2011; Morrison & Crosland, 2000). Busza et al. (2004) emphasized that the trafficking of women is a global public health concern, with a focus on women's sexual and reproductive health. However, health issues faced by trafficked women extend beyond sexual and reproductive health; poor working environments, inadequate living conditions, poor sanitation, inadequate nutrition, and limited healthcare access create a multitude of health issues. Health risks, including permanent physical injuries, post-traumatic stress, a wide range of diseases (including sexually transmitted infections), substance abuse, and malnutrition begin at recruitment, continue through the exploitation period, and persist post-trafficking. In Sri Lanka, the Sri Lanka Bureau of Foreign Employment (SLBFE) (2020) data indicates that the highest number of complaints per a single reason logged in the year 2020 is regarding health (sickness). This is one indication of the importance of focusing on the health issues of the trafficked in Sri Lanka.

Health issues of the trafficked are exacerbated as individuals are often reluctant to seek medical assistance due to their status as illegal migrants, captivity, and lack of financial resources. When care is sought, it is often of sub-standard quality and provided under assumed or false identities, complicating follow-up processes. Therefore, a comprehensive analysis of trafficked women's health is essential, emphasizing the urgent need to address and prioritize their health.

### 2.1.1 Human Trafficking Profile in Sri Lanka

Data on exploitation forms in human trafficking and several female cases detected in South Asia, with particular reference to India, Nepal, and Sri Lanka, indicate that victims who are taken for forced labour constitute more than half of the identified trafficked cases in this sub-region. Following forced labour, forced marriage emerges as a significant exploitation form, alongside sexual exploitation. Additionally, instances of trafficking people for exploitative begging and forced criminal activity have been reported in the region (International Labour Organization, 2004).

Human trafficking is pervasive in Sri Lanka. Siddhisena and Ranasinghe (2016) highlight that in Sri Lanka, labour migration is a significant factor contributing to trafficking. Since the 1970s, international labour migration flows have been prominent in Sri Lanka. Data from the SLBFE indicate a rapid increase in labour migrants between 1986 and 2019. Initially, in 1986, the number of male migrants exceeded that of females. However, this trend reversed after 1988, with female migrants outnumbering their male counterparts. The pattern shifted again after 2006, and since 2008, male migrants have consistently outnumbered female migrants. This change can be attributed to various policies and programs implemented by the Sri Lankan government over the years. By 2019, 122,257 males and 80,830 females migrated as labour migrants and as shown in Fig. 2.3, a significant portion of Sri Lankan labour migration is directed towards the Gulf countries (Information Technology Division-SLBFE, 2020).

Among the total Sri Lankan labour migrants, the majority were reported in Kuwait, Qatar, Saudi Arabia, and UAE. Jayatilaka (2008) as well as Siddhisena and Ranasinghe (2016) investigated the trafficking issue in Sri Lanka and says that most of the Sri Lankans are trafficked in the Gulf region. It is also noted that men and women who migrate on their own will to Kuwait, Jordan, Saudi Arabia, Qatar, Lebanon, the UAE, Oman, Bahrain, and Singapore to work as construction workers, domestic helpers, or garment factory workers are trafficked in numerous forms, such as exploitation of labour, violation of human rights and fundamental freedom,

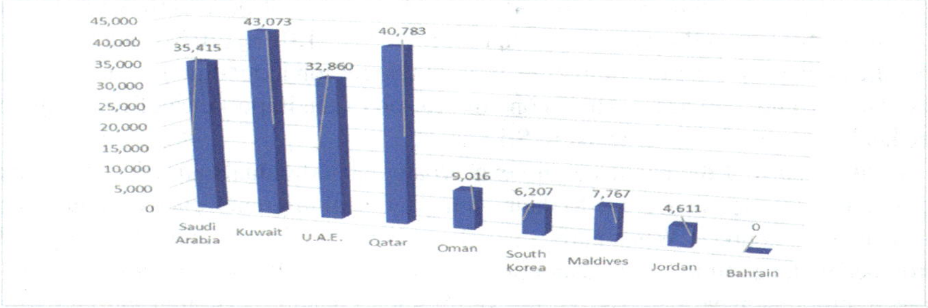


**Fig. 2.3** Total departures of Sri Lankans for foreign employment by destination country, 2019. *Source* Information Technology Division-SLBFE (2020)

**Table 2.1** Complaints received by the SLBFE (2015–2020) from migrant workers according to gender

| Year | Male | Female | Total |
|---|---|---|---|
| 2015 | 1735 | 6305 | 8040 |
| 2016 | 1830 | 4320 | 6150 |
| 2017 | 1010 | 3364 | 4374 |
| 2018 | 596 | 2944 | 3540 |
| 2019 | 1133 | 3781 | 4914 |
| 2020[a] | 1641 | 3489 | 5130 |

[a] Provisional
*Source* Information Technology Division-SLBFE (2020)

forced labour, violence and discrimination against women, sexual exploitation, and forced prostitution (Amirthalingam et al., 2013; Siddhisena & Ranasinghe, 2016). The SLBFE data demonstrates the number of complaints by migrant workers from 2015 to 2020 by gender (Table 2.1) which indicates their situation.

Table 2.1 indicates that the number of complaints by females is more than that of males for all the given years. More importantly, the figures are at least twice that of males for any given year. These complaints are diverse and can directly or indirectly impact the health of the woman. By 2020, the highest number of complaints per a single reason is regarding health (sickness) indicating the importance of health issues as a consequence of trafficking in the country (Table 2.2).

**Table 2.2** Complaints received by nature of complaint—number of complaints (2015–2020)[a]

| | Nature of Complaints | Year | | | | | |
|---|---|---|---|---|---|---|---|
| | | 2015 | 2016 | 2017 | 2018 | 2019 | 2020[a] |
| 1 | Breach of employment contract | 1443 | 1314 | 1092 | 894 | 1090 | 802 |
| 2 | **Sickness** | **1151** | **838** | **621** | **605** | **816** | **1046** |
| 3 | Non-receipt of wages | 1011 | 1041 | 640 | 473 | 611 | 462 |
| 4 | Not sent back after completion of contract period | 1059 | 618 | 529 | 418 | 406 | 560 |
| 5 | Harassment | 990 | 516 | 334 | 401 | 544 | 342 |
| 6 | Lack of communication | 681 | 452 | 399 | 299 | 429 | 365 |
| 7 | Beings Stranded without employment | 134 | 126 | 89 | 103 | 36 | 117 |
| 8 | Overworked | 152 | 62 | 61 | 44 | 59 | 72 |
| 9 | Premature termination | 115 | 110 | 53 | 31 | 48 | 22 |
| 10 | Employee missing (Run Away) | 63 | 27 | 70 | 80 | 132 | 83 |
| 11 | Problem at employee's home (Sri Lanka) | 146 | 71 | 33 | 37 | 225 | 189 |
| 12 | Other | 1095 | 975 | 436 | 155 | 518 | 1070 |
| | Total | 8040 | 6150 | 4374 | 3540 | 4914 | 5130 |

[a] Provisional
*Source* Information Technology Division-SLBFE (2020)

Analysing Table 2.2 reveals that health issues are a major concern faced by international migrants subjected to trafficking. This is a significant problem not only in Sri Lanka but also globally and it remains an under-documented aspect of trafficking (Zimmerman et al., 2011; Morrison & Crossland, 2000). This global public health concern (Busza et al., 2004) impacts the entire life cycle of affected individuals from recruitment to exploitation and even after they are freed from trafficking (Zimmerman et al., 2011). These health issues encompass a wide range, from physical and sexual to mental health problems. However, there is a tendency to view the health issues of trafficked individuals as purely health-related, often overlooking its connection to trafficking. This research aims to connect the two, and investigate the impact of trafficking on women victim's health and thereby emphasize the critical need to address and document this area comprehensively.

### 2.1.2 *Objective of the Study*

The primary and first objective of this research is to comprehensively investigate the impact of human trafficking on women's health. To achieve this, the study focuses on two stages in the trafficking process—the recruitment stage and the exploitation stage at the destination. Secondly, the research aims to analyse the factors contributing to the health status of the women at the destination and the specific types of health issues that they encounter. By uncovering these underlying factors, the study aims to highlight the complex elements that lead to women's health due to trafficking. Through these goals, the research aims to provide a thorough analysis of the multifaceted relationship between human trafficking and the health of trafficked women, ultimately contributing to the broader understanding of this critical issue and informing policy and intervention strategies.

## 2.2 Materials and Methods

This study is based on primary data collected from the family members of trafficked women who visited the 'Repatriation Section' of the Ministry of External Affairs (MEA) in Sri Lanka to lodge complaints about trafficking. The participants comprised spouses, parents, children, siblings, or close relatives of the trafficked women. Both quantitative and qualitative data were gathered from these family members to address the research problem.

Quantitative data collection was conducted through a structured questionnaire survey, while qualitative data were obtained via in-depth interviews and case studies. The study population consisted of ninety-four (94) individuals who lodged complaints related to trafficking at the MEA between 5th September 2016 and 21st November 2016. These participants were selected using a purposive sampling method based on their agreement to partake in the questionnaire survey. The quantitative data were analysed using the Statistical Package for the Social Sciences (SPSS), employing both univariate and bivariate analyses. This data predominantly facilitated a descriptive analysis of the study sample. Conversely, the qualitative data were analysed using content analysis, focusing on the main themes outlined in the in-depth interview guidelines, which were aligned with the study's objectives. This dual approach allowed for a comprehensive examination of the impact of trafficking on women's health, combining statistical rigour with detailed, thematic insights.

## 2.3 Results and Discussion

Rescue and Restore (2019) indicated that inhumane living conditions, poor sanitation, inadequate nutrition, poor personal hygiene, severe physical and emotional assaults by traffickers, dangerous workplace conditions, occupational hazards and general lack of quality health care, etc. affect the health of the trafficked. Literature highlights that these conditions occur throughout the three stages of the trafficking process—i.e. (i) recruitment stage (ii) transportation stage; and (iii) exploitation stage. The present study will discuss the health issues of the trafficked according to two stages of the trafficking process: (i) pre-migration (recruitment) stage; and (ii) destination (exploitation) stage, where migrants are primarily exploited under sexual exploitation and labour exploitation.

### *2.3.1 Pre-Migration Stage: The Hidden Health Issues Among Trafficked Migrants*

Attention to the health conditions of the migrants should start at the pre-migratory stage but are not given priority. The dominant issues focused in analysing this stage are the demographic and socio-economic status of the migrants or the determinants for migration. When it comes to trafficking, health is deliberately hidden by both the trafficker and the trafficked. Potential migrants may not divulge their health condition as it would be an obstacle to migration. On the other hand, as UNODC (2023) notes, trafficking is exploiting people for profit and when exploitation is the aim, the health of the victim is compromised. The health of the migrant at the recruitment stage is however important as health conditions can aggravate due to trafficking. Further, new health issues can also emerge due to situations and methods of trafficking.

In this study, family members of four victims reported pre-migratory multiple psychological health issues; these included sleepiness (3.1%), mental disquietude (2.1%), declined self-aggrandizement (2.1%) and mental issues (1.1%). Further, three women were identified to have suffered from physical illnesses like high blood pressure (1.1%), joint pain (1.1%), heart issues (1.1%), and diabetes (2.1%). One woman was pregnant and reported pregnancy-related health concerns (1.1%).

**Table 2.3** Reasons for Women's migration

| Reasons | Responses | |
|---|---|---|
| | Number | Percentage (%) |
| Economic hardships in the family | 90 | 95.7 |
| Unemployment | 41 | 43.6 |
| Escape domestic violence | 9 | 9.6 |
| Total responses | 140 | [a] |

[a] Multiple responses
*Source* Present study

Though reports of illnesses were very few, indirect information allowed us to conclude that health issues were more prevalent. In the study, 98.9% migrated illegally (using illegal documents or overstaying at the destination). Among those who made illegal documents, 18.1% provided forged medical documents. This can be because the trafficker or the trafficked did not want their true health conditions to be exposed. It could also mean that the victims were poor and could not afford medical investigations. Besides, the traffickers may have forced/advised and helped the victims to forge documents to achieve their aim. The fact that migrants hide their health status is proved by the below example.

> My mother migrated to the country'Z'.[1] because she wanted to free the family from poverty. When she migrated, she was suffering from high blood pressure and had joint pains. But she did not reveal that illness because she wanted to migrate. (Janu[2] [daughter of trafficked])

Another indirect understanding can be obtained by analysing the reasons for migration (Table 2.3). Three main reasons for migration were identified, and most of the migrants indicated multiple responses. Nearly all mention economic hardships, and around half state unemployment. Rathnayaka (1999) also notes that poor economic conditions and unemployment significantly influence female migration.

A minority (9.6%) had migrated to escape domestic violence. There is ample literature on the physical and psychological health issues resulting from domestic violence (8.5%). Though such issues were not reported in the study specifically, it is possible to conclude that at least a portion of the victims had health issues. However, since domestic violence is mentioned here as an escape route, people elaborate more on the positives of the escape than the negatives of health issues.

Vulnerability due to domestic violence and poverty makes women easy prey for traffickers. In this study, 67% of the women migrated through agency persons and agency personnel take advantage of their vulnerability, especially by providing financial and material incentives to the women and creating debt bondage. This situation has significant impacts on the mental health of the trafficked at the recruitment stage as noted by Pavi.

[1] Names of countries are withheld.

[2] Pseudonyms are used.

> The family was objecting to my sister migrating. Domestic violence and economic hardships created push factors for her decision. But at one point she wanted to refrain from migrating. However, the agency person threatened saying the lack of rupees was spent on her and if she does not want to go she must pay back 6 lacks. Sister was frightened and she went through a lot of mental stress. She was caught between the family who did not want her to migrate and the agency threat. Finally agency person took her to Colombo without telling us. We have not heard from her for 6 months. (Pavi [sister of trafficked])

Situations such as those elaborated by Pavi are many, and these leave the victims no alternative but to migrate and be trafficked.

However, a detailed analysis of the health conditions in the pre-migratory stage cannot be done as only a few family members report the health conditions of the women prior to migration. However, many women have reported health issues at the destination. The second section of the analysis delves into the health issues that migrants face at their destinations, highlighting the connection of these to the trafficking process.

### *2.3.2 Destination Dangers: Health Challenges Faced by Trafficked Women*

The health conditions of trafficked individuals encompass physical (including disabilities), mental, and sexual aspects. This study focuses only on physical (including disabilities) and mental health and collected information on the trafficked individuals' health under five categories: 'very good,' 'good,' 'moderate,' 'bad,' and 'very bad'. According to the family members, the majority of the trafficked women's health status was reported as 'very bad' (60.6%). Thirty-two (31.9%) percent reported that the health status was 'bad.' Thus, the health status of 92.5% can be described as negative. Only 6.3% of the female migrants are reported to have 'good' health conditions, and just 1.0% are reported to have moderate health conditions.

Figure 2.4 shows the distribution of the women according to their health conditions under the three broad areas that were focused on. Very few suffered from a stand-alone physical or disability condition. However, nearly one-fifth of the women (19.1%) suffered from only mental issues.

Figure 2.4 clearly shows that under trafficking conditions the majority face multiple health issues. Most of those who had physical illnesses and disabilities also suffered from mental issues. This is to be expected as mental health is common to most who have physical or disability issues. Thus, among the trafficked mental health is a high concern.

Table 2.4 provides details as to the proportions suffering under each of the broad areas either as a single cause or combined with another. Among the victims, most suffer from psychological issues, followed by physical illnesses.

Specific illnesses suffered under each of the three broad categories of health discussed are given in Table 2.5. Multiple responses show that the victims have more

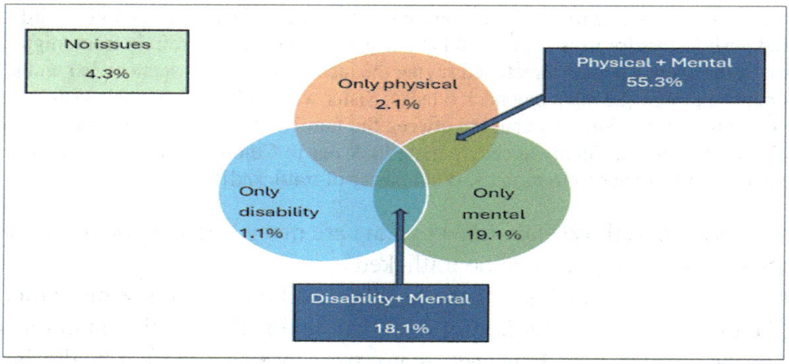


**Fig. 2.4** Multimorbidity conditions among trafficked women

**Table 2.4** Type of health issues as single cause or in combination with another

| Nature of illnesses | N | (%) |
|---|---|---|
| Physical illnesses | 54 | 57.4% |
| Psychological difficulties | 87 | 92.6% |
| Disabilities | 18 | 19.1% |
| Total responses | 159 | [a] |

[a] Multiple Responses

than one illness. For example, just above half of those reporting a physical illness had a skin disease, while 61.1% who reported a physical illness had blood pressure.

Table 2.5 presents only the most prominent illnesses, but the victims have also reported other multiple issues as depicted in the stories below.

**Table 2.5** Specific types of illness suffered by the trafficked women

| Physical (%) | | Psychological (%) | | Disabilities (%) | |
|---|---|---|---|---|---|
| Asthma | 38.9 | Sleeplessness | 98.9 | Hand | 83.3 |
| Pressure | 61.1 | Hopelessness | 92 | Leg | 55.6 |
| Skin disease | 53.7 | Short memory loss/ severe forgetfulness | 2.4 | Backbone | 5.6 |
| Heart problems | 35.2 | Anger | 1.1 | Join pain | 61.1 |
| Diabetes | 13 | Distorted mental state | 2.3 | | |
| | | Low self -esteem | 92 | | |
| Total number of trafficked women | 54 | | 87 | | 18 |

[a] Multiple Responses

*Note* Only the most prominent three diseases have been noted

> Mother migrated to the country 'X' for a period of 2 years as a housemaid one and a half years ago. But she has not been paid for six months and is suffering from a serious stomach illness. The employers do not treat her illness. She has to work in a three-storied house and is not able to eat properly due to having a huge workload. This has led to a malnutrition condition. (Vigneshwari [daughter of a victim])

> My wife went to country 'M' in 2014, as a housemaid. She was being tortured by her employer. She had been suffering from diabetes and now has started bleeding when passing urine. (Indika [husband of trafficked])

It shows the complex nature of the health conditions of the trafficked, which includes different illnesses covering both physical and mental aspects.

### 2.3.3 *Reasons for Health Status: Issues of the Working Environment*

Traffickers give cheap promises of lucrative employment when offering the job, although, in reality, they are "3 D" jobs. According to Tyuryukhanova, migrant women are employed in highly unregulated and corrupt sectors of employment. Similar findings are presented by Siddhisena and Ranasinghe (2016) when they show that high numbers of Sri Lankan migrant women are employed in the informal sector where working conditions are poor. However, brokers (i.e. traffickers or allies of traffickers) disguise this as a good job. The bad working conditions can be identified as the primary reason for health issues faced by the trafficked.

Table 2.6 reveals the employment category of the trafficked and their health status. Women engage in three main job categories at the destinations. The majority work as domestic helpers, followed by 6 women engaged as prostitutes and 1 as a labourer.

The majority of individuals across all job categories have either 'bad' or 'very bad' health statuses. A minority of domestic helpers and one engaged in prostitution reported good health. Since this is a very small number, this group is actually an anomaly and not the norm. However, it is widely reported that the possibility of

**Table 2.6** Employment category of the trafficked and their health status

| Employment category | Health status | | | | |
|---|---|---|---|---|---|
| | Good | Moderate | Bad | Very bad | Total no of women |
| | N | N | N | N | |
| Domestic work | 5 | 1 | 25 | 52 | 83 |
| Prostitution | 1 | - | 2 | 3 | 6 |
| Labour | - | - | - | 1 | 1 |
| Total | | | | | 90[a] |

[a] Information on the employment of 4 women who migrated for reasons other than work (i.e. on the pretence of shopping) is not available

*Notes* Since no one reported 'very good' health conditions the category is removed from the table

contracting sexually transmitted infections and illnesses such as urinary tract infections is high for prostitutes. Prostitutes can also be subject to physical harassment and harm by their clients. Further, sexual exploitation connected to trafficking is associated with violence and a range of other serious health issues.

According to the present study, the primary reason for the negative health status is exploitation at the destination (93%). According to UNODC (2014), exploitation is mainly divided into (i) labour exploitation and (ii) sexual exploitation. The exploitation of the migrants takes diverse forms. Table 2.7 indicates the types of labour exploitation and harassment the trafficked faced at the workplace or by the agency personnel at the destination.

When analysing the findings of Table 2.7, it is seen that the exploitation of women takes two forms. One is to impose harassment on them. The other is depriving them of their rights. In this study, five types of imposing—i.e. physical harassment, mental harassment, rape/sexual harassment, overworked and abuse are reported, and while four types of deprivations—i.e. not giving basic needs, non-payment of salary, not allowed to return home after contract period and not allowed to communicate are reported. The highest number of exploitations is reported as physical harassment and deprivation of communication with family. Deprivation of basic needs comes to a close second. Siddhisena and Ranasinghe (2016) note that trafficked women face various difficulties without inadequate food and facilities. According to the 2019 records of the SLBFE, 611 complaints from women were regarding non-payment of agreed wage (Table 2.7). In this study, 72.6% reported the same reason.

Some examples of exploitation are stated below.

> My daughter worked as a housemaid in country 'P'. Though she works for nearly 20 hours per day, she is not paid a monthly wage by the employer. She is now having a skin disease on her leg and it was reported as very painful. But they didn't give any treatment. (Jefa [mother of trafficked])
>
> My wife migrated to the country 'Q' as a housemaid through a visit visa. She informed the agency that she needed to return as she had developed severe panting while working. The agency informed us that they want five lakhs to send her back. She was injured by the agency

**Table 2.7** Type of exploitation at the workplace or by agency personnel

| Type of exploitation | N | % |
|---|---|---|
| Physical harassment | 71 | 78 |
| Mental harassment | 62 | 68.1 |
| Overworked | 19 | 20.9 |
| Rape/ Sexual harassment | 23 | 25.3 |
| Deprivation of basic needs | 69 | 75.9 |
| Non-receipt of wages | 66 | 72.6 |
| Not allowed to return after completion of contract period | 28 | 30.2 |
| Lack of communication with family | 71 | 78 |
| Total | 94 | [a] |

[a] Multiple Responses

> person and they frightened her through phone calls by saying that they were going to kill her. (Suba [husband of trafficked])

> My daughter travelled to country 'W' to work as a housemaid in 2015. Though the first few months were okay, after that she was punished for the smallest mistake she made as time passed by. Now she is having difficulties in walking as she had been whipped on her feet by the employer. (Anu [mother of trafficked])

> Though my wife migrated to the country 'L' for an employment period of two years, the employer is not allowing her to leave that house even after the completion of service. When she complained to the agency regarding this problem, the agency said that the wife had signed a paper which extended the period of the contract. If she needs to go back home she has to pay Rs.180000. The agency officer has also poured hot oil to her body. (Gam [husband of trafficked])

> My daughter migrated to the country 'P' as a housemaid where she worked happily in the first couple of months. But after some time the occupants of the house have burnt her back and cut her hair. She is suffering from severe back pain because she is being kicked on her spine while she is asleep. (Neeka [mother of trafficked])

> My mother departed to Dubai to work as a housemaid without informing any of the family members. As she was an attractive woman who was timid, the man of the house had gotten attracted to her. The wife of the employer has chopped her hair off and she is suffering mentally as she is being physically harassed. She has lost her identity as a woman. (Shan [daughter of trafficked])

The multiple answers provided by the women in Table 2.7 and the quotes above indicate that women's exploitation is multifaceted. The diverse types of exploitation can impact health status in very complex ways. For example, as Beyrer and Stachowiak (2003) show, physical harassment against migrants impacts their mental health. The examples indicate some of these complexities. Additionally, the study revealed that sexual exploitation at the destination directly contributes to various health issues for women, including physical health problems, psychological issues, and injuries. The following section briefly discusses this scenario further.

### *2.3.4 The Special Case of Sexual Exploitation*

The present study revealed that out of the total migrant women, 23 were sexually abused (Table 2.7) at the workplace and at the agencies. Neupane and Kallestrup (2015) citing the Global Report on Trafficking data released in 2014 (UNODC, 2014), note that sexual exploitation is the commonest form of human trafficking (53%), followed by forced labour (40%). They however state that this figure of forced labour may be incorrect because it is hidden and not reported frequently or detected.

Similar to other exploitation, Siddhisena and Ranasinghe (2016) noted that migrant women are also being abused by the brokers. According to the present study, 16% of the trafficked were abused by brokers. Laki's case study can be taken as an example.

> My daughter departed for country 'R' in 2014 in order to work as a housemaid. She was kept at the agency for about one week after she complained about the first house she worked at where they harassed her. When she had stated that she wanted to go back home the lady at the agency had 'sold' her to a different man. She tried to commit suicide several times. (Laki [mother of trafficked])

Taylor (1986) noted that migrants often face significant difficulties when choosing their options, sometimes becoming so vulnerable that they commit suicide. This study confirms that harassment at the workplace and subsequent house arrest by agencies negatively impact migrants' health. Similarly, Basu (2003) highlighted that sexual and physical exploitation leads to mental depression in women. Scholars also reported that deteriorated mental health is a prevalent and persistent negative effect of human trafficking, with psychological consequences including depression, post-traumatic stress disorder, other anxiety disorders, suicidal thoughts, and somatic conditions such as disabling physical pain or dysfunction. According to the present study, among the migrants, 23 women experienced sexual abuse, including rape and sexual harassment at their destination. As a result of this sexual exploitation, 11 women suffered from physical illnesses, 23 women endured psychological disorders, and 10 women sustained various injuries. In this context, the families of these women were asked to pay agencies or employers at the destination to repatriate the migrants to Sri Lanka for proper medical treatment or to save their lives. In the present study sample, 18% of the families paid substantial sums to various individuals to free their family members from violence and bring them back to Sri Lanka. The following three scenarios illustrate this situation in further detail.

> I am a father of three children and 33 years old. My wife migrated to the country 'N' on a two-year work contract. But the owner of the house (employer) is not allowing her to leave, and he uses my wife as a sex provider. The employer has increased the validity of her medical reports for three years by force. I asked him to send her back. But the employer asked me to send a replacement or pay six lacks if I wanted her returned. Six lacks is a dream for me …. (Perumal [husband of the trafficked])

> My wife migrated to the country 'L' as a housemaid through a visit visa. She is always sexually harassed by the owner of the house and she went to the agency as she developed panting. Agency persons told them they want rupees five lacks to send her home. If we don't pay, they are planning to 'sell' her to another country. She was injured by them and frightened by phone calls saying that they were going to kill her. (Suresh [husband of the trafficked])

By analysing these scenarios, the study reveals that many family members at the origin attempted to save the lives of trafficked migrants. During the study, it was found that many migrants were detained in prisons, and agencies due to illegal migration and physical and mental harassment in their workplaces, which severely impacted their health. In this context, family members had to pay substantial sums hoping to bring the migrants back to Sri Lanka to save their health and lives.

## 2.4 Conclusion

Trafficking is a global health issue which surpasses sexual health and includes all aspects of the physical and mental health of the trafficked. This study elaborates on the mental and physical (including disability) health of 94 trafficked women from Sri Lanka and highlights the complexities of health issues of the trafficked from recruitment to exploitation at the destination. During recruitment, women often hid health issues and used forged medical documents. Further, forced migration and false promises significantly impacted their mental health. At destinations, women suffered physical health problems, psychological disorders, disabilities, and injuries due to labour and sexual exploitation and harassment from both the agencies and the employers.

The health of the trafficked women is still an under-researched area, mainly because of limitations in reporting due to the vulnerability of the trafficked because of illegal migration, threats from the employer or the traffickers, and sheer helplessness in the form of poverty, etc. The findings underscore the need for public awareness programs on trafficking, stricter laws against middlemen (i.e. agency personnel/ brokers), and improved standards for employment agencies. Mechanisms should be in place for legal security, and embassy operations must be transparent and efficient. Governmental support should also extend for health care seeking including proper counselling and legal and financial assistance for the currently trafficked. Immediate measures are required for the protection of the mental and physical well-being of the trafficked and the facilitation of repatriation without lengthy procedures.

## References

Amirthalingam, K., Jayatilaka, D., Liyanage, N. (2013). *Victims of human trafficking in Sri Lanka. Narratives of women, children and youth.* ILO Study.

Basu, R. (2003). Trafficking of women: confused responses. *Combat Law*, August–September.

Beyrer, C., & Stachowiak, J. (2003). Health consequences of trafficking of women and girls in Southeast Asia.

Busza, J., Castle, S., & Diarra, A. (2004). Trafficking and health. *BMJ (Clinical research ed), 328*(7452), 1369–1371.

Disrupt Human Trafficking. (2024). https://www.disrupthumantrafficking.com/

International Labour Organization. (2004). *Review of Sri Lankan Laws on the trafficking women, by the center for the policy alternative.* ILO.

International Labour Organization. (2020). *World employment and social outlook.* ILO, Geneva. www.ilo.org/sites/default/files/wcmsp5/groups/public/@dgreports/@dcomm/@publ/documents/publication/wcms_734455.pdf

Jayatilaka, R. (2008). *Women migrant workers and trafficking in Sri Lanka.* Women's Education and Research Center, Colombo.

Morrison, J., & Crosland, B. (2000). *The trafficking and smuggling of refugees, the end game in European asylum policy* (145).

Neupane, D., & Kallestrup, P. (2015). *Human trafficking: An emerging global health problem.* Available via DIALOG http://www.globalhealthminders.dk/wp-content/uploads/2015/01/GHM-HumanTrafficking-Brief.pdf

Rescue & Restore. (2019). *Victims of human trafficking regional program* (pp. 1–12). Available via DIALOG www.acf.hhs.gov/sites/default/files/documents/otip/rescue_and_restore_data_fact_sheet_fy2008_2017.pdf

Siddhisena, K. A., & Ranasinghe, M. A. (2016). Women on the move: Human trafficking in Sri Lanka. *Sri Lanka Journal of Population Studies,* 15–16.

Sri Lanka Bureau of Foreign Employment. (2020). *Statistics 2020, Si Lanka Bureau of Foreign Employment*. Colombo, Sri Lanka:

Taylor, E. J. (1986). Differential migration, networks, information and risk. *Research in Human Capital and Development, 4,* 147–171.

United Nations Office on Drugs and Crime. (2014). *Global report on Trafficking in persons.* United Nations.

United Nations Office on Drugs and Crime. (2020). *Global report on Trafficking in persons.* United Nations.

United Nations Office on Drugs and Crime. (2023). *Global report on Trafficking in persons.* United Nations.

Zimmerman, C., Hossain, M., Watts, C. (2011). Human trafficking and health: A conceptual model to inform policy, intervention and research. *Social Science and Medicine, 73*(2), 327–335.

# Chapter 3
# Women's Health in the Wake of Disasters: Investigating the Outcomes of Natural Disasters on Women's Health and Gender Sensitivity in Bangladesh

**Naema Fatima**

**Abstract** The impacts of natural disasters worldwide are apparent, with vulnerable groups bearing a disproportionate brunt. Many of these challenges, when combined with the gender disparity impacts on health systems, make it doubly difficult for women to access healthcare. In this brief essay, we explore the meeting of inequities and women's health—especially those particular to disaster-prone areas in Bangladesh, where natural vulnerabilities are pushing risk toward the environment. Being a country in the deltaic area, Bangladesh is highly vulnerable to natural disasters like cyclones, floods, river erosions, and droughts, exposing existing gender disparities. The research examines how entrenched gender norms, structural inequalities, and societal discrimination impede women's capacity to be prepared for disasters, respond effectively when a disaster occurs, and progressively recover from disasters. Women have to rise above this, and the statement further calls for gender-sensitive disaster policies that support the socioeconomic status and resilience of women. The paper concludes by recognizing the need for women to frame an understanding of disaster vulnerability, preparedness, risk management, and response strategies if detailed knowledge is provided regarding unique issues faced by them during disasters. In addition, it provides the ways gender-based impacts influence women's preparedness directly or indirectly on women's health during natural disasters. The results support women's engagement in disaster risk reduction efforts and appropriate measures to be taken to protect their rights and welfare. Overall, this study expects to contribute to the gendered impacts of natural disasters and policy advocacy work—emphasizing the importance of gender-responsive disaster management in Bangladesh.

**Keywords** Women's health · Natural disasters · Gendered impacts · Cyclones · Floods · Mental health

---

N. Fatima (✉)
Environmental Sciences and Bioinformatics Program, Asian University for Women, Chittagong, Bangladesh
e-mail: naimafatima0319@gmail.com



P. Chouhan et al. (eds.), *Women's Health Dynamics in South Asia*, Asian Perspectives on Public Health, https://doi.org/10.1007/978-981-95-2321-4_3

## 3.1 Introduction

The events or threats that act as catalysts for natural disasters and catastrophes are known to be environmental hazards. Environmental hazards can come in different forms, for example, geophysical, hydrological, meteorological (fog, storms, and extreme temperature), climatological, biological (insect infestation, diseases, etc.), and extraterrestrial (space weather). For countless years, the earth's terrain has been formed by natural calamities such as flooding, earthquakes, hurricanes, thunderstorms, drought, landslides, forest fires, and volcanic explosions. When such natural phenomena engage with artificially created elements, including buildings, farming, and communities, they culminate in disasters of nature (Chaudhary & Piracha, 2021). 11,360 natural disasters unfolded from 1995 to 2022, with an average of 398 annually. Asia has witnessed 4390 natural disasters and 918,198 natural disaster deaths, the greatest number of disasters and victims among the continents (Tin et al., 2024). Nearly 4969 hydrological disasters constituted the highest occurrences among the types of disasters, with geophysical disasters accounting for the greatest mortality of 770,644. Biological disasters generated the majority of injuries in 2544 individuals (Tin et al., 2024). Many natural disasters claim the lives of 40,000 – 50,000 individuals annually, the mean, throughout the prior several decades (Ritchie et al., 2024). 399 natural hazard-related incidents were reported in 2023 by the Emergency Events Database (EM-DAT), according to the Center for Research on the Epidemiology of Disasters (CRED). These incidents killed 86,473 individuals and impacted 93.1 million others (Centre for Research on the Epidemiology of Disasters (CRED), 2024).

South Asia comprises 8 countries: Afghanistan, Bangladesh, Bhutan, India, the Maldives, Nepal, Pakistan, and Sri Lanka. These nations constitute roughly 3.2% of the globe's surface area and 10% of Asia (Shrestha, 2008). Although having abundant natural assets, over 70% of people in South Asia live in poverty due to political unrest, bad governance, and natural calamities. More than half of the world's impoverished people reside in Asia, specifically South Asia (Kafle, 2017). Given its geographic location, socioeconomic and political circumstances, and entrenched disparities caused by caste, economic status, faith, and ethnic background, South Asia is exceedingly susceptible to climate change and natural disasters. The issue becomes more challenging because of the reality that women are less able to mitigate the effects and adjust to environmental disasters due to sexist prejudice and pervasive gender inequalities. These elements increase the domain's susceptibility to the impact of climate change (Sangwan & Brahmachari, 2023). The World Bank in Washington has collated data showing that a minimum of a single disaster has impacted 750 million South Asian individuals (Siddiqui, 2023). The likelihood of death from disasters is fourteen times greater for women and children than for males (Okai, 2022). Natural disasters have increased in frequency, and because of structural issues like poverty, inequality, and fast population expansion, women are especially exposed. Women are more likely to be displaced, lack preparedness plans for disasters, and experience resilience problems (Fatema et al., 2021). Disasters have a gendered effect on people, with an increased incidence of chronic sickness, mental disorders, poverty, reliance, familial disputes, and disabilities. The well-being of women is a major concern during disasters, particularly in lower-income nations, as they are particularly vulnerable to violence and exploitation (Fatema et al., 2021).

Bangladesh is one of the most vulnerable countries in South Asia. The country is in a highly hazardous region with strong seismic and hydrometeorological risks. South Asia's Multiple Mortality Risk Index (MMRI) is greatest in Bangladesh, followed by India, Pakistan, and Sri Lanka (Kafle, 2017). In a study of natural disaster patterns and repercussions from 1995 to 2022, Bangladesh ranked 8th out of 10 nations with the most natural disasters in a total of 192 natural disasters (Tin et al., 2024). Cyclones, floods, and droughts are among Bangladesh's most common natural disasters (Kafle, 2017). Moreover, Bangladesh, a riverine nation, frequently experiences severe riverbank erosion (Akter et al., 2019). Table 3.1 shows the names of the natural disasters, the timelines, and the number of victims of the natural disasters mentioned below.

Natural disasters provide distinct obstacles and issues, such as certain disaster forms, displacements, family involvement in trauma mitigation, psychological responses, and coping mechanisms, all of which can have a bearing on an individual's capacity to adjust (Lazarus et al., 2002). Natural disasters can impact family well-being in 3 forms: destruction of health, resources, and earnings. Injuries, deaths, and disease outbreaks all negatively impact the standard of living (Gaihaet al., 2012). Bangladesh, a developing country, is extremely vulnerable to catastrophes such as floods, cyclones, droughts, and riverbank erosion, given its smooth landscape, shallow weather, and scarcity of assets. The nation also needs more availability of healthcare services and adequate prevention systems. This vulnerability is worsened by the nation's distinct seasons, rainfall patterns, and weather characteristics (Fatema, 2020). Women are more susceptible than men beforehand, during, and following natural catastrophes in Bangladesh, as it seems prevalent (Akter et al., 2019). Natural disasters occur commonly on Bangladesh's coastlines, inflicting substantial harm to the people living there. Women, teenage girls, and youngsters are thought to be at greatest risk after natural catastrophes, comprising over 75% of those displaced (Alam & Rahman, 2014). In the following sections, this paper will discuss the detrimental impacts on women's health induced by natural disasters like cyclones, floods, droughts, and river erosion in Bangladesh. The paper includes gender-based impacts or influences that affect women in terms of their preparation, vulnerability, risk handling, and awareness before, during, and after natural disasters.

## 3.2 Materials and Methods

This chapter uses a secondary data analysis to examine the effects of natural disasters on women's health in Bangladesh. The latter is an approach that is designed to obtain, but also systematically analyze and synthesize all the available literature and data from different sources on a topic of interest.

**Table 3.1** The types of disasters and numbers of victims

| Name of the Disaster | Year | Affected/Death | Source |
|---|---|---|---|
| Cyclone | 1970 Bhola Cyclone | Death: 300,000–500,000+ people<br>Affected: 20 million people | (Hossain & Mullick, 2020)<br>(Kafle, 2017) |
| | 1985 Cyclone | Death: 11,069 people | (Saha, 2017) |
| | 1988 Cyclone 04B | Death: 5,708 people | (Dhaka Tribune, 2024) |
| | 1991 Cyclone | Death: 139,000 people<br>Affected: 15 million people | (Rahman & Bennish, 1993)<br>(Kafle, 2017) |
| | 1997 Cyclone | Death: 155 people | (Hossain & Mullick, 2020) |
| | 2007 Cyclone Sidr | Death: 3,363 people | (Saha, 2017) |
| | 2009 Cyclone Aila | Death: 150 people | (Hossain & Mullick, 2020) |
| | 2013 Cyclone Mahasen | Death: 17 people | (Saha, 2017) |
| | 2016 Cyclone Roanu | Death: 27 people | (Saha, 2017) |
| | 2017 Cyclone Mora | Death: 7 people | (Hossain & Mullick, 2020) |
| | 2019 Cyclone Fani | Death: 12 people | (Hossain & Mullick, 2020) |
| | 2020 Cyclone Amphan | Death: 30+ people | (Dhaka Tribune, 2024) |
| | 2022 Cyclone Sitrang | Death: 20+ people<br>Affected: a million people | (Dhaka Tribune, 2024) |
| | 2023 Cyclone Mocha | Death: 3 people | (Dhaka Tribune, 2024) |
| | 2023 Cyclone Midhili | Death: 7 people | (Dhaka Tribune, 2024) |
| Floods | 1971 Flood | Death: 120 people | (Shaibur et al., 2017) |
| | Floods During 1972–2017 | Death: 42,279 people<br>Affected: 304,256,323 people | (Baten et al., 2018) |
| Droughts | Droughts During 1972–2017 | Death: 18 people<br>Affected: 25,002,000 | (Baten et al., 2018) |
| River Erosion | 1996 | Affected: 10,103,635 people | (Islam & Rashid, 2012) |
| | 1997 | Affected: 173,090 people | (Islam & Rashid, 2012) |
| | 1998 | Affected: 321,000 people | (Islam & Rashid, 2012) |

(continued)

Table 3.1 (continued)

| Name of the Disaster | Year | Affected/Death | Source |
|---|---|---|---|
| | 1999 | Affected: 899,275 people | (Islam & Rashid, 2012) |
| | 2000 | Affected: 415,870 people | (Islam & Rashid, 2012) |
| | Yearly | It affects millions of people annually | (Billah et al., 2023) |

### 3.2.1 Source of Data

The research uses a variety of secondary sources, including scientific articles, government reports, organizational publications, and relevant books. The key databases were searched, including Google Scholar, BMJ Journals, Springer, PubMed, Elsevier, ResearchGate, and MDPI for relevant studies describing the impacts of natural disasters on women's health in Bangladesh.

### 3.2.2 Literature Review

An extensive literature review was performed to summarize research studies conducted on the health consequences associated with natural disasters and women. The review was based on experience with published studies in the past two decades to limit outdated information. It was conducted to identify and summarize the evidence, along with key themes/emerging trends in the published literature on women's health outcomes post-disasters.

### 3.2.3 Data Extraction and Organization

Details were extracted systematically from the included sources, focusing on types of natural disasters (floods, cyclones, river erosions, and droughts), health outcomes (physical injuries, mental health issues, reproductive health, etc.), as well as socioeconomic implications for women. The data were then clustered according to themes for analysis and synthesis.

### 3.2.4 Data Analysis

Thematic analysis revealed similar and unique patterns across the different types of natural disasters and the effects of natural disasters having specific impacts on women's health. Major themes focused on the disparate impacts of disasters, including cyclones, flooding, river erosion, and droughts on women. It also identified gender differences in at-risk and resilience factors, availability of resources, coping strategies, health services utilization, and institutional response that were affected by socially imposed roles or expectations before, during, and after disasters.

### 3.2.5 Synthesis of Results

The results were synthesized to present a unified storyline on the health effects for women in Bangladesh due to natural disasters. This synthesis aimed to demonstrate the complexity and how intertwined various determinants for women's health were, as well as inform on the necessity of incorporating gender-sensitive approaches within disaster management and public health responses.

The approaches employed in this chapter can help contribute to the knowledge of links between natural disasters and women's health in Bangladesh, while providing insights into the intersection of gender considerations in disaster risk reduction within a national framework. These insights, in turn, will inform the leaders of tomorrow as they chart a course around this monumental issue.

## 3.3 Results

Because of the geographical, climatic, and environmental conditions, natural calamities like cyclones, floods, droughts, and river erosions are a recurrent phenomenon in Bangladesh. The aftermath of these calamities greatly affects the health status of women in Bangladesh. These impacts may be direct (e.g., injury or death) in the short term or result as a consequence of disruptions and stressors that originate from a disaster. Table 3.2 illustrates the different types of natural disasters and their negative effects on women's health in Bangladesh.

Natural disasters have differential impacts on both men and women, with suggestions of aspects in terms of unequal exposures to catastrophes and a "gender-based terrain of disasters." The increased frequency of natural catastrophes and people affected theoretically and practically supports this argument. Bangladesh experiences concurrent forms of gender challenges and frequent natural disasters. This exposes the interplay of gender and natural disasters to be rather vivid (Juran & Trivedi, 2015). Natural disasters have far-reaching impacts on women, penetrating every sphere of their lives and often accentuating other imbalances, which can prolong impacts on

**Table 3.2** The impacts on women's health due to various natural disasters in Bangladesh

| Natural Disasters | Impacts on Women's Health | Sources |
|---|---|---|
| Cyclones | 1. Gendered impacts include death, injuries, disabilities, chronic conditions (with associated psychosocial health problems), poverty, increased dependency on men for income, unemployment, and family breakdowns<br>2. Women are particularly vulnerable to harm and violence in emergencies—especially when pre-existing inequalities expose them to exploitation that has dangerous repercussions for their health and rights<br>3. Women after cyclones are reported to experience depression, Post-Traumatic Stress Disorder (PTSD), Common Mental Disorder (CMD), psychosocial and mental health problems, anxiety, and poor physical health<br>4. The healthcare issues faced by pregnant women are transportation problems, lack of health facilities and sanitation for themselves, and tragedies while hurrying to cyclone shelters when natural disasters emerge<br>5. Women face extra work demands and potential assaults or sexual violence from temporary accommodation sites, with the phenomenon being enhanced in numbers through cyclone-induced displacement<br>6. Trauma, genito-urinary infections, as well as post-natal medical conditions during and after natural disasters, further deteriorate the general health of women | (Fatema et al., 2021)<br>(Shamsuddoha et al., 2024)<br>(Chowdhury et al., 2022) |
| Floods | 1. Women face numerous problems when displaced, including sanitation, hard physical labor, indecent acts such as sexual assault or abuse, and their susceptibility to the consequences of floods<br>2. Women's rights are violated by sudden-onset disasters like floods, which cause injuries and fatalities<br>3. Affecting both women and girls during floods and cyclones, gender-based & domestic violence forces them into searching for jobs, thus exposing them to different forms of mistreatment<br>4. Child marriages increase due to financial stresses and school closures after flood levels rise. Burden-sharing inequities, violence against women, and child marriage significantly affect women's mental health, leading to chronic anxiety disorders, PTSDs, severe depression episodes characterized by nightmares, as well as lack of self-esteem and happiness<br>5. In one study, women in extreme floods faced various threats, including animal attacks, harassment, and food shortages that disrupted their lives<br>6. Women can be infected with skin infections, diarrhea, fever, and cholera during a flash flood outbreak. Physical injuries consist of hand-leg-finger fractures and head–waist injuries<br>7. The floods also affect the health of women in matters concerning their reproductive health, since limited spaces make it hard to change their menstrual garments<br>8. Pregnant women suffer from nutritional deficiencies, physical damage, and even miscarriages due to serious wounds and delayed visits to the hospital | (Shamsuddoha et al., 2024)<br>(Afrin, 2021)<br>(Nahar et al., 2021) |

(continued)

**Table 3.2** (continued)

| Natural Disasters | Impacts on Women's Health | Sources |
|---|---|---|
| Droughts | 1. Vector-borne infections and drought-related disorders can increase in rainfall-deficient situations and affect reproductive health and fetal development<br>2. Poor earnings make it difficult for women to get enough nourishment during pregnancy, boosting the possibility of impairment of fetal development along with decreased birth weight<br>3. Droughts can increase the amount of labor needed by pregnant women due to traveling long distances in search of water, physically straining them, and leading to lower birth weight<br>4. Drought can increase the possibility of illness in mothers and children, early marriage, and violence against women | (Le & Nguyen, 2022)<br>(Khan, 2022) |
| River Erosions | 1. Women, victims of erosion, are exposed to all sorts of challenges, including sanitary concerns, heavier workloads, unfriendly behavior, violence, sexual abuse, and exposure to dangers related to climate change<br>2. It impacts severely on women's mental and physical well-being by destroying housing and other resources, leading to debt, domestic abuse, family disintegration, and an increased workload | (Shamsuddoha et al., 2024)<br>(Akter et al., 2019) |

their health and well-being since every type of impact or effect is interrelated. Here are some gender-based impacts that befall women and influence their preparedness, directly and indirectly impacting women's health before, during, and after natural disasters.

### 3.3.1 Economic Status

Women are more highly affected by climate change because of economic, social, and governmental disparities. Analyzing disaster data for 141 countries, higher rates of female mortality can be linked back to their social and economic disadvantage. When everybody is equal within a society, the mortality rate varies less. According to the Asian Development Bank analysis, human impact from natural disasters could be reduced by enhancing women's economic status (Sangwan & Brahmachari, 2023).

### 3.3.2 Education

Poor education for women contributes to the lack of female doctors in times of natural crises. There is a claim that most women prefer not to be examined by male doctors just to avoid embarrassment and humiliation during such medical checkups (Sangwan & Brahmachari, 2023). Poor infrastructure, low literacy levels, and insufficient understanding put the South Asian area in a debtor position to an epidemic (Kafle, 2017). A good number of studies also reveal that women who were less educated or illiterate had significantly higher effects of PTSD, depression, CMD, disability, and morbid physical concurrence (Fatema et al., 2021).

### 3.3.3 Family Dynamic

For cultural, social, and economic purposes, South Asian women usually rely on men. They have limited mobility, are excluded from decision-making processes, and experience violence from family members—especially from men. A son is seen as someone of value, while a daughter is considered a financial burden under the paradigm of dowry. Moreover, the short-term concerns of women are beside the point; invariably, their decision-making power is compromised. In many such cases, women's voices get drowned amidst the household responsibilities, taking care of elderly parents and children, especially after a disaster, making it hard to leave the affected area (Sangwan & Brahmachari, 2023). The lack of familial support and economic factors, coupled with men having to leave behind their families for money-making purposes, presents a problem for women seeking safer ground to live in disaster situations. Women have to be more responsible for taking care of their families while men are away from home (Akter et al., 2019). Health complications are a consequence of low family and social assistance after natural disasters; on the other hand, sufficient exposure to family and health care protects individuals against the destructive effects of stressful experiences (Fatema et al., 2021).

### 3.3.4 *Difficulty in Accessibility*

Women find it difficult to access food preparation, water, and relief materials after natural disasters, which limits them further from pursuing their education and other employment opportunities outside their home setting (*Women & Girls in Disasters—Center for Disaster Philanthropy*, 2022). Studies indicate that Bangladeshi women have limited access to all resources that may be used for reducing risk, including land, financing, leadership positions, agricultural supplies, technological advances, and educational services. The coastal communities are the worst affected by this crisis (Islam, 2012).

### 3.3.5 *Policy Implementation*

Despite the policy statements from relief groups emphasizing gender issues, women's responsibilities in manufacturing, and progress remain underrepresented in development and disaster execution. Novel responsibilities for women emerge, and daily routines become challenging in crises. To improve the socioeconomic status of women who stand at risk of disasters, policymakers, NGOs, and researchers must address the gender-based aspect of these issues (Ashraf & Azad, 2015).

By examining these topics, it is possible to gain a thorough understanding of the various ways that natural disasters affect women as well as the demands and difficulties that are unique to women in the oversight and aftermath of natural disasters. These settings influence more or less the preparedness of women in natural disaster-prone regions, eventually impacting their mental and physical health. It is evident that by examining gender disparities beforehand, during, and in the aftermath of natural disasters, we can recognize the connections underlying women's vulnerability, preparedness, risk-handling, and awareness.

## 3.4 Discussion

Bangladesh, at the bottom point of the Ganges, Brahmaputra, and Meghna Basin, is a gently sloping, shallow delta (Islam, 2012). It is particularly vulnerable to river erosion, floods, tropical storms, droughts, and other natural disasters yearly. The nation's distinct geographical characteristics mostly bring on disasters. These entail a great deal of worldly and human damage. Bangladesh is one of the biggest targets of disasters since many people live along the shores (Islam, 2012). Conventional gender-specific work divides, uneven availability of resources, and discrimination against women all worsen natural disasters. Due to organizational prejudices, restricted movement, and gendered socializing, women are disadvantaged when it comes to receiving help and compensation benefits, which makes it more difficult for them to grapple with and heal from crises (Akter et al., 2019). If women are fortunate enough to escape natural disasters, there can be longer-lasting, unseen "secondary" effects, like an increase in abuse committed against women or increased job instability (Akter et al., 2019). Bangladesh's natural disaster casualties, which include 90% of fourteen thousand and 80% of the ten thousand female deaths following cyclones in 1991 and 2007, demonstrate that women are frequently more severely impacted than men. Higher incidence of accidents, disabilities, chronic illnesses, mental disorders, impoverishment, reliance, familial disputes, unemployment, and the possibility of being exploited and mistreated as a result of natural disasters are some examples of the gendered effects (Fatema et al., 2021). When racing to cyclone shelters, pregnant women frequently encounter difficulties like limited mobility, dangerous situations, climate change-related risks, inadequate medical care and sanitation, and injuries. Pregnant women are left without access to immediate medical attention, leading to catastrophic repercussions like miscarriage (Shamsuddoha et al., 2024). Health problems that affect women in cyclone shelters before and afterward their confinement include trauma, panic attacks, depression, PTSD, genito-urinary infections, and postpartum health difficulties (Chowdhury et al., 2022). For floods, rapid-onset natural hazards have the potential to cause casualties and harm that endanger the lives of women (Shamsuddoha et al., 2024). Like cyclones, domestic violence has a severe effect on women in floods, driving them to look for work and subjecting them to harassment. Bangladesh's rates of child marriage increased in the wake of extreme weather and flooding because of the shutdown of schools and financial turmoil. Dowries encourage impoverished families to swiftly arrange weddings against the girl's approval, which has a detrimental effect on the emotional and physical well-being of women (Afrin, 2021). Floods put women in danger of food shortages, discrimination, and assaults by animals. Women become vulnerable to wounds, infections, and illnesses, including cholera, diarrhea, and skin problems. Floods can have an impact on reproductive health and pregnant women, causing miscarriage because of delayed medical appointments, inadequate nourishment, and injuries to their bodies (Nahar et al., 2021). River erosion, like other disasters, can destroy resources and financial obligations, cause domestic violence, family dissolution, and additional load, jeopardizing women's mental and physical wellness (Akter et al., 2019). Natural disasters like cyclones, floods, and river erosion have caused displacement. The most frequent places for people to make temporary homes or shelters after displacement are beside embankments or roads. Women are particularly affected by displacement, as they often deal with issues related to hygiene, heavier workloads, abuse, and sexual harassment (Shamsuddoha et al., 2024). Droughts are a common meteorological hazard, although Bangladesh is primarily affected by hydrological disasters. Lack of rainfall increases the incidence of drought-related sicknesses and vector-borne infections, leaving an impact on pregnant women and the development of the fetus (Le & Nguyen, 2022). Due to the negative effects of insufficient rainfall on aquaculture, forest production, and cultivation, droughts are capable of resulting in reduced earnings and nourishment. In addition to the difficulty in women accessing enough nourishment throughout pregnancy, there is a higher chance of birth weight loss and fetal underdevelopment. Pregnant women may strain themselves as they are more likely to commute to faraway destinations to obtain water (Le & Nguyen, 2022). Moreover, droughts in Bangladesh have been associated with a surge in child marriages and violence against women (Khan, 2022).

Natural disasters affect women and men differently, indicating that they are not equally exposed. The rising frequency of these events in Bangladesh highlights the relationship between gender and natural disasters. Disasters have a significant influence on women in every aspect of their daily lives and frequently exacerbate other imbalances that may worsen the consequences on their health and well-being. As discussed in the results section, women's health and preparedness are impacted by specific gender-based factors before, during, and following disasters. These effects can be either direct or indirect. Economic status, education, family dynamics, disability in accessing services, and policy implementations can influence a woman's preparedness and awareness during a natural disaster. Women's preparedness is affected in disaster-prone locations, which in turn affects their physical and mental health. Women's vulnerability, preparedness, risk management, and awareness are all correlated with gender disparities during disasters.

Some of the recommendations for women and their health and gendered disparities caused by natural disasters are given below:

- Knowing the significance of emergency preparedness, growing training initiatives to address medical issues, executing research regarding suitable women's healthcare methods, and striving for government panels to form disaster policies are some suggestions for women's health and gendered disparities caused by natural disasters (International Confederation of Midwives, 2024).
- The initial progression to gender-sensitive risk control is the involvement of women as the main players in policies of natural disaster mitigation (Sangwan & Brahmachari, 2023).
- Hazard education and awareness must be implemented throughout administrative levels, especially local, regional, national, and global. It must be customized to various populations and situations (Chaudhary & Piracha, 2021).
- Government and non-governmental organizations must work together during natural disasters to lower the risk of disasters and protect women from harm. To support women's coping mechanisms, this entails offering separate housing, sanitary facilities, and health services in addition to promoting awareness, putting early warning systems, and developing job prospects for women (Nahar et al., 2021).
- People impacted by disasters, especially women, can benefit from a partnership between disaster prevention and healthcare. Exposure to female doctors can lower mental disorders, and health consequences can be mitigated by health experts

actively participating before, during, and following disaster recovery initiatives (Fatema et al., 2021).

- Climate change increases the severity of droughts, with grave implications for pregnant women in regions prone to drought. Assistance with finances and nutrition can lessen the detrimental effects on the mother's and the offspring's health. To mitigate the disorder, government assistance for healthcare for expectant mothers could additionally be taken into consideration (Le & Nguyen, 2022).
- During natural disasters, women must have access to different facilities within multifunctional shelters. Networks of transportation should be established for quick mobility and rescue. Additionally, facilities must guarantee an adequate supply of water to use (Islam, 2012).
- Effective measures must be implemented by authorities to prevent burglary, hijacking, violence against women, and other unforeseen incidents (Islam, 2012).
- Organize workshops and conferences to enhance community-based awareness-raising activities while guaranteeing women's involvement (Islam, 2012).

### *3.4.1 Limitations of the Study*

It is essential to recognize the limitations of this approach since it uses secondary data, which can introduce certain biases that may be linked with original implementations and research in different contexts. Also, data may differ in various cases, hence the influence on the completeness of the analysis.

## 3.5 Conclusion

Topographical features make Bangladesh a shallow delta, which is prone to floods, storms, river erosion, and droughts. These, in turn, are further compounded by uneven resource availability and gender discrimination. In this regard, it is the impact of natural disasters on the health of women in Bangladesh that underlines an imperative approach of sensitizing disaster management and recovery efforts on a gender basis. It is a complex interplay of factors in the social, economic, and cultural arenas that determines the unique vulnerabilities women face during and after disasters. Some of the examples include floods, cyclones, and river erosions, all of which entail population displacement to a new location where they have to settle temporarily in makeshift shelters along highways or embankments. In such conditions, women will have to contend with inadequate personal hygiene, heavier workloads, violence, and sexual assault. Droughts impact pregnant women and fetal development through an increased burden of diseases and vector-borne infections, as particularly shown in the case of Bangladesh. Women face decreased support and compensation owing to institutional biases, reduced mobility, and gendered socialization, all of which make it hard for women to bounce back from crises. Even when women do survive disasters, they can have continued implications. It is informed that women are more likely to bear the direct physical effects of disasters, such as injuries and fatalities, in addition to indirect health effects associated with long-term challenges to health, including mental health problems, trauma, increased domestic violence, reproductive and maternity health complications, economic instability, and educational deprivation.

The key findings of this paper underline the importance of integrating women's views into strategies for disaster preparedness and response. Active involvement of women in decision-making at all levels will ensure that their specific needs and concerns are addressed in coming up with more effective and fair ways to manage disasters. Besides, promoting women's access to resources, education, and healthcare services is very vital in building resilience and empowering them to cope with preparedness and aftermath stages of any natural disaster.

Improved health outcomes associated with women's economic empowerment emphasize the necessity of targeted interventions that promote gender equality in disaster-prone areas. Efforts, such as skills training to survive, financial support, and employment opportunities, help a lot in reducing the negative impacts of disasters on the physical bodies and minds of women. These involve collaboration between government agencies, non-governmental organizations, and local communities to create a comprehensive framework for reducing disaster risks and prioritizing women's health. For example, to develop early warning systems, build gender-sensitive health facilities, promote the mitigation of social gender disparities (child marriages, dowries, domestic abuse, and sexual harassment), and ensure a safe space for women during emergencies.

Ultimately, gendered natural disasters present issues of social justice and are one step to creating community resilience and recovery in Bangladesh and other places. With rising intensities and more frequent recurrence of disasters as a result of climate change, there is an immediate need to embrace an all-inclusive approach to disaster management. By recognizing these challenges unique to women, we can work toward a more equitable and sustainable future for all that leaves no one behind in the face of adversity.

## References


Afrin, S. (2021, July 10). *Impacts of cyclones on women and girls and the way forward*. Dhaka Tribune.https://www.dhakatribune.com/science-technology-environment/climate-change/252027/impacts-of-cyclones-on-women-and-girls-and-the-way

Akter, K., Dey, S., & Hasan, S. (2019). Riverbank erosion and its impact on rural women: Case study of Ulania village in Bangladesh. *Asian Journal of Women S Studies, 25*(1), 76–95. https://doi.org/10.1080/12259276.2019.1577343

Alam, K., & Rahman, M. H. (2014). Women in natural disasters: A case study from southern coastal region of Bangladesh. *International Journal of Disaster Risk Reduction, 8*, 68–82. https://doi.org/10.1016/j.ijdrr.2014.01.003

Ashraf, M. A., & Azad, M. A. K. (2015). Gender issues in disaster: Understanding the relationships of vulnerability, preparedness and capacity. *Environment and Ecology Research, 3*(5), 136–142. https://doi.org/10.13189/eer.2015.030504

Baten, A., González, P. A., & Delgado, R. C. (2018). Natural disasters and management systems of Bangladesh from 1972 to 2017: Special focus on flood. *OmniScience: A Multi-disciplinary Journal, 8*(3), 35–47. https://sciencejournals.stmjournals.in/index.php/osmj/article/view/753

Billah, M. M., Majumdar, A., Rahman, S. M. A., Alam, M. S., Hossain, M. J., Talukder, J., Islam, M. M., & Khanam, T. (2023). Riverbank erosion and rural food security in Bangladesh. *World, 4*(3), 528–544. https://doi.org/10.3390/world4030033

Centre for Research on the Epidemiology of Disasters (CRED). (2024). 2023 Disasters in numbers—World. *ReliefWeb.* https://reliefweb.int/report/world/2023-disasters-numbers

Chaudhary, M. T., & Piracha, A. (2021). Natural disasters—Origins, impacts, management. *Encyclopedia, 1*(4), 1101–1131. https://doi.org/10.3390/encyclopedia1040084

Chowdhury, T. J., Arbon, P., Gebbie, K., Muller, R., Kako, M., & Steenkamp, M. (2022). Lived-experience of women's well-being in the cyclone shelters of coastal Bangladesh. *Prehospital and Disaster Medicine, 37*(4), 437–443. https://doi.org/10.1017/s1049023x2200070x

Dhaka Tribune. (2024, May 26). *Deadliest cyclones in Bangladesh's history.* https://www.dhakatribune.com/bangladesh/347566/deadliest-cyclones-in-bangladesh%E2%80%99s-history

Gaiha, R., Hill, K., & Thapa, G. (2012). Natural disasters in South Asia 1. In *Routledge handbook of South Asian economics* (pp. 109–128). Routledge. https://crawford.anu.edu.au/acde/asarc/pdf/papers/2010/WP2010_06.pdf

Fatema, S. R. (2020). Women's health-related vulnerabilities in natural disaster-affected areas of Bangladesh: A mixed-methods study protocol. *British Medical Journal Open, 10*(11), Article e039772. https://doi.org/10.1136/bmjopen-2020-039772

Fatema, S. R., East, L., Islam, M. S., & Usher, K. (2021). Health impact and risk factors affecting South and Southeast Asian women following natural disasters: A systematic review. *International Journal of Environmental Research and Public Health, 18*(21), 11068. https://doi.org/10.3390/ijerph182111068

Hossain, I., & Mullick, A. R. (2020). Cyclone and Bangladesh: A historical and environmental overview from 1582 to 2020. *International Medical Journal, 25*(6), 2595–2614. https://www.researchgate.net/profile/Irin-Hossain-2/publication/344321172_Cyclone_and_Bangladesh_A_Historical_and_Environmental_Overview_from_1582_to_2020/links/5f677120a6fdcc00862f3e42/Cyclone-and-Bangladesh-A-Historical-and-Environmental-Overview-from-1582-to-2020.pdf

International Confederation of Midwives. (2024, May 13). *Health of Women and Children in Disasters | International Confederation of Midwives.* https://internationalmidwives.org/resources/health-of-women-and-children-in-disasters/

Islam, M. F., & Rashid, A. B. (2012). Riverbank erosion displacees in Bangladesh: Need for institutional response and policy intervention. *Bangladesh Journal of Bioethics, 2*(2), 4–19. https://doi.org/10.3329/bioethics.v2i2.9540

Islam, M. R. (2012). Vulnerability and coping strategies of women in disaster: A study on coastal areas of Bangladesh. *Arts Faculty Journal*, 147–169. https://doi.org/10.3329/afj.v4i0.12938

Juran, L., & Trivedi, J. (2015). Women, gender norms, and natural disasters in Bangladesh. *Geographical Review, 105*(4), 601–611. https://doi.org/10.1111/j.1931-0846.2015.12089.x

Kafle, S. K. (2017). Disaster risk management systems in South Asia: natural hazards, vulnerability, disaster risk and legislative and institutional frameworks. *Journal of Geography & Natural Disasters, 7*(3). https://doi.org/10.4172/2167-0587.1000207

Khan, N. (2022, August 25). Reproductive health management in the climate change affected areas in Bangladesh. *Dhaka Tribune.* https://www.dhakatribune.com/epaper/292938/reproductive-health-management-in-the-climate

Lazarus, P. J., Jimerson, S. R., & Brock, S. E. (2002). Natural disasters. In *Best practices in school crisis prevention and intervention* (pp. 435–450). https://citeseerx.ist.psu.edu/document?repid=rep1&type=pdf&doi=3913c32b90ab8e9ea6f532d24bff2242b5331bbd

Le, K., & Nguyen, M. (2022). Droughts and child health in Bangladesh. *PLoS ONE, 17*(3), Article e0265617. https://doi.org/10.1371/journal.pone.0265617

Nahar, N., Islam, S., &Mahiuddin, S. (2021). Flash flood impacts on the life and livelihood of women at haor areas in Bangladesh. *National Geographical Journal of India, 67*(3), 322–333. https://doi.org/10.48008/ngji.1780

Okai, A. (2022, March 24). *Women are hit hardest in disasters, so why are responses too often gender-blind?* UNDP. https://www.undp.org/blog/women-are-hit-hardest-disasters-so-why-are-responses-too-often-gender-blind

Rahman, M., & Bennish, M. (1993). Health related response to natural disasters: The case of the Bangladesh cyclone of 1991. *Social Science & Medicine, 36*(7), 903–914. https://doi.org/10.1016/0277-9536(93)90082-f

Ritchie, H., Rosado, P., & Roser, M. (2024, March 12). *Natural disasters*. Our World in Data. https://ourworldindata.org/natural-disasters

Saha, S. K. (2017). Cyclone, salinity intrusion and adaptation and coping measures in coastal Bangladesh. *Space and Culture, India, 5*(1), 12–24. https://www.researchgate.net/publication/318058294_Cyclone_Salinity_Intrusion_and_Adaptation_and_Coping_Measures_in_Coastal_Bangladesh

Sangwan, G., &Brahmachari, D. (2023). Climate change disasters and impact on women in South Asia. In *International Handbook of Disaster Research* (pp. 1–14). https://doi.org/10.1007/978-981-16-8800-3_146-1

Shaibur, M. R., Khan, M. H., & Rashid, M. S. (2017). Climate change may cause natural disasters in Shyamnagar, Satkhira: the southwestern parts of Bangladesh. *Bangladesh Journal of Environmental Science, 32*, 101–110. https://www.researchgate.net/publication/340778803_CLIMATE_CHANGE_MAY_CAUSE_NATURAL_DISASTERS_IN_SHYAMNAGAR_SATKHIRA_THE_SOUTHWESTERN_PARTS_OF_BANGLADESH

Shamsuddoha, M., Jabed, M. A., Islam, M. S., Sultana, N., Imran, A., Rabbi, S. N. A., Jenat, T. U., Shams, S., & Sharif, M. M. (2024). Impacts of climate change-induced natural hazards on women and its human rights implications: A study in the southwest coast of Bangladesh. *Journal of Migration and Health, 9*, Article 100221. https://doi.org/10.1016/j.jmh.2024.100221

Shrestha, M. S. (2008). Impacts of Floods in South Asia. *Journal of South Asia Disaster Studies, 1*(1), 85–106. https://www.researchgate.net/profile/Mandira-Shrestha/publication/259484329_Impacts_of_flood_in_South_Asia/links/0c96052c28501ea59b000000/Impacts-of-flood-in-South-Asia.pdf

Siddiqui, U. (2023, July 8). What makes South Asia so vulnerable to climate change? *Al Jazeera*. https://www.aljazeera.com/news/2023/7/8/what-makes-south-asia-so-vulnerable-to-climate-change

Tin, D., Cheng, L., Le, D., Hata, R., & Ciottone, G. (2024). Natural disasters: A comprehensive study using EMDAT database 1995–2022. *Public Health, 226*, 255–260. https://doi.org/10.1016/j.puhe.2023.11.017

*Women and Girls in Disasters—Center for Disaster Philanthropy*. (2022, April 20). Center for Disaster Philanthropy. https://disasterphilanthropy.org/resources/women-and-girls-in-disasters/#:~:text=This%20can%20include%20lining%20up,to%20education%20or%20outside%20employment

# Chapter 4
# Surviving in the Margins: Addressing the Health Issues of Homeless Women in NCT Delhi

**Nirupama Singh, Aradhya Singh, and Menka Rai**

**Abstract** India has one of the largest homeless populations in the world. Due to the unavailability of recent census data on the homeless population in India, this study will employ an empirical approach to develop a holistic understanding of the health status of homeless women in NCT of Delhi. The homeless urban women experience homelessness due to poverty and unemployment and are often denied their fundamental constitutional and human rights. The transition to homelessness is often associated with physical and mental abuse, social and personal issues, and failure in the implementation of existing government policies. The ill effect of homelessness is not restricted to the absence of a roof, food, and clean water but also extends to chronic health issues ranging from minor diseases like malnourishment, anaemia, diabetes, and malaria, to life-threatening diseases such as HIV, tuberculosis, Sars-CoV2, parasitic infections, and venereal diseases, etc., however, only common diseases were encountered during the survey for the chapter. Exposure to extreme environmental conditions frequently taking place increases the mortality rate of such homeless women adding to their plight. As per the study, an absence of bodily hygiene, food security, maternity benefits, and well-managed habitation increases their physical and psychological vulnerability. This study will thus, end with recommendations to address the issue of degrading health status of urban homeless women and the gap in implementation of the existing legislative policies.

**Keywords** Homeless · Women · Health · Diseases; · Urban

N. Singh (✉)
Content Manager - Historian, Tagbin Services Pvt. Ltd., Gurgaon, Haryana, India
e-mail: nirupamasingh52@gmail.com

A. Singh
School of Law, UPES, Dehradun, Uttarakhand, India

M. Rai
Amity Law School, Amity University, Noida, Uttar Pradesh, India

 
P. Chouhan et al. (eds.), *Women's Health Dynamics in South Asia*, Asian Perspectives on Public Health, https://doi.org/10.1007/978-981-95-2321-4_4

## 4.1 Introduction

In densely populated and fast-growing economies like India, homelessness is emerging as a severe issue that is often aggravated by poverty and the migration of people from rural to urban areas in search of work. Thus, urban areas in India face a high number of homeless populations which comes to around 9.38 lakh out of 17.73 lakh (Census of India, 2011). In metropolitan cities like Delhi, many people flock from nearby states like Uttar Pradesh and Bihar or nearby small towns in search of work. These people end up sleeping on streets in a dearth of housing facilities and increased living expenses. Thus, adding to the existing homeless population in the city. As per, the census of India 2011, the NCT Delhi accommodates 47,076 houseless people out of 46,724 who live in urban areas of Delhi. The share of homeless women in Delhi comes near nine thousand (Table 4.1), and at the pan-Indian level, there are 726,169 homeless women which is less in comparison to men. However, the impact of homelessness is severe on homeless women who must bear the burn of domestic violence, and mental, physical, or sexual abuse in addition to the absence of basic sanitary facilities. Less number of females on the streets is also indicative of human trafficking for sexual and commercial exploitation (Roy & Chaman, 2017). The literacy rate of homeless people is low in Delhi (46.13%) which further disables them from exercising their rights and finding employment ("Delhi is homelessness", 2017).

Contrary to the figures presented in the census of 2011, the Indo-Global Social Service Society (IGSS) conducted an independent survey in which the number of homeless in Delhi was found to be 246,800 (Roy & Chaman, 2017). In addition to this, an article in Hindustan Times has reported that three districts namely central Delhi, New Delhi, and north Delhi in the NCT of Delhi have higher rates of homeless people (Stevens, 2017). Roy and Chaman (2017), based on the Mission Convergence program's survey also highlighted that Hanuman Mandir and Connaught Place in central Delhi, Yamuna Pushta in east Delhi, and Nizamuddin and Kalkaji Mandir in south Delhi have a higher concentration of homeless population.

At the onset of this chapter, it becomes important to define the term homeless. The 2011 Census of India describes the homeless as the "houseless people" who do not reside in the "census houses", which means a structure with a roof. Therefore, people who are not adequately housed—that is, without even a rudimentary roof over their heads, not even a "*kuccha*" (unfinished) slum or shanty house are considered homeless (Chaudhry et al., 2014). The Census recorded that there are 4.5 lakh houseless families without a roof over their heads in India (Census of India, 2011).

**Table 4.1** Houseless population in NCT Delhi

| Union Territory | Total | Urban | Rural | Male | Female | Literacy |
|---|---|---|---|---|---|---|
| NCT of Delhi | 47,076 | 46,724 | 352 | 37,836 | 9240 | 46.13% |

*Source* Census of India (2011)

However, most scholars engaged in the subject believe that defining homelessness is more complex than the above definition. Every country in the world has a different method for classifying its homeless citizens. Therefore, given the relativity of meaning and historical variance across different locations or communities, no single definition of home is adequate (Sattar, 2014; Singh et al., 2018). According to IGSSS, homelessness in India is an urban phenomenon emerging from the lack of basic provision and employment running parallel with urban development and migration (IGSSS, 2018). Moreover, the causes of homelessness in India have been discussed into two broad categories; first are immediate factors and second are structural reasons (Bhatt & Jamil, 2012). The immediate factors include drug abuse, mental illness, and domestic disputes which affect the individual and convert them into homeless (Bhatt & Jamil, 2012). The structural reasons include unemployment, lack of social security and affordable housing, and deinstitutionalization (Bhatt & Jamil, 2012). Similarly, seasonal homelessness consists of people migrating interstate and intrastate during a specific time of the year for informal employment. Bhattacharya (2024) suggests that the causes of homelessness in the modern era are numerous, intricate, and unclear. The vagueness around the concept of causes arises from the fact that they differ in a broad range of dimensions, ranging from individual incidents of homelessness against aggregate homelessness, or distal to proximal in terms of predisposing factors. Chaudhry et al. (2014) considers violence to be an intrinsic part of homelessness for women. Lack of housing for women inevitably means that they also must go through various forms of violence such as verbal and physical abuse, sexual violence and exploitation, risks to security and personal safety, risks to health and difficulty in accessing healthcare, lack of access to government schemes and livelihood opportunities, increasing vulnerability and hunger (Chaudhry et al., 2014). Therefore, risk to health and lack of access to health services is considered a form of violence. Additionally, they argue that all homeless women face violence, however, certain groups are even more vulnerable. These groups include especially abled women, those affected by mental illness, victims of substance abuse, women with AIDS, and pregnant and lactating mothers (Chaudhry et al., 2014), thus, mostly including those women dependent on the health system.

Despite existing surveys and literature on urban homeless women, there remains a gap in understanding the concerns and barriers to accessing healthcare and remedial measures. There is still a lack of data as to how often and in what ways homeless women use existing healthcare services and identify issues in service delivery and there is a lack of study in identifying and addressing the barriers that prevent homeless women from accessing healthcare services, such as lack of identification, address proof, financial constraints, or stigma.

Therefore, it becomes crucial to take up empirical research on this glaring matter of homelessness among women which is influenced by economic, social, and health-related factors. The objectives of this chapter are to identify the health issues of urban homeless women who reside in makeshift arrangements or on streets which exposes them to high-risk environments with limited access to healthcare services. Hence, addressing their health needs requires a targeted approach that considers their specific circumstances and vulnerabilities. This chapter further elaborates not only on the existing legal frameworks but also on the governmental policies for the betterment of urban homeless women. In this direction, collaboration and advocacy would be required from civil societies, community organisations, healthcare providers, and policymakers to advocate for better health services and support for urban homeless women. The study highlights how, despite their severe inadequacy, temporary shelters provide critical relief to the destitute and homeless who would otherwise endure extreme deprivation without any form of support.

### 4.1.1 The Legal Landscape of Homelessness

The issue of homelessness is not unidimensional, it entails the most basic human right that is guaranteed under the Indian constitution, International Declaration, and Conventions ratified by the South Asian countries and can be promised by a developing state to its citizens. India is one of the signatories to the UDHR (1948) which grants the basic right to a standard of living that is adequate for the well-being of humans including clothes, food, shelter, medical care, and other necessary services.

It was in the year 1948 when the right to health originated through the international organisation, i.e. World Health Organisation (WHO) which formulated health terms as a basic inherent human right. Since then, WHO has continuously strived to promote health and safeguard vulnerable and marginalised populations all over the globe. As per WHO, health is a state of wholesome and complete physical, mental, and social well-being, and not merely an absence of a disease. In the same timeline, in response to the traumatic effects of World War II that outraged the inner conscience of mankind; a declaration (Universal Declaration of Human Rights) was signed by various nations to put an end to atrocities and to recognise the most basic and inherent human rights. Article 25 of UDHR covered a wide range of rights, including the right to sufficient food, water, sanitation, shelter, clothing, and health services. Children and mothers are also given special attention in the declaration.

The issues raised by Article 25 are further expounded upon in Article 12(1) of the International Covenant on Economic, Social, and Cultural Rights (ICESCR) which states that "everyone has the right to the enjoyment of the highest attainable standard of physical and mental health" (Brown, 2016). Although extreme poverty is not specifically mentioned in the UDHR, the latest Sustainable Development Goals (SDG) aim to "eradicate extreme poverty for all people everywhere, by 2030", and it should be interpreted as an expansion of the issues raised in Article 25, which deals with the standard of living. Goal 3 of the Sustainable Development Goals talks about universal health coverage and equal distribution of healthcare services and assistance to all persons irrespective of their gender, it also talks about preventive measures that can be taken to curb the death of infants' newborns, and children under five therefore it aims to stop child mortality. Looking at the recent past wherein the pandemic COVID-19 made us realise the lack of medical help and assistance throughout the globe, therefore Goal 3 becomes of utmost importance yet difficult to achieve (Filip et al., 2022).

In India, the right to health which is recognised and established by the honourable apex court of the country is also protected under various legislation, primarily under the Constitution of India. Though, unfortunately, social and economic justice to the citizen falls under Part IV of the constitution of India which is the directive principles of state policy and hence are unenforceable in the court of law.

The Indian Constitution and various legislations address the issue of homelessness, including the specific challenges faced by homeless women. Article 21 guarantees the right to life and personal liberty, which has been interpreted by the Supreme Court to include the right to shelter. This provision can be leveraged to argue for the protection and support of homeless individuals, including women. The Directive Principle of State Policy (DPSP) under Part IV of the Constitution mandates the state to perform inter-alia duties. Article 38 talks about promoting the welfare of its people, Article 39, clause (e) talks about protecting the health and strength from abuse, Article 41, which provides public assistance in case of sickness, disability, or "undeserved want", Article 47, focuses on raising the nutrition level, improving the standard of living, and considering improvement of public health as the state's primary duty. The DPSP though unenforceable in the court of law sets a social obligation over the state to provide above above-enumerated directive policies in the favour of public health. After the 73rd and 74th Amendments, 1992 respectively the panchayats and municipalities have also been bestowed the duty to provide clean drinking water, sanitation, promotion of social welfare, health care centres, and dispensaries for the local people inclusive of the destitute.

It must be noted that the Constitution of India does not expressly address or protect the right to health as a fundamental right under Part III of the Constitution. However, it has provided the right to health inclusive of clean water, adequate food, medical assistance, and sanitation, as an integral part of the right to life that is enshrined under Article 21. This article is an umbrella of such inherent rights impliedly guaranteeing the right to health, as one of the most important rights under the right to life and personal liberty. The right to live connotes a deep meaning and it is not confined to animal existence but also includes human dignity and decency. In this chapter, it has been seen that the homeless population even if residing in shelters provided by government agencies or non-governmental organisations is living in a dire state.

The National Human Rights Commission (NHRC) also plays an important role in defending the basic human rights of homeless people and addressing the human rights violations faced by them. Also, the right to a livelihood and a place to dwell is guaranteed under Article 21 of the Indian Constitution, as determined by a five-judge Supreme Court panel in the Olga Tellis case in 1985 (ESCR-Net, 2023). It acknowledged that the right to housing included two sets of rights: the right to rehabilitation through already-existing programs and the right to notice and hearing before eviction.

Despite these frameworks, upholding landmark judgments and the wide implications of various laws the implementation remains a significant challenge. Issues such as inadequate infrastructure promised by the state and central government, lack of resources, and social stigma affect the efficacy of these measures. Moreover, specific needs of homeless women, such as safety, healthcare, and protection from violence, require specific intervention by the addressing agencies.

Homeless women become vulnerable due to a range of factors which include extreme poverty, lack of affordable housing, changes in the industrial economy leading to unemployment, forced eviction/demolition of homes without adequate resettlement, displacement from land/home, inadequate income support, ostracization of women due to physical and mental health problems, lack of family and social support, disability, substance abuse, domestic violence/family abuse, stigmatisation of illness, and abandonment by family. Homeless women suffer altogether more during their pregnancy and after childbirth. The law claiming the beneficial provisions for mothers in their employment, i.e. The Maternity Benefit Act does not directly cover homeless women as it targets employees of establishments covered under the Act. This means that homeless women who do not have formal employment may not be able to claim benefits under this Act.

## 4.2 Materials and Methods

This chapter draws from a quantitative study comprising in-depth interviews with homeless women in Delhi (Fig. 4.1). The inclusive criterion for this survey included homeless women aged between 15 and 80 years. The research team for the study comprised authors who have experience in qualitative research.

This study proceeded in various stages; in the first stage, the organisations working with homeless people were identified out of which only one NGO named Jamghat responded. Then, an attempt was made to understand and define the urban homeless women. For this purpose, the definition of Indian Census, 2011, was adopted and a homeless woman was defined as homeless if she stayed without a roof over her head for more than 6 months. She could be staying at a homeless shelter, rehabilitation centre, footpath, pipes, traffic signals, railway platforms, etc. In the second stage, sampling categories were created and a range of factors causing homelessness were also mentioned.

For this chapter data was obtained from 1st May to 28th June 2024, through a self-structured bi-lingual (English and Hindi) questionnaire, and verbal consent was taken from the participants. To maintain the confidentiality of participants their identity is kept anonymous, and their lived experiences are discussed with changed names. The inductive thematic analysis approach is adopted which provides fresh insight into the narrative of homelessness with the help of a collected data set.

The interviews were carried out at the convenience of the participants and the method of respondent-driven sampling was adopted. Through this method, approaching homeless women in Delhi became much easier. For connecting with the respondents residing in the shelter homes and streets help of Jamghat was taken. While conducting the survey, are presentative of Jamghat familiarised the team with the respondents. After this, the duration of the interview was between half an hour to

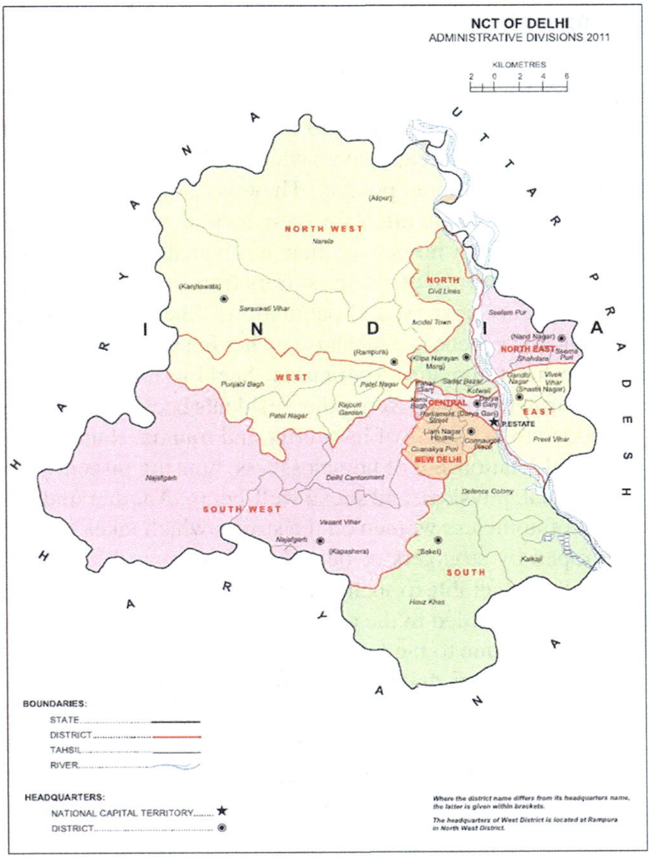


**Fig. 4.1** Administrative division map of Delhi. *Source* Census of India (2011)

an hour. The topics covered during the interaction ranged from the reason for homelessness, vulnerability status, accessibility to any services received by the government and non-governmental organisations, prevalent diseases, psychological issues, awareness of the policies and schemes, and access to healthcare services. For this survey, a preliminary sample size of 50 homeless women was taken from central, and New Delhi, since these areas have a higher number of homeless populations. Some of the samples collected were specifically from women's shelter homes as the scope of the research is strictly restricted to homeless women's health. Other samples were taken from women dwelling on the roadside, footpath, and pavements.

## 4.3 Results and Discussion

As suggested before, there are various factors leading to homelessness. Some of the factors that caused homelessness have also been highlighted in the current survey. Participants had generational homelessness which affected their physical and mental health and led to intergenerational poverty. They were often estranged from family even after receiving medical attention for their mental and physical ailments, and they ended up living in shelter homes for their survival, as can be seen in the case of Rani (changed name). At the age of 40, she suffers from various mental health issues, such as severe depression, anxiety, and palpitations. She also has been a victim of physical, emotional, and psychological abuse by her husband and his relatives which have contributed to her traumatic experiences. Seeking refuge in a shelter home, Rani encountered further violence from other residents because of her psychological condition. This added to her sense of insecurity and trauma. Rani's case thus, highlights the intertwined relationship of homelessness, housing insecurity, poverty, and poor health with mental, physical, and social well-being. Another underlying issue is sexual harassment of homeless women on the streets which takes many forms, from being groped to raped by strangers or other homeless men. Mentally ill homeless women are especially vulnerable to such assaults (Bhattacharya, 2024). However, no such occurrences were recorded in the current study because women were reluctant to answer such questions due to the fear of stigmatisation.

The study thus underscores that the participants had a complex history of homelessness. In many cases, women depended on a sole breadwinner hence when the head of the household abandoned his wife or family due to death or separation, the family's condition deteriorated, and they became homeless. In the current survey, most of the women were homeless for more than a year, and many experienced generational homelessness. The main reasons for homelessness were the breakdown of a relationship or family, physical or mental health issues, and domestic violence. It has emerged that homelessness was often a result of gender inequality. Most of the participants were living with various health issues which worsened due to the stress of being homeless. The participants reported physical health problems like pain in joints, back, and muscles, dental issues, weak eyesight, rapid heartbeat, panic attacks, and allergies.

During the survey, Heena (name changed) 25-year-old woman, became homeless along with her two children due to abuse and abandonment by her husband. In addition to intimate partner violence, she was a victim of child marriage due to which she lacked formal education. Thus, she had limited economic opportunities and worked as a cleaner which provided her modest income. After the separation from her husband, she moved into the shelter home where her sister lived. The shelter home too was a temporary refuge and not a permanent solution. After she transitioned to homelessness, she suffered from anxiety and chronic depression which rendered her unemployed and contributed to her precarious financial situation. The case thus, underscores the long-term challenges faced by women who have been victimised. Despite the safety offered by the shelter home, the lack of permanent solutions highlights the need for comprehensive support such as legal assistance, employment opportunities, stable housing, and mental health services to homeless women for their recovery and future stability.

Homelessness thus is a multifaceted challenge faced by individuals or families. It does not have a single form and is affected by socio-economic and political factors such as employment, income, calamities, violence, demographic factors, etc. Thus, homelessness can be categorised into generational homelessness, temporary homelessness, and transitional homelessness. Generational homelessness is marked by generational poverty. It refers to the kind of homelessness when the situation is repeated across many generations of the same family. In other words, it is a cyclic phenomenon as the individual has inherited homelessness from his/her parents (individually or family), and in turn, their parents have also been homeless at some point in their lives (Flatau et al., 2013). This cycle of homelessness is also marked by poverty as individuals/families cannot afford a permanent dwelling unit. Lack of affordable housing and finances are the most important causes of intergenerational homelessness. Temporary Homelessness, on the other hand, is when people are forced from their regular homes due to natural or man-made disasters or ailments ("Homelessness, Health", 1988, p. 23). In the context of Delhi, many people visit hospitals like AIIMS for their treatment. When the treatment period is prolonged, due to a lack of financial resources people are forced to live near the medical institutions in tents or on pavements. Similarly, many migrants who come to the capital in search of menial jobs also stay in tents as working in the unorganised sector does not pay them sufficient money to afford a proper residence.

Lastly, transitional homelessness which is also prevalent in India is a state of homelessness that results from major life changes or catastrophic events. These life transitions may include job loss, health crisis, substance addiction, domestic abuse, and divorce, among others. These conditions leave people without a place to live ("What are the", 2021). In India, one can observe that there is an overlap between temporary and transitional homelessness. Anyone who becomes homeless finds it nearly impossible to reintegrate into the society. The local job scenario is not favourable, thus these relocated people often have little income from their employment which makes it difficult for them to find new accommodation. It is made even more difficult by inter-related circumstances such as scarcity of employment, experiencing relationship conflicts, abandonment by family, experiencing reactive depression, or substance abuse, etc.

Homelessness turns a person into a miserable state, yet it is often criminalised in India. As per the Delhi Police Act 1978 if a person is found under suspicious circumstances between sunset and sunrise, lying and loitering in any street, yard, or other place and is unable to furnish a satisfactory account of himself will end up being apprehended by the police officials. Due to these circumstances, they are always under the apprehension of arrest which in turn devoid them from Article 21. In 2016, a bill named Persons in Destitution (Protection, Care and Rehabilitation) Model Bill was tabled to provide protection, comfort, care, and support to persons in destitution and it defines destitution as a state of poverty or abandonment arising from economic or social deprivation including age and infirmity, homelessness, disability, and prolonged unemployment.

The right to health forms the most essential part of human dignity and becomes the responsibility of the policymakers and legislators to ensure that the right to health is protected for all individuals despite of their religion, race, ethnicity, gender, or socio-economic status Accessing healthcare system is one of the most prominent barriers for homeless and destitute. Many shelter homes provided by the government and non-governmental organisations do not offer any prompt and sufficient medical care to homeless people. These people must visit government healthcare centres for treatment. As per our survey when the condition of homeless women deteriorates, they can't access ambulance services due to narrow and dingy streets leading to the centres.

Homeless people lack adequate clothing, bedding, food, and shelter, making them susceptible to extreme weather conditions. This condition decreases their inbuilt immunity and makes them more vulnerable to mortality and permanent ailments. In this scenario, homeless women due to their biological construct of menstruation, pregnancy, childbirth, breastfeeding issues, infant mortality rate, post-partum, menopause, and other conditions suffer to an unmeasurable extent. There have been innumerable circumstances where destitute have been turned away from capitalist medical centres and the ever-growing population of the country makes it difficult for such homeless people to get the help and assistance, they need from a government medical college or hospital they need. This status quo extends to the children that are born on the streets keeping them away from the basic needs that our constitution and various international conventions guarantee for a growing child.

The government of India has implemented various schemes and policies for sustaining the people on the margins. Since 2015, the Ministry of Housing and Urban Affairs (MoHUA) has been supporting the States' and Union Territories' efforts to provide pucca houses in urban areas nationwide by offering Central Assistance under the Pradhan Mantri Awas Yojana—Urban (PMAY-U). According to the official report, 1.8 crore dwelling units have been sanctioned based on the project proposals out of which 85.04 lakh have been handed over to the qualified recipients. Further, the implementation period of PMAY-U has been extended to 31st December 2024, which was originally aimed at 31st March 2022. The Deendayal Antyodaya Yojana—National Urban Livelihoods Mission (DAY-NULM) and the Shelter for Urban Homeless (SUH) schemes are some of the other initiatives that guarantee the availability and accessibility of permanent shelter, along with essential infrastructure amenities like safety, security, regular water supply, and sanitation. Under this program, 1986 shelter homes with room for more than 1.41 lakh people have been established for the nation's urban homeless to date (Homeless People, 2024).

The Government of Delhi runs 17 women-only shelters (Table 4.2) established in different districts, which have a capacity of around 50–300 women. These districts include central, southeast, southwest, northeast, northwest, New Delhi, etc. Housing and Land Rights Network's report mentions that in 2021 due to COVID-19, 10 temporary shelters and four isolation centres were also established for the homeless population. Delhi thus has the highest number of shelter homes in India despite this it only caters to 10 percent of the city's total homeless population (Housing & Land Rights Network, 2021).

The following Table 4.2, gives the details of 17 women-only centre in Delhi with the type of buildings whether permanent (RCC Buildings) or temporary (Porta Cabin), along with the organisations associated with them. The RCC Building made of Reinforced Cement Concrete is a permanent structure with a maximum capacity of 300 women. On the other hand, the portable cabins, are often used as temporary shelters with a constant occupancy of 50 women.

The spread of these shelters across different locations in Delhi highlights a decentralised approach of the government in providing community support and services. Every shelter is associated with a specific organisation that manages and operates its activities. These organisations facilitate various social welfare activities like community gatherings, educational programs, health services, etc. This set of data thus provides information not only on the living conditions of homeless women but social welfare and health assistance for homeless women which provides a necessary base for this chapter.

The 2024 data on homeless shelters show a mixed trend compared to 2017: a decline in some areas, an increase in others, and new additions in shelter capacity. The decline can be seen in the closure of the shelters at Jama Masjid, Akshardham temple, and two shelter homes for destitute pregnant and lactating mothers in Sarai Rohilla and Jahangirpuri respectively. The capacity of Nizamuddin Basti was increased from 50 to 300 when the porta cabin was converted into an RCC building. The Community Hall at Karol Bagh was added to the 2024 list as a permanent building (Table 4.3).

The following are other initiatives and programs that the government is putting into place to help these women and give them employment, educational opportunities, empowerment, and rehabilitation.

Swadhar Greh Schemes provides basic requirements to women facing challenging circumstances. These circumstances included being pushed to prostitution, crime, violence, mental trauma, and social ostracism. The program seeks to rehabilitate women economically and emotionally through housing, food, clothes, counselling, vocational and skill enhancement training, clinical support, and legal aid (Ministry of Women and Child Development).

A Home for Widows is a social scheme under which shelter is provided to the widows that are set up in Vrindavan Uttar Pradesh that provides a safe place with additional services of health, nutritional food, free legal aid, and psychological counselling to cope with the present.

One Stop Centres (OSCs), also known as Sakhi Centres aids and various facilities to women who are affected by assault and violence including domestic and intimate partner violence. Under this centre, legal aid and access to police are also being provided for coping with the atrocities and harassment and reporting such criminal acts through the state machinery with the help of these agencies. Under these centres, legal aid becomes of prime importance as the women who have suffered any kind of harassment or have been a victim of any heinous crime but are unaware of the

**Table 4.2** District-wise shelters list for homeless women in Delhi

| S. No | Name of the Shelter | District | Type | Capacity | Agency |
|---|---|---|---|---|---|
| 1 | Nizamuddin Basti near Hazrat Nizamuddin Dargah (F.F.) | Southeast | RCC Building | 300 | SPYM |
| 2 | Community Hall, Regharpura, Karol Bagh | Central | RCC BUILDING | 110 | Jyoti Samajik Sewa Sanstha |
| 3 | Community Centre Hanuman Mandir Yamuna Bazar | Central | RCC BUILDING | 210 | Sadik Masih Medical Social Servant Society |
| 4 | Kharian Mohalla, Roshanara Road | Central | RCC BUILDING | 210 | Jyoti Samajik Sewa Sanstha |
| 5 | Sector-3, PH-II, Dwarka | Southwest | RCC BUILDING | 70 | Safe Approach for Nascent Termination of Social Hazard |
| 6 | 2819/VIII, Turkman Gate, Gali Shanker | Central | RCC BUILDING | 20 | Sofia Educational and Welfare Society |
| 7 | Bangla Sahib-1 | New Delhi | PORTA CABIN | 50 | SPYM |
| 8 | Lodhi Road near the Indian Social Institute | Southeast | PORTA CABIN | 50 | SPYM |
| 9 | Munirka near Masjid Sec.- 4, R. K. Puram | New Delhi | PORTA CABIN | 50 | SPYM |
| 10 | Jama Masjid-1 | Central | PORTA CABIN | 50 | Sofia Educational and Welfare Society |
| 11 | Raja Garden-119 | West | PORTA CABIN | 50 | Safe Approach for Nascent Termination of Social Hazard |
| 12 | Mansarover Park-2, Lal Bagh | Northeast | PORTA CABIN | 50 | Rachna Women's Development Association |
| 13 | Kalkaji Mandir | Southeast | PORTA CABIN | 50 | Janpahal |
| 14 | Pushta Usmanpur Opp. Jag Pravesh Hospital | Northeast | PORTA CABIN | 50 | Rachna Women's Development Association |
| 15 | Kali Mandir, Sec-3, Rohini | Northwest | PORTA CABIN | 50 | Maa Astha Samajik Vikas Sewa Sansthan |
| 16 | Bangla Sahib Gurudwara Site-6 | New Delhi | PORTA CABIN | 50 | SPYM |
| 17 | Anand Vihar -2 | Shahdara | PORTA CABIN | 50 | Rachna Women's Development Association |

*Source* Delhi Urban Shelter Improvement Board

**Table 4.3** District-wise capacity of women's shelter homes in Delhi

| Districts | Capacity of women's shelter homes |
|---|---|
| Southeast Delhi | 400 |
| Central Delhi | 600 |
| Southwest Delhi | 70 |
| New Delhi | 150 |
| Northwest Delhi | 50 |
| Northeast Delhi | 100 |
| West Delhi | 50 |
| Shahdara | 50 |
| Total | 1470 |

*Source* Primary survey

legal remedy available, are being helped by these centres to achieve justice. Meanwhile, these centres provide temporary shelter psycho-social counselling, and other integrated services available.

Women Helpline (WHL) scheme is a 24*7 emergency helpline number that works in both public and private spaces by interlinkage with police authorities, medical facilities, and legal services. This helpline number assists in an automated response to traumatised women who are affected by violence and atrocities. It also provides information regarding social welfare schemes for such women to give them a better life ahead.

However, even after the existence of various schemes and policies of the government for the welfare of homeless people due to the lack of timely implementation of these policies homeless people suffer. Recent coverage of The Hindu highlighted this issue. It showed that a total number of 192 homeless people died in Delhi in 2024. This was the highest recorded death in Delhi in the past 22 years. However, the data from the Zonal Integrated Police Network and Ministry of Home Affairs indicated that 14 people died in Delhi between 11 and 19th June due to heat stroke. Ministry of Home Affairs further stated that the homeless people who died were suffering from pre-existing ailments. The Centre for Holistic Development an NGO maintained that the number stated in the government records was much less in size because many homeless people do not get the required medical attention, and they die even before hospitalisation ("Record number of deaths", 2024).

In Table 4.4, it is observed that only 60% of homeless women who resided in shelter homes could access the health care system freely. Access to healthcare or an ambulance was difficult for women staying on the roadside.

Table 4.4 revealed that most women were found to be homeless for more than a year (40%) and many were very homeless by birth (25%). Distinct reasons responsible for their homelessness included abandonment (14%), relationship conflict (20%), temporary homelessness (40%), and generational homelessness (26%). Many of these women are victims of intimate partner violence (22%), violence by relatives of husbands (34%), and child marriage (44%) (Fig. 4.2).

**Table 4.4** Data received from the questionnaire of the primary survey

| Questions | Options | Number of women | Percentage |
|---|---|---|---|
| Area of dwelling | Shelter homes | 30 | 60% |
| | Roadside | 20 | 40% |
| Duration of Homelessness | 6 months | 7 | 14% |
| | 1 year | 10 | 20% |
| | More than a year | 20 | 40% |
| | By birth | 13 | 26% |
| Reason for homelessness | Abandonment | 7 | 14% |
| | Relationship conflicts | 10 | 20% |
| | Temporary homelessness | 20 | 40% |
| | Generational homelessness | 13 | 26% |
| Employment status | Working | 17 | 34% |
| | Not working | 33 | 66% |
| Financial aid received | Nil | Nil | Nil |
| Conditions affecting the health status of women | Lack of food availability | 20 | 40% |
| | Water scarcity | 20 | 40% |
| | Lack of sufficient sleep due to rough living conditions | 20 | 40% |
| | Lack of sanitation facilities | 20 | 40% |
| | Lack of menstruation hygiene | 50 | 100% |
| Prevalent diseases among homeless women | Malnourishment | 40 | 80% |
| | Anaemia | 40 | 80% |
| | Hyperglycemia and diabetes | 20 | 40% |
| | Hypertension | 36 | 72% |
| | Dental issues | 13 | 26% |
| Psychological issues faced by women because of homelessness | Increased anxiety | 40 | 80% |
| | Palpitations | 30 | 60% |
| | Suicidal tendencies | 2 | 4% |
| | Substance abuse | 1 | 2% |
| | Depression | 11 | 22% |
| | Post-traumatic stress disorder (PTSD) | 2 | 4% |
| | Bipolar disorder | 1 | 2% |
| Victimisation and vulnerability of women | Intimate partner violence | 11 | 22% |
| | Violence by relatives of husband | 17 | 34% |
| | Child marriage | 22 | 44% |

(continued)

**Table 4.4** (continued)

| Questions | Options | Number of women | Percentage |
|---|---|---|---|
| Help received during pregnancy by any organisation | Nil | 1 | 2% |
| Awareness of government policies and schemes | Janani Suraksha Yojana (JSY) | 1 | 2% |
| | Ayushman Card | 0 | 0 |
| | Ayushman Bharat Health Account | 0 | 0 |
| | Pradhan Mantri Jan Arogya Yojna (PM-JAY) | 0 | 0 |
| | Rashtriya Swasthya Bima Yojana | 0 | 0 |
| Free access to the health care system | Government health and wellness centres | 30 | 60% |
| | Private health centres | 0 | 0 |
| | Access to ambulance | 0 | 0 |

*Source* Primary survey

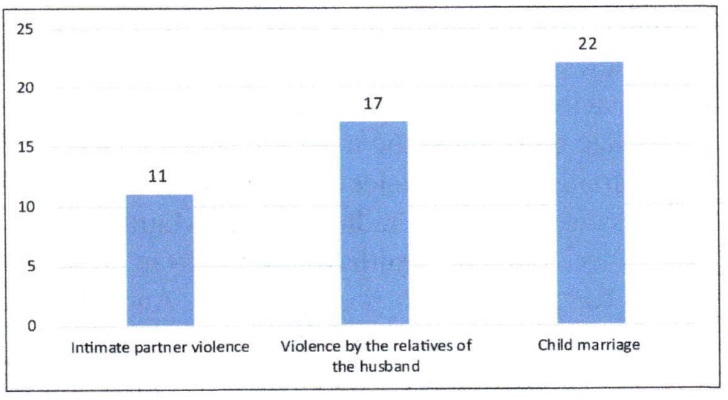


**Fig. 4.2** Victimisation and vulnerability of women

Out of 20 women facing temporary homelessness, 11 were found to have been victims of intimate partner violence. Women had to go through various health issues because of their poor living conditions (Fig. 4.3), such as lack of food, water, sleep, sanitation, and menstrual hygiene. Despite the location of these homeless women all of them faced difficulty in maintaining menstrual hygiene. Though, the National Health Mission has adopted various schemes for the Promotion of Menstrual Hygiene by providing access to high-quality sanitary napkins at Janaushidhi Kendras under the Pradhan Mantri Bhartiya Janausadhi Pariyojna (PMBJP) at a subsidised rate of one rupee per pad (PIB Delhi, 2022). The menstrual health condition of homeless women is still in grave condition as many cannot afford, access, or are unaware of these facilities.

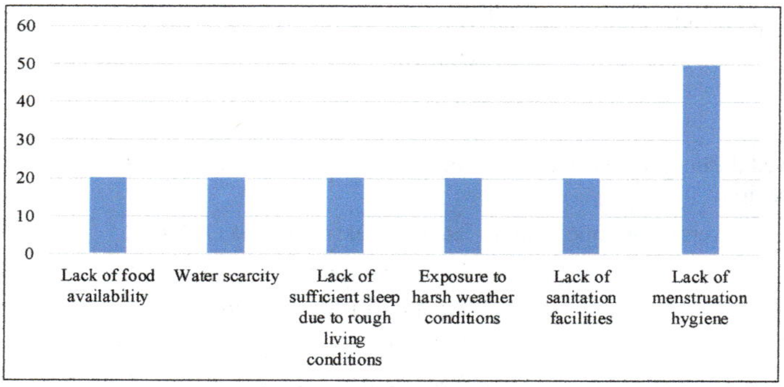


**Fig. 4.3** Conditions affecting the health status of women

Seventy–two to eighty percent of women, in both shelter homes and outside were suffering from malnourishment, anaemia, and hypertension. Twenty-six to forty percent of women were also suffering from diseases like hyperglycaemia and diabetes, as well as dental issues (Table 4.4, Fig. 4.4). The lack of employability, violence, and victimisation faced by homeless women also affected their mental health and self-worth. Most of them were suffering from anxiety (80%), and palpitations (60%); few of them were suffering from depression (22%), PTSD (4%), substance abuse (2%), and bipolar disorder (2%) (Fig. 4.5).

Homeless women face severe challenges when it comes to maternity care, with issues that include lack of access to healthcare inclusive of prenatal and postnatal care, inadequate nutrition to the newborn, and safety concerns. There are various government initiatives and policies created for the welfare of pregnant women, extended to homeless women. The Pradhan Mantri Matru Vandana Yojana (PMMVY) under the aegis of the National Health Mission aims at providing financial support to pregnant women for prenatal and postnatal care. Another scheme, Janani Suraksha Yojana focuses on reducing maternal and infant mortality by promoting institutional deliveries. Efforts are made to ensure that this program reaches vulnerable populations, including the homeless. However, accessing these schemes can be challenging for

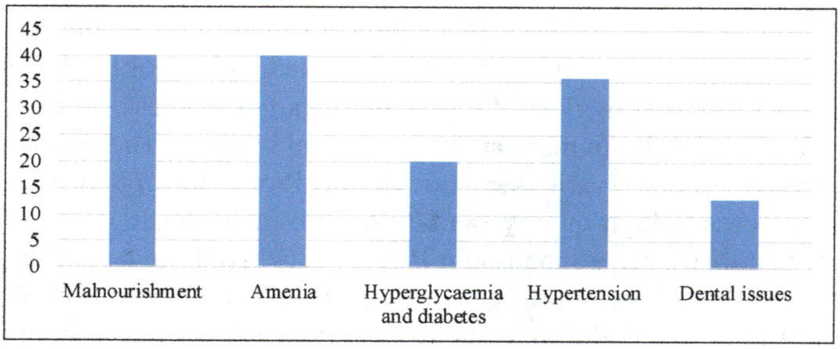


**Fig. 4.4** Prevalent diseases among homeless women

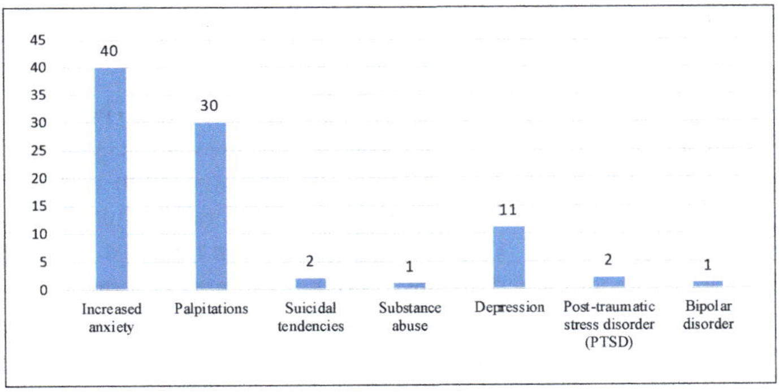


**Fig. 4.5** Psychological issues faced by women

homeless women without a permanent address. In this context, the Delhi High Court initiated a *Suo moto* action on the reports of the death of a homeless woman on a pavement in Shankar market in Connaught Place after childbirth. The court directed to establishment of two shelter forms, especially for destitute pregnant women equipped with all medical facilities ("HC wants shelter", 2011). Adhering to this decision, two shelter homes for pregnant and lactating (destitute) women were established at Sarai Rohilla and Jahangirpuri which were functional till January 2014 (Department of Women and Child Development) and were listed in the shelter home list of the Delhi Shelter Board of 2017. In 2022, a tender was issued for running and managing these shelter homes by the Department of Women and Child Development, Government of NCT of Delhi. However, the 2024 list of shelter homes in Delhi does not include them suggesting the closure of the shelter homes (Table 4.2).

It was also found in the survey conducted for this chapter that women had no awareness regarding the policies and schemes of government to assist them in accessing health care services such as Janani Suraksha Yojana (JSY), Ayushman Card, and Pradhan Mantri Jan Arogya Yojna (PM-JAY). In addition to this lack of specialised shelter homes for pregnant destitutes exasperated the issue. Only 1 out of 50 women was able to access Janani Suraksha Yojana during her pregnancy.

The existing survey unveiled that necessities were available for the homeless women, though not in abundance. There was still a lack of sanitation, menstrual hygiene, food, and water. Homeless women pointed out that access to food was restricted due to unfriendly staff and middlemen corruption. The food, beverages, stationeries, medical facilities, etc., that they had access to were provided by the civil societies. Apart from government interventions, various non-governmental organisations, and civil society extend their hand of help to these homeless women.

### 4.3.1 Limitations of the Study

The investigation in the chapter is limited to the NCT of Delhi. The chapter investigates the health status of urban homeless women. The survey was conducted during the daytime, and it was difficult to trace the homeless women as they were out in search of work, etc. Many women were reluctant to talk about their issues and incidents of sexual harassment. Due to a lack of hope in terms of repeated surveys conducted before they maintained distance and they did not elaborate on their issues. The relevant data set of this chapter was primarily taken from two districts of Delhi having a higher concentration of urban homeless population. Therefore, the data set may not be generalised for the present conditions of homeless women in NCT Delhi.

## 4.4 Conclusion

This chapter aims to investigate the barriers to healthcare access for homeless women in NCT Delhi and assess the effectiveness of current intervention strategies. Addressing the health issues of urban homeless women requires a multifaceted approach that integrates healthcare provision, education, community engagement, social policies, and advocacy. By identifying their specific health needs and providing targeted support, one can contribute to improving the overall well-being and quality of life for homeless women in urban areas. The chapter revealed in the key findings that the primary barriers to healthcare access include lack of identification documents, lack of awareness about the existing legislative policies, and address proof. Additionally, existing legislative intervention programs were found to be inadequate in addressing the specific needs of such homeless women, especially the maternity benefits comprising of childbirth benefits, post-partum support, and childcare, that are provided in the legislation and policies. The recommendations for policymaking for the upliftment of the social conditions of these women will include improving shelter home conditions for homeless women, enhancing legal protection by the legal machinery and administration of the state, and promoting community engagement by raising awareness about the issues faced by homeless women. Though India has various policies addressing homelessness as discussed in the chapter, such as a national shelter strategy and a national urban homelessness policy, irrespectively, the implementation and effectiveness of such policy frameworks for homeless women often fall short. Since, the chapter employs empirical research of a limited sample, future researchers are suggested and recommended to conduct surveys to assess the specific health needs and conditions prevalent among homeless women from a larger sample. This could include chronic illness, mental health issues, and reproductive health needs. Also, compare the health issues faced by homeless women with those of homeless men and the general population to highlight the disparities and unique needs keeping the intersectional perspective on gender role construct in homelessness.

**Acknowledgements** The authors would like to thank and appreciate Jamghat and its team for their support during the survey and for every homeless woman who participated and contributed their valuable time and opinion.

## References

Advocate Khoj. (n.d.). *Being found under suspicious circumstances between sunset and sunrise.* Retrieved 21 June, 2024 from https://www.advocatekhoj.com/library/bareacts/delhipolice/102.php?Title=Delhi%20Police%20Act,%201978&STitle=Being%20found%20under%20suspicious%20circumstances%20between%20sunset%20and%20sunrise

Butani, A. (2024, June 22). Record number of deaths of homeless in capital due to heat, lack of amenities. *The Hindu.* https://www.thehindu.com/news/cities/Delhi/record-number-of-deaths-of-homeless-in-capital-due-to-heat-lack-of-amenities/article68318075.ece

Bhatt, S., & Jamil, G. (2012). Temporary shelters for the homeless in Delhi: A study-based reflection. *Social Work Chronicle, 1*(2), 14–30.

Bhattacharya, P. (2024). *Homeless individuals with serious mental illnesses.* Routledge.

Brown, G. (2016). *The universal declaration of human rights in the 21st century: A living document in a changing world.* Open Book Publishers.

Census of India. (2011). Primary Census Abstract data for Houseless, India & States/UTs – district level. Office of the Registrar General & Census Commissioner. Government of India. https://censusindia.gov.in/nada/index.php/catalog/5047

Chaudhry, S., Joseph, A., & Singh, I. P. (2014). *Violence and violations: The reality of homeless women in India.* Housing and Land Rights Network. http://hlrn.org.in/documents/Violence_and_Violations_Homeless_Women_in_India_2014.pdf

Chronicle Publications Pvt. Ltd. (n.d.). *Persons in destitution (protection, care and rehabilitation) model bill, 2016.* Retrieved 25 June, 2024 from https://www.chronicleindia.in/year-book/chronicle-year-book-2023/persons-in-destitution-protection-care-and-rehabilitation-model-bill-2016#:~:text=Preparation%20Tips%2FTricks-,Persons%20in%20Destitution%20(Protection%2C%20Care%20and%20Rehabilitation)%20Model%20Bill,the%20objectives%20identified%20there%20under

Comic Relief US. (2021). *What are the four types of homelessness?* https://www.comicrelief.org/posts/what-are-the-four-types-of-homelessness

Delhi Urban Shelter Improvement Board (DUSIB). (n.d.). *District wise night shelters list.* Retrieved 19 July, 2024 from https://delhishelterboard.in/occupancy-report/index-ag2.php

Department of Women and Child Development. (n.d.). *List of short stay institutions in Delhi for women.* Retrieved 21 July, 2024 from https://wcd.delhi.gov.in/wcd/list-short-stay-institutions-delhi-women

Department of Women and Child Development. (n.d.). Shelter Institution for Pregnant and Lactating Destitute Women. Retrieved 7 August 2024 from https://wcd.delhi.gov.in/wcd/shelter-institution-pregnant-and-lactating-destitute-women

Filip, R., Gheorghita Puscaselu, R., Anchidin-Norocel, L., Dimian, M., & Savage, W. K. (2022). Global challenges to public health care systems during the COVID-19 pandemic: A review of pandemic measures and problems. *Journal of Personalized Medicine, 12*, 1–22.

ESCR-Net. (2023, August 29). *Olga Tellis & Ors v Bombay Municipal Council [1985] 2 Supp SCR 51.* ESCR-Net. https://www.escr-net.org/caselaw/2006/olga-tellis-ors-v-bombay-municipal-council-1985-2-supp-scr-51/

Flatau, P., Conroy, E., Spooner, C., Edwards, R., Eardley, T., & Forbes, C. (2013). *Lifetime and intergenerational experiences of homelessness in Australia.* Australian Housing and Urban Research Institute.

Goel, K., Tarique, M., Anand, M., & Munyoka, E. (2024). Homelessness in India: A state legislative and civil society perspective. In C. Bevan (Ed.), *The Routledge handbook of global perspectives on homelessness, law & policy*. Routledge.

HC wants shelter for destitute pregnant women. (2011, January 12). *Times of India*. https://timesofindia.indiatimes.com/city/delhi/hc-wants-shelter-for-destitute-pregnant-women/articleshow/7270830.cms

Housing and Land Rights Network. (2015). *The human rights to adequate housing and land in India: Report for the United Nations Human Rights Council*. http://hlrn.org.in/documents/UPR_Recommendations_Housing_and_Land_India_HLRN_Sept_2015.pdf

Housing and Land Rights Network. (2021). *Housing and land rights network, impacts of the second wave of the pandemic on Delhi's homeless population: Findings of a rapid assessment survey*. https://www.hlrn.org.in/documents/Homelessness_Delhi_Pandemic_Second_Wave.pdf

India Filings. (n.d.). *Women helpline (WHL) scheme*. Retrieved 21 July, 2024 from https://www.indiafilings.com/learn/women-helpline/

Indo-Global Social Service Society. (2018). *Understanding homelessness in Delhi: Rethinking perspectives, policy and practice*. https://igsss.org/wp-content/uploads/2022/06/Understanding-Homelessness-in-Delhi.pdf

Institute of Medicine (US) Committee on Health Care for Homeless People. (1988). *Homelessness, health, and human needs*. Washington (DC): National Academies Press. https://www.ncbi.nlm.nih.gov/books/NBK218240/

Ministry of Housing and Urban Affairs. (n.d.). *Homeless people*. Retrieved 4 July, 2024 from https://pib.gov.in/PressReleseDetail.aspx?PRID=2035215

Ministry of Law and Justice. Govt. of India. (n.d.). *Constitution of India*. Retrieved 20 June, 2024 from https://legislative.gov.in/constitution-of-india/

Ministry of Women and Child Development. (n.d.). *SWADHAR Greh (A Scheme for Women in Difficult Circumstances)*. Retrieved 21 July, 2024 from https://wcd.nic.in/schemes/swadhar-greh-scheme-women-difficult-circumstances

Ministry of Women and Child Development. (2022). *Scheme for Promotion of Menstrual Hygiene*. https://pib.gov.in/PressReleasePage.aspx?PRID=1846147

National Human Rights Commission, India. (2023). Brochure. https://nhrc.nic.in/sites/default/files/Overview%20of%20National%20Human%20Rights%20Commission%2C%20its%20functions%20and%20various%20activities_0.pdf

Press Information Bureau. (2024, July 22). *Homeless people*. Ministry of Housing & Urban Affairs. https://www.pib.gov.in/PressReleasePage.aspx?PRID=2035215

Roy, S., & Chaman, C. (2017). Homelessness in Delhi: Roots, rhetoric and realities. *International Physical Medicine & Rehabilitation Journal, 1*(1), 1–6. https://medcraveonline.com/IPMRJ/homelessness-in-delhi-roots-rhetoric-and-realities.html

Sattar, S. (2014). Homelessness in India. *Shelter: A HUDCO Publication, 15*(1), 9–15.

Singh, N., Koiri, P., & Shukla, S. K. (2018). Signposting invisibles: A study of the homeless population in India. *Chinese Sociological Dialogue, 3*(3). https://www.ihrn.org.in/files/editor/Signposting%20invisibles%20-%20a%20study%20of%20the%20homeless%20population%20in%20India.pdf

Stevens, H. (2017, May 24). Delhi is homelessness capital with three districts among India's worst six. *Hindustan Times*. https://www.hindustantimes.com/delhi/homelessness-census-data-shows-three-of-india-s-worst-six-districts-in-delhi/story-xwTd5kl2R3eEFs4TJyLOoM.html

United Nations. (1948). Universal Declaration of Human Rights. https://www.un.org/en/about-us/universal-declaration-of-human-rights

# Chapter 5
# Assessing the Impact of Forced *Refugeehood* on Women's Health in South Asia

**Prashna Samaddar**

**Abstract** Forced displacement and refugeehood is a significant problem all across the globe and South Asian countries play a pivotal role in accommodating this issue to a greater extent. Women, young girls, and adolescent children cover a significant portion of the population who unabatedly get stuck in the constant process of forced migration. One of the pertinent challenges that they face significantly is their health concerns. A healthcare regime is considered as a basic rubric of a society but when it comes to the context of refugee women and girls, such a regime becomes quite a far-reaching concept. Health issues like, menstrual health, puberty issues, sexual health, schematic use of contraception, sexually transmitted diseases, pregnancy complexities, UTIs, anaemic issues, psychological distress, and other mental health-related concerns are pertinent among refugee women. These issues get aggravated due to the highly challenging environment through which they have to survive in their entire transit time and even when the host states accommodate them in the makeshift, dilapidating camps which are overcrowded and are in want of hygienic surroundings. The scanty toilets and sheer dearth of private spaces for them to deal with these health issues often lead to virulent diseases for them which they themselves remain unaware of due to non-accessibility towards such awareness camps and non-assimilation with the mainstream population. The chapter is dedicated to highlighting the backdrop of some such healthcare challenges and areas that are quite grey for the 'she refugee' population in the South Asian region.

**Keywords** Forced displacement · South Asia · Women · Refugees · Health factors

P. Samaddar (✉)
Xavier Law School, St. Xavier's University, Kolkata, West Bengal, India
e-mail: samaddarprashna@gmail.com



P. Chouhan et al. (eds.), *Women's Health Dynamics in South Asia*, Asian Perspectives on Public Health, https://doi.org/10.1007/978-981-95-2321-4_5

## 5.1 Introduction

As of July 2024, the South Asian population is estimated to be 2,050,323,496 (as of July 19, 2024) based upon the up-to-the-minute United Nations survey (Population of Southern Asia, 2024—Worldometer, n.d.). The sub-continent is characterized by a rich migration and refugee group-yielding region in past centuries. People have been associated with long-standing migration patterns since time immemorial due to variety of reasons that have worked as catalysts for the human population in South Asia (India, Nepal, Bhutan, Bangladesh, Pakistan, Afghanistan, Sri Lanka, and Maldives).

Out of the earlier quoted approximate population of South Asian nations, an approximate female population in South Asia is reported as 947,313,755 persons in 2023 (World Bank collection of development indicators) (South Asia—Population, Female—2024 Data 2025 Forecast 1960–2023 Historical, n.d.). Hence, the rubric is quite clear that nearly 46.6% of the total population who are residing in South Asia are females. Figure 5.1 depicts the extent of refugee density across the globe. Red colour showcases the highest number of refugees globally; South Asian countries majorly fall in that list. Bringing in the issue of refugeehood, the region accommodates more than 3.6 million refugees as reported by the end of 2019(Migration Data in Southern Asia, n.d.) and women form a significant part of this population (Migration Data in Southern Asia, n.d.). Figure 5.1 depicts the highest refugee-hosting States spread across the globe as per the 2010 UNHCR report (which also includes internally displaced). Refugeehood brings with it self my riads of issues that come along with its forced nature and jeopardizes a lot of basic human rights elements among the affected ones. As women comprise the majority of the affected population, it is needless to say that they are quite relevant and invincible bearers of the challenges thrown by the entire refugee process. Although forceful movement includes both internal displacement and beyond the borders; internationally the problem of refugees is recognized as people who leave their habitual place of stay owing to challenges making them impossible to stay there further and leading to cross the borders of their state. The present chapter chiefly deals with the impact of forceful refugeehood on the women population who are forced to cross the international borders of one or more states in South Asia and maybe with their other family members or might be alone. While dealing with such forced displacement there lies a multitude of issues that they face at varied stages. Challenges like, dreadful climatic conditions, compromised physical protection and mental peace, private toilets and clean lavatories, and a range of health issues analogous to these challenges become quite consequential to these movements. Many times, women are left with no choice but to use men's washrooms during these movements or even open fields. These pervasive environments which the majority of them are to face bring unprecedented health challenges to them.

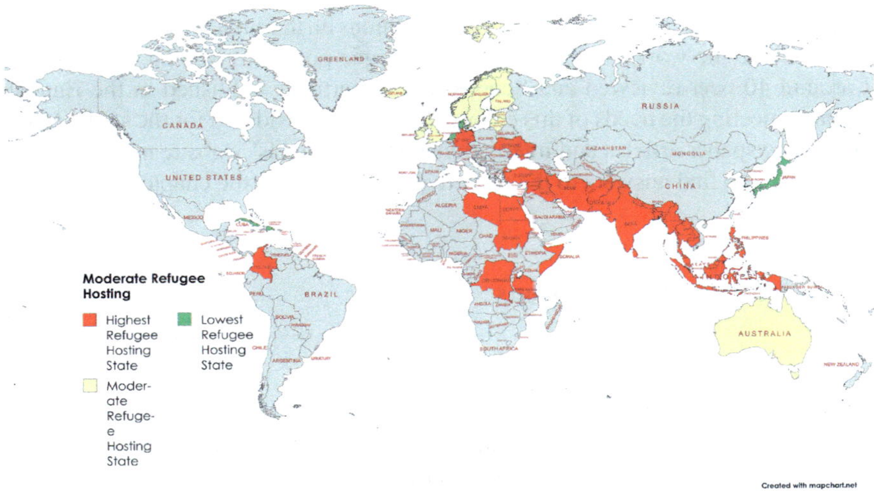


**Fig. 5.1** Extent of refugees hosting states in the Globe

### 5.1.1 *Rationale of the Study*

The present chapter has picked up a niche area of addressing the health challenges faced by the women who are subjected to forceful refugee displacement across the borders of South Asian countries. The main objective of the chapter is to, highlight the effects of forced refugeehood on the female population in South Asia in general; find out the chief impact on their health quotient while being involved in movements attached to such forced displacement, and trace the main areas on which any step has been taken already to address those pertaining and locatable health challenges (specifically; regionally or particularly by any member nation of South Asia).

## 5.2 Materials and Methods

The methodology adopted for this chapter is parentally an extensive doctrinal study of existing literature related to the area. An in-depth analytical, logical, diagnostic, and quality analysis method has been adopted for shortlisting the area's contemporary literature. A thematic literature review has been carried on to explore knowledge, gather the chief findings and experiences, and extract qualitative insights to comprehend the understanding of the target population group of South Asian women in the refugee camps of South Asia. Databases like; Elsevier, PubMed, National Clinical Database, Web of Science, National Institute of Health (NIH), National Library of Medicine, United Nations High Commission for Refugees (UNHCR), World Health Organisation (WHO), and UNICEF were searched thoroughly to acknowledge the real data gathered and preserved by the organizations on this area. Map Chart has been used to create the world map for depicting refugee population extent. Publications of around 40 peer-reviewed and Scopus-indexed articles published in the English language meeting the needs of this chapter have been considered for the study. Many leading newspaper articles and international news channels' website materials have been studied to find answers to the objectives laid down for the chapter.

## 5.3 Results and Discussions

### *5.3.1 Augmenting Reality*

Women as said earlier, comprise a huge part of the refugee population in South Asia naturally or consciously. Refugees in that section of society that in the first place doesn't form voluntarily but owing to such situational glitches faces a lot of hurdles at various stages of their forceful displacement. It is a fact that the apathy attached to refugeehood starts from their place of habitual stay itself, as the reasons (whatsoever it is) compromise their safe and peaceful stay over there and make them open to choose displacement over any other option. In many such cases, choosing displacement is not left as an option but becomes an inadvertent necessity. According to Article 1(a), a refugee is a person who;

> Owing to well-founded fear of being persecuted for reasons of race, religion, nationality, membership of a particular social group or political opinion, is outside the country of [their] nationality and is unable or, owing to such fear, is unwilling to avail [themselves] of the protection of that country. (Convention Relating to the Status of Refugees, 1951)

This phrase "owing to a well-founded fear of being persecuted" leaves a lot of people irrespective of their gender, in a position of dismemberment from their habitual place of stay and crossing their home borders to start an unknown journey full of unplanned and unprecedented events. The South Asian region of the globe is chiefly characterized by an overwhelming refugee population augmented with quite relentless relocation owing to their living conditions (Nair, 1997).

Figure 5.2 depicts the fact that more than 3 lakhs of the population have been in a constant flow of seeking asylum owing to refugeehood since the 1990s in the forced refugeehood process in South Asia (Refugee Population by Country or Territory of Asylum for South Asia, 2024). The women population takes up a lot of stakes in these movements. They are subjected to many unseen challenges that affect their health quotient in many ways. Health condition is not just limited to physical features and their related attributes, it has much to do with mental health conditions and psychological factors as well. The forced refugeehood in itself brings tons of challenges in the lives of the affected ones and when it is about the 'she' gender, the challenges escalate to a much higher degree. Women are the worst sufferers when it comes to weighing the horrors of ethnic violence, marginalization, and wars (San Suu Kyi, n.d.). The most striking effect that these outbreaks of violence carry is on

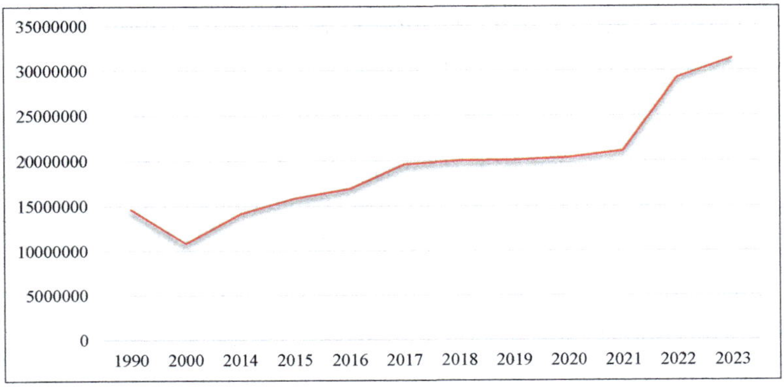


**Fig. 5.2** Global Refugee Population (1990–2023). *Source* Refugee Population by Country or Territory of Asylum for South Asia (2024) and World Development Indicators | DataBank (n.d.)

the health factor of those women sufferers. They bear the pain of major war crimes in the form of brutal rape, trafficking, sex slavery, etc. which leaves them in a quirky situation than what is imagined. Due to being a part of any persecuted community, it anyway becomes tough to address the harsh outcomes of physical or mental brutalities women face. This is a common global habit and South Asia being one of the highest refugees producing regions, is not an exception to this. Approximately more than half of the women refugee population succumbs to the unprecedented health challenges that they face during forced displacement.

Some theories have emerged over time to study the pattern of transboundary migration although it is witnessed that hardly any of them have given importance to its gender-oriented perspectives (Oishi & The Center for Comparative Immigration Studies, 2002). Theories like; Neo-classical economic theory, Structurist Theory, and Household Strategy theory, are some of the popular theories that reflect on the economic, social, and cultural impediments that come along with cross-border migration however as mentioned, they all fell short of describing the gender-oriented migrational challenges. In recent times though gender as a variable has been considered quite often to highlight the complexities, attached to it (Pessar & Mahler, 2003). However, the same studies identify that these studies are quite overlapped with the geometrical matrices like; geographical, social, political, and structural. The famous author Patricia Collins has also highlighted this matrix through the lens of the human diaspora in her celebrated work on migration (Collins, 2008). The work has dealt with 'women of colour' as migrants in the first world and its related impediments. Impediments associated with forced immigration of women folk like; poverty, slavery, lack of education, reproductive concerns and the sex trade have been addressed in the writing as recurring issues of such migrations. Some of the impediments have a nexus with health concerns and their impact has contributed to the normative understanding of the common challenges experienced transitionally in the context.

### 5.3.2 *Major Health Care Challenges Among Refugee Women in South Asia*

As per Fig. 5.3, it can be seen that although the refugee convention internationally doesn't strike out 'gender' specificity as a matter of concern to be addressed it has been realized by and large that women often end up facing the worst after-effects of refugeehood (Afghanistan Humanitarian Crisis, n.d.; "Nepal/Bhutan: Refugee Women Face Abuses," 2020; Maldives Islands—Migrants & Refugees Section, 2023; Bangladesh, n.d.).

Their oppression becomes double as they face ostracization not only of being persecuted and unwelcomed in majority States but also owing to the sensitivity attached to their gender (Kumari, 2012). The vulnerability that they carry in the majority of cases puts a heavy burden on their health quotient. Their well-being is compromised in several stages starting from where the process gets its inception. As refugee situation arises out of persecuting factors in their homeland, women refugees in the majority of cases are treated as soft targets. They face unabated rapes and other sexual violence which leaves them with a heavy traumatic mental condition and no medical protection. It has been reported by UNICEF that, the majority of the women and girls belonging to the Rohingya community who got refuge from Myanmar have faced multiple rapes or at least sexual assaults while feeling from their home State (Bonefeld, 2018). There have been reported factsheets which reflect that, that the Rohingya Muslim women in the Rakhine state of Myanmar have been systematically raped leading to their degrading mental and physical well-being to a higher extent (Manchanda, 2004). It has been claimed by UNHCR that the 1991 mass exodus from Myanmar got triggered due to mass rapes of adolescent girls. These incidents often leave them so traumatized that they feel uncomfortable opening up about these

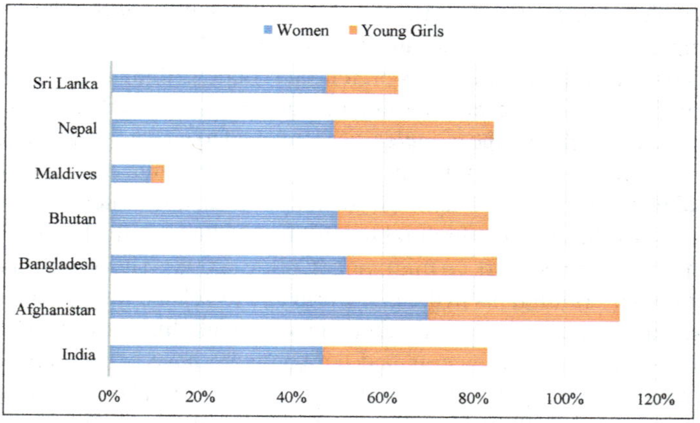


**Fig. 5.3** Percentage of women and girl refugees in South Asian countries by 2023. *Source* Afghanistan Humanitarian Crisis (n.d.), "Nepal/Bhutan: Refugee Women Face Abuses" (2020), Maldives Islands—Migrants & Refugees Section (2023), and Bangladesh (n.d.)

incidents to any such authority which probably takes up their responsibility in the host State. The majority of the host states, in addition, consider them as 'illegal aliens' and the consequential treatment becomes no less horrifying in the garb of providing protection. The adolescent girls and widowed women become primary targets of the traffickers as they are in high want of legal protection and amidst all these no satisfactory medical recourse is made accessible to them. They are largely exposed to 'transactional sex' which makes it more difficult for them to cope both physically and psychologically (Erhardt-Ohren & Lewinger, 2020). Even when they successfully manage to reach any host State that accommodates them for that time, its temporariness fails them to give any kind of safety towards their mental or physical health. In most cases, these unabated sexual atrocities bring in unwanted and untimely pregnancies among women refugees. Many of them remain in their age of minority when they assume such kinds of unexpected pregnancies (Nagesh et al., 2023). The United Nations Women have time and again highlighted the laxity and the poor maternal and neonatal care received by refugee women in South Asia. The process is not so straightforward to understand this involves a lot of layers and complexities. Often the host States where the refugees are allowed to take shelter stand out as completely unable or incapable of providing them with proper localities and houses. They are left with no options but to reside in those makeshift camps or cordoned areas choicelessly. These houses or rather dilapidating structures are often populated more than expected. Under these circumstances, women who get pregnant are needed to adjust themselves without any other opportunity. These unwanted pregnancies not only bring physical barriers for them but as they are major outcomes of violence, they are often found very vulnerable both physically and mentally. Also, even those who are not pregnant mothers owing to any accidental mishap are left separated from their husbands or left alone in many instances. Incidences of brutal killings in the form of genocide at their home state or in transit leave a heavy scar on their mental well-being that reflects on their health and of course, impacts their foetuses as well.

There lies an approach called the 'intersectional feminist approach to migration' which acknowledges the challenges faced by the female population facing migration profoundly (Division for the Advancement of Women et al., n.d.). The approach mainly targets the multiple oppressions faced by women while they are subjected to transboundary migration. The intersectionality feminist approach extends to the facets of rape and other sexual atrocities faced by women migrants at various phases of migration. Their vulnerability often pushes them to what is most popularly known as, 'identity politics' which makes it more complex to address the variety of challenges they face during forceful displacement (Crenshaw, 1991). Present-day feminism and studies on intersectionality highlight the fact that one of the most virulent women atrocities happens while they are in inter-border transit. However, due to the paucity of relevant emphasis and consequential studies, there lies a void and irreparable space to address those aspects.

Illegal and unintended abortions invite another set of healthcare challenges for the forced-displaced population in the region. It has been reported by an American research organization named, Guttmacher which conducts studies concerning sexual and reproductive health rights around the world, reported that countries like; India,

Nepal, and Bangladesh have one of the highest ranges of illegal abortions ranging from 58% to 90% (Kamdar, 2021). Among these, the majority of subjects are from refugee settlements in these countries. Only a few member nations in South Asia have proper laws to address the victimizing aspects involved in the process of abortion. Among the recent studies conducted by non-profit organizations, it is found that more than 50% of illegal and unassisted abortions take place in the refugee settlements of India, Pakistan, and Bangladesh (Hossain & Dawson, 2022). The SHR (sexual health rights) are compromised to the highest possible extent due to lucid or no legal compliance requirements. As per the data of the United Nations Population Fund, approximately 25–50% of maternal deaths in refugee settings are due to complications from unsafe abortion. These deaths are hardly documented on an official portal due to the related complexities and the status of the affected ones. With a very scanty post-abortion care and medications, these vulnerable are pushed to further vulnerabilities. Due to the sheer absence of research and data updation in the refugee settlements, the present conditions in the context of unsafe and home-based abortions are fairly made known to the people at large and to the notice of the regulatory authorities.

Parturition is another facet of health challenges faced by the women of South Asian refugee camps. In most camps, which are hard to live in, adequate medical facilities are a hard dream to imagine. As per Fig. 5.4, the unabated child births at the refugee camps of the South Asian region make it quite challenging for many analogous health risks for the concerned stakeholders to address (South Asian Association for Regional Cooperation and United Nations Call for Commitment to Support Millions of Pregnant Girls and Young Mothers in South Asia, 2024; "Midwifery Programme Tackles Afghanistan's High Maternal and Infant Mortality Rates," 2023). The findings of 'Save the Children' provide that, "48,000 Rohingya babies are set to be born in overcrowded refugee camps in Bangladesh in 2018" (Cook & Bhatnagar, 2019). The majority of the camps due to these overcrowded places make it impossible to cater to the neonatal care and the post-partum care for the new mothers. The use of home-based labour mechanisms and childbirth are widespread and are opted over for assisted medical attention. Refugee women continue to face higher maternity risks due to complicated pregnancy times, unavailability of pre-natal healthcare, and inaccessibility of required medication during these times (Yeo et al., 2023). Another challenging aspect is the steeply low participation in the decision-making in terms of childbearing which increases short-interval births and more adverse maternal and child health concerns (Khan & Khanam, 2023). These pertaining challenges not only compromise the existing health matrix of the populates but also impact largely on the future health regime that they will be subjected to.

As per the study, the South Asian countries are the producers of around 2.2 million adolescent mothers in the world on an annual basis out of whom nearly 5000–6000 such mothers die in the process of child rearing (South Asian Association for Regional Cooperation and United Nations Call for Commitment to Support Millions of Pregnant Girls and Young Mothers in South Asia, 2024). As per the joint analysis of UNICEF, UNFPA, and SAARC, "babies born out of such adolescent mothers face significantly higher risks of death compared to babies born out of adult women

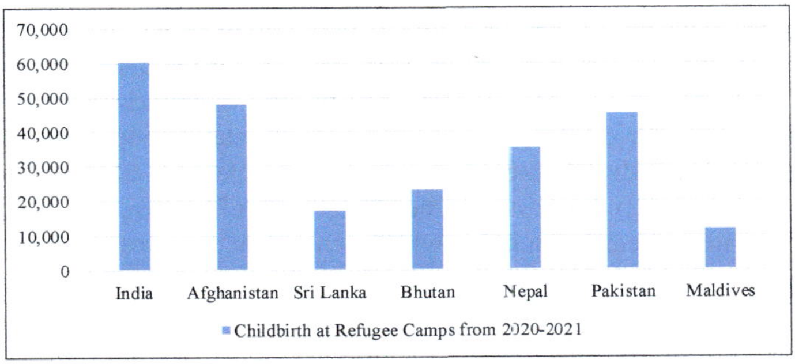


**Fig. 5.4** Extent of childbirths in refugee camps of South Asian countries. *Source* South Asian Association for Regional Cooperation and United Nations Call for Commitment to Support Millions of Pregnant Girls and Young Mothers in South Asia (2024) and "Midwifery Programme Tackles Afghanistan's High Maternal and Infant Mortality Rates" (2023)

in refugee camps" (South Asian Association for Regional Cooperation and United Nations Call for Commitment to Support Millions of Pregnant Girls and Young Mothers in South Asia, 2024). With scanty or no midwifery system in the camps, child rearing in inexperienced hands leads to a lot of labour and neonatal deaths.

The use of contraception and its availability for safe sexual health is another bottleneck challenge for women refugees in the region. As the majority of the women population shares a history of traumatic forced displacement coupled with rapes and forced sexual intercourse followed by no contraception mechanism available for them invites huge health risks. Contraception is a cost-effective and efficient way to prevent deaths from pregnancy or childbirth-related complications, as well as health problems related to unintended pregnancies (IRC, 2022). However, the minimum economic status which is required for adopting contraception methods is found absent in the majority of situations. Often contraception and emergency pills are treated as safer processes over illegal and unsafe abortions but owing to many existing reservations and traditional approaches, relying on those contraceptive measures becomes a guest of few women victims. The strictly rooted religious and regional customs make their ways so deeply connected with the emotional upbringing of the said population, that even when many women do realize that contraception may help them to get rid of unwanted pregnancies, owing to unsafe intercourse, their acceptability to resort to those measures becomes very limited. In addition, the knowledge and understanding of using contraception among young and adolescent girls are quite rare. They hardly understand the utility and the positive health impact of using contraception to stop unwanted pregnancies. Adolescent girls seemed to be the easy targets of sexual violence both in their home country and potentially in the camps as well. Yet, it could be extremely problematic and risky for them to access and obtain SRH services, given the perceived bias from service providers and the community stigma (Casey et al., 2019).

Malnutrition among the women and young girls who are refugees is another very pertinent health concern in South Asia. As per UNICEF data revelations, a soaring rate of women especially lactating mothers are due to extreme malnutrition among them. The majority of this population belongs to countries like; Bangladesh and Afghanistan (Wylie, 2023). Around half of the world's malnourished women live in three developing countries; Bangladesh, India, and Pakistan and despite decreasing in recent years, malnourished women remain high across Bangladesh, India, and Nepal (Waghmare et al., 2022). Interestingly, nearly 63% of refugee women in South Asia are among the mainstream population who belong to the total malnourished women of the region (Mahat, 2023). These health conditions percolate to a large extent to discourage proper mental and physical growth of young and adolescent girls in the camp lives. UNICEF's research in addition reflects that the regions with the highest levels of maternal undernutrition also contain the highest numbers of child undernutrition. The relatable low malnutrition is due to a plethora of reasons like; limited food accessibility during transit, locational differences percolating to food availability, climatic limitations pouring down to the productivity and availability of food at the camp areas, and limited or no accessibility to basic health supplements and drinks, etc. (Corbett et al., 2006).

Another major challenge area is the post-refugee psychological traumas causing mental health issues among the women refugee populations. Approximately, 80% of Rohingya women are reported to have depressive and emotional distress symptoms, and 60% had post-traumatic stress disorders after fleeing violence in their home country (Islam et al., 2024). Discriminatory behaviour and ill-treatment by the near ones and the co-inhabitants of the refugee camps pose a serious threat to their psychological quotient. The crisis period of refugeehood at varied levels starting from seeing heinous crimes with their near ones, human trafficking, organ trafficking, eloping their near ones, and sending them to such locations which are not in their knowledge are some of the very often witnessed wrong done by the women refugees which acts as catalysts towards degrading their mental well-being to a higher extent. Their questionable mental conditions percolate highly onto their progenies and the existing relatives for whom treating such conditions is an almost impossible task. The anomaly leads to escalating analogous challenges, which act as a precursor among the young generations to grow in a healthy environment.

Menstruation hygiene during the cycles among adolescent girls is another hard face challenge among the young refugee girls staying in makeshift camps. It is provided that, around 67% of Rohingya girls have improper or no access to the toilets during their menstruation days (Akter et al., 2023). Only 37.7% girls of in the camps in Bangladesh reportedly use sanitary pads and soaps or other lather agents after using toilets or cleaning their private parts. It is also found that many menstrual hygiene-related issues crop up not only due to the unavailability of menstrual products or medications but also unawareness and lack of education about maintaining hygiene during menstruation (Akter et al., 2023). The stigma attached to it and in many groups, the ethnic traditional practices act as prohibitive means to reach emancipation and access to medical attention and hygiene. Also, the unavailability of proper private spaces to maintain cleanliness and change sanitary pads in due intervals is highly absent among refugee girls in their dilapidating camps. In the wake of finding a proper country for safe shelter, food, and a little peace, these bodily challenges which are inevitable for women's lives go unnoticeable (Pandit et al., 2022). These results in the infliction of many menstrual-related diseases like; bacterial vaginosis, yeast infection in the urinary tracts, menorrhagia, etc. which are commonly communicable among the girls who normally get affected in post-menstrual days and get escalated to a higher degree when they are exposed to unclean and shab by vicinity prevalent among refugee women and girls (Hossain & Dawson, 2022).

An array of sexually transmitted diseases among women refugees in South Asia is another predominant challenge that the region faces rampantly. It is provided by the National Library of Medicine that, nearly 95% of the infiltrating refugee population always carry a threat of STDs like; Syphilis, Chlamydia, Gonorrhea, and HIV positive cases (Stauffer et al., 2012). These diseases are most commonly found equally among men and women with varied degrees. And due to unabated rapes and sexual violence taking place against women population in the process of refugeehood, the chances of women having these transmitted diseases become very high. Their complex humanitarian crises make it quite easy for these diseases to be perpetrated among the female refugee population and expose them to these risks to a higher extent (Hossain et al., 2018).

### *5.3.3 Addressed Challenges and Policy Heterogeneity*

The previous parts have highlighted some of the existing threats to the health conditions of refugee women and young girls in the South Asian refugee population which are serious enough to be addressed as an obligation of majority states under international law on a customary basis or either as an obligatory act. Globally health issues related to refugee women are something which has been taken quite seriously. There are such global organizations especially NGOs who are working collectively for the growth and amelioration of the health condition of refugee women on a global basis. At SEMA the reproductive health and sexual well-being of the women at the refugee camps are addressed very seriously (Health Program | SEMA International, 2024). Through various pilot camps and awareness missions, raising consciousness among the sufferers to address the issue with more promising solutions. Due to health camps being organized in some refugee camps, they are enabled to understand the array of reasons behind their existing condition of refugeehood which allows them to stay apart from healthcare access. International Organisations like; UNHCR (United Nations High Commissioner for Refugees) are in high order to understand the quality of sexual and reproductive healthcare services to be provided to the refugees in the camps within their reach (Sexual and Reproductive Health | UNHCR, n.d.). All the major arenas of health concerns highlighted above, ranging from birth time precautions to reproductive care services, from pre-natal to post-natal care, from skilled birth attendants to nurses for initial care and first-aid, from contraception to family planning, from addressing various contagious diseases to sexually transmitted diseases, all are kept under the realm of UNHCR to work for their address and proper mitigation

(Sexual and Reproductive Health | UNHCR, n.d.). Moreover, their range of protection extends to people of the LGBTQIA+ community people who face the wrath of refugeehood with the additional responsibility of getting their health rights protected or lest get attacked by ill-managed circumstances. International NGOs are taking very sporadic interests in these sectors to ameliorate people of their existing apathy. The RESPOND program instituted by the International Planned Parenthood Federation is a classic example of such undertaken efforts (Empowering Afghan Refugees Through Medical Camps in Pakistan | IPPF East & South East Asia & Oceania, 2023). They are working tirelessly for the amelioration of women's health conditions. The medical camp that is conducted by the Rahnuma-Family Planning Association of Pakistan (R-FPAP), a Member Association of the International Planned Parenthood Federation (IPPF), provides a lot of awareness missions in the camp areas concerning sexual health and SRH services (Empowering Afghan Refugees Through Medical Camps in Pakistan | IPPF East & South East Asia & Oceania, 2023). Menstrual well-being is another area that has been intervened a lot for the women of refugee camps. Although the patriarchal, heterosexual, religiously traditional, and metastatic societal fabric doesn't allow them to shun their shyness and come up openly about the problems they face while in transit or at the camp lives of the host country, many such actors are paving their ways to crack through these prohibitions and reach in the baseline crises zone to address the health plights. Making young girls aware of their menstrual hygiene, and dealing with their white discharges and black bleeding during these days due to the anaemic condition of their bodies gives them a lot of relief and related information (Ussher et al., 2017). In a recent study conducted at the Geneva camp in Bangladesh, it was encountered that, approximately 59.4% of women have some know-how about menstrual health, around 27% use sanitary napkins, and in contrast, 73% use old clothes, 4.27% use toilet tissue papers, 9.4% uses cotton and 25.64% uses reusable cotton cloths during their cycles (Huda et al., 2022). Often the linguistic disparities and cultural differences among the refugee resettles, and the prohibitive notions of gender equality hold them away from getting enlightened by the steps taken by the initiators to ameliorate. The studies showcase that, certain refugees in Bangladesh refugee camps near Mohammadpur Geneva camp in Dhaka are highly ignored groups in terms of MHM (menstrual hygiene management) (Huda et al., 2022).

Child immunization programs which have been conceived by UNICEF for the refugee population across the world have spread in many refugee camps in India and Bangladesh over the years (Selim & English, 2022). Routine vaccination centres at these camps like (Bhasan Char Camp) for the children a boon for these populations who cross multiple borders and are at high risk of getting infected with virulent diseases. Even for the COVID-19 vaccines as well, WHO has joined hands with local actors in spearing the vaccination facilities for the inhabitants of refugee camps through properly regulated mechanisms (COVID-19 Vaccination: WHO Supports an Effective Campaign in Bangladesh While Strengthening Vaccine Roll-out Preparedness for Rohingya, 2021). There are many experiences which have been gathered by field researchers which reflect the fact that nursing care and midwifery have escalated a lot in recent years. The new mothers and the ones who are mothers to their second or third child are sharing experiences wherein they have encountered betterment facilities and health care provisions for parturition times. UNICEF in recent years launched a very interesting Radio Listeners Club which has created interest among young girls to listen to various inputs on a global basis and this impacts not only their awareness but also advances their mental well-being (Ekka, 2024). BITA is an NGOs that has joined hands with WHO to bring together Rohingya women and girls together to form groups that have been entrusted with the task of providing knowledge and raising know-how about the female-trafficking, sex slavery, sexually transmitted diseases, problems of multiple partners, gender-based violence, and other similar intimate and sensitive issues which only females can address in a better manner (Jean, 2020). Concepts like, 'model mother' have been initiated whereby they are made to speak to pregnant women about their pre and post-natal care and their health protection mechanisms which they can adopt to avoid many pregnancy-oriented infections and related miscarriages (Jean, 2020).

UNHCR has made a remarkable breakthrough in the field of raising awareness about mental and psychological health at the refugee camps of the Cox Bazar area of Bangladesh (Majumdar, 2023). UNHCR's MHPSS (mental health and psychosocial support) program currently reaches over 150,000 Rohingya refugees, they not only provide individual counselling but also offer group counsellors for group stress relief and distress mechanisms at refugee camps (Majumdar, 2023). They are also planning to provide Refugee Medical Assistance (short-term medical insurance) to include pre-natal and post-natal cures and other medical distresses as well. Some qualitative interviews have reflected that the availability of healthcare providers is a key element in the positive assimilation of refugees to open up about their health issues (Ahmed et al., 2020). The cases of malnutrition in the Kuttupalong camps of Cox Bazar in Bangladesh have been constructively addressed by community nutrition volunteers through MUAC (mid-upper arm cases) taping (Kruglinski, 2023). The MUAC taping is the colour-coding system done for the malnourished kids and young girls in the refugee camps to identify their degree of malnourishment and address accordingly (Kruglinski, 2023). The awareness camps designed by WHO for the advanced countries have models to engage refugees and migrants in understanding the paradigm of accessibility to medical aid, their availability, and their attainability (Essén et al., 2018). They are planning to extend those models as per the varying needs of the South Asian region for better healthcare services that can be catered to them. The strategic designing of healthcare tools like; the Integrated Refugee Health Information System (IRHIS), UNHCR is trying to achieve a very sporadic approach to ensure quality health services for the refugee camps in India (Strategic Health Information | UNHCR India, n.d.). They have designed strategies like; Health Access and Utilization Surveys (HUAS), Standardized Expanded Nutrition Surveys (SENS), Balanced Score Card (BSC), and Surveys on the Inclusion of Refugees in National Systems, etc. to ensure, healthcare access to non-camp refugees, locating the levels of anaemia in children and women, tracking feeding practices among infants and young children, tracking access to food assistance, safe drinking water, sanitation and hygienic toilets and use of long-lasting, insecticide-treated mosquito nets at the camps, providing balanced score care cards which helps in identifying gaps in healthcare inputs and existing infrastructure so that UNHCR and other partners can attain targeted references and monitor progresses over a span, and inclusion of these refugee population in the existing national healthcare regime to make them accessible to those without extra infrastructural involvements (Strategic Health Information | UNHCR India, n.d.). Activities and efforts of many NGOs and locally based organizations are quite commendable in achieving many of these targets along with international organizations. For instance, the Organisation for Eelam Refugees Rehabilitation (OERR), is acting in the direction of improving the quality of health care across many refugee camps in India (Improving Healthcare for Refugees in India—India, 2018). These camps accommodate more than 60,000 Tamil Sri Lankans in India (Improving Healthcare for Refugees in India—India, 2018). From providing healthcare awareness sessions to even providing financial support for urgent medical assistance, the organization is working tirelessly for the betterment of the health quotient among its target population in a gender-neutral approach (Improving Healthcare for Refugees in India—India, 2018). Plans like installing pad vending machines and BIOSAN toilets in the camps are getting stronger day by day to cater to the needs of menstrual hygiene and proper sanitation (Makhanu & Raja, 2016; Waswa, 2018). However, it also needs to be understood that, there lies an underlying approach discrepancy amidst many efforts which are designed for attending the healthcare reasons among refugees on a country basis. The developed countries treat their inhabiting refugees in a far better and more schematic manner than that of the refugees in South Asian states. They are understood as quite an 'othered' group of the society whose medical needs could be handled tertiary than that of the civilians in the mainstream population. However, this is important to understand that among the South Asian populations, the treatment is more or less quite on the same platform its horizontal application of policies more or less than being vertical in terms of applying the health regime on the women refugee congregation of the region.

### *5.3.4 Limitations of the Study*

The study is chiefly doctrinal and is limited to the challenge of accessing the women refugee population who are languishing with health concerns to reach up to them for interviewing and addressing their challenges on a first-hand basis. So much reliance had to be placed on the data and research of the leading international organizations and research groups.

## 5.4 Conclusion

While there is a plethora of issues that take centre stage while refugee studies are undertaken, often health care issues assume a backseat in comparison to others on offering protection and safe shelter to the refugee population for a host country.

Women refugees especially young girls who are the most highly susceptible victims of these health challenges find themselves in an absolute quagmire when it comes to their health concerns. The stakeholders in some instances do understand the underpinning effects of neglecting physical and mental health and hygiene factors that play a pivotal role in integrating refugees into the mainstream population many times, however, in the majority of cases these health concerns are kept stale and given hardly any regard. The theorists who have invested time and done extensive research on trends of women migration have also agreed that forced migration coupled with the matrix of feminine gender faces many complexities compared to other genders. The recurring atrocities that they face include a huge challenge associated with the particularities of the migration trend. The region of diaspora, the transit distance, the extent of migration, the international borders, and the reason for such migration all impact their health and well-being. But if the existing measures are treated seriously then the women refugee population (including young and adolescent girls) who are just now stepping towards puberty and are facing huge precursors towards assimilating societally due to health reasons, may get a lot of support and aid towards better assimilation and healthy lives. The combined efforts of nations, international organizations and NGOs working in this field may raise the health risks prevalent among the women refugees of South Asia towards a better direction.

## References

*Afghanistan Humanitarian Crisis.* (n.d.). UNHCR. Retrieved August 3, 2024, from https://www.unrefugees.org/emergencies/afghanistan/#:~:text=The%20impact%20of%20the%20conflict,Afghanistan%20are%20women%20and%20children

Ahmed, R., Aktar, B., Farnaz, N., Ray, P., Awal, A., Hassan, R., Shafique, S. B., Hasan, M. T., Quayyum, Z., Jafarovna, M. B., Kobeissi, L. H., Tahir, K. E., Chawla, B. S., & Rashid, S. F. (2020). Challenges and strategies in conducting sexual and reproductive health research among Rohingya refugees in Cox's Bazar, Bangladesh. *Conflict and Health, 14*(1). https://doi.org/10.1186/s13031-020-00329-2

Akter, M., Jamil, S., & Kabir, H. (2023). Recognizing Rohingya adolescent girls' menstrual hygiene in Bangladesh to enhance reproductive health: A commentary. *Annals of Medicine and Surgery, 85*(4), 1304–1305. https://doi.org/10.1097/ms9.0000000000000283

*Bangladesh.* (n.d.). Global Focus. https://reporting.unhcr.org/operational/operations/bangladesh#:~:text=As%20of%2031%20December%202023%2C%20971%2C904%20Rohingya%20refugees%20have%20been,cent%20comprise%20women%20and%20girls

Bonefeld, A. S. (2018, March 21). *When going to the bathroom takes courage.* UNICEF. Retrieved August 3, 2024, from https://www.unicef.org/rosa/stories/when-going-bathroom-takes-courage

Casey, S., Puls, C., Jacobi, L., Krause, S., Quick, D., & Rich, S. (2019). A clear case for need and demand: Accessing contraceptive services for Rohingya women and girls in Cox's Bazar. *Women's Refugee Commission.* https://www.womensrefugeecommission.org/wp-content/uploads/2020/04/Contraceptive-Service-Delivery-in-the-Refugee-Camps-of-Cox-s-Bazar-Bangladesh-05-2019.pdf

Collins, P. (2008). *Black feminist thought: Knowledge, consciousness, and the politics of empowerment* [Print]. Routledge Publications. https://www.routledge.com/Black-Feminist-Thought-Knowledge-Consciousness-and-the-Politics-of-Empowerment/HillCollins/p/book/9780415964722?srsltid=AfmBOop15Kfb6riSRGtqdrlix4yHIk7M0mUs83Yfjd09n10TSD2Sdla2

Cook, D., & Bhatnagar, B. (2019, September 9). Rohingya babies born in refugee camps | Save The Children UK. *Save the Children*. Retrieved August 3, 2024, from https://www.savethechildren.org.uk/news/media-centre/press-releases/48-000-rohingya-babies-set-to-be-born-in-overcrowded-refugee-cam#:~:text=New%20figures%20reveal%20that%20more,made%20of%20plastic%20and%20bamboo

Corbett, A. O., Corbett, A. O., Bajulaiye, O., Guterres, A., & Morris, J. (2006). *Malnutrition in protracted refugee situations: A global strategy*. https://www.unhcr.org/sites/default/files/legacy-pdf/45fe62642.pdf

*COVID-19 vaccination: WHO supports an effective campaign in Bangladesh while strengthening vaccine roll-out preparedness for Rohingya*. (2021, May 20). https://www.who.int/bangladesh/news/detail/20-05-2021-covid-19-vaccination-who-supports-an-effective-campaign-in-bangladesh-while-strengthening-vaccine-roll-out-preparedness-for-rohingya

Crenshaw, K. (1991). Mapping the margins: Intersectionality, identity politics, and violence against women of color. *Stanford Law Review, 43*(6), 1241. https://doi.org/10.2307/1229039

Division for the Advancement of Women, Department of Economic and Social Affairs, & United Nations. (n.d.). *Women and International Migration*. https://www.un.org/en/development/desa/population/migration/events/coordination/3/docs/P01_DAW.pdf

Ekka, A. (2024, April 8). *World Health Day: Women's healthcare challenges in Bangladesh*. Médecins Sans Frontières (MSF)/Doctors Without Borders. https://msfsouthasia.org/world-health-day-womens-healthcare-challenges-in-bangladesh/

Erhardt-Ohren, B., & Lewinger, S. (2020). Refugee and internally displaced women's abortion knowledge, attitudes and practices: Addressing the lack of research in low- and middle-income countries. *International Perspectives on Sexual and Reproductive Health, 46*(Suppl. 1), 77. https://doi.org/10.1363/46e1120

Essén, B., Mosselmans, L., & Salzmann, T. (2018). *Improving the health care of pregnant refugee and migrant women and newborn children: Technical guidance on refugee and migrant health*. WHO, Europe. Retrieved August 4, 2024, from https://iris.who.int/bitstream/handle/10665/342289/9789289053815-eng.pdf?sequence=1&isAllowed=y

*Health Program | SEMA International*. (2024, July 29). SEMA International. https://sema-sy.org/our-programs/health/

Hossain, M. M., Sultana, A., Mazumder, H., & Munzur-E-Murshid, N. (2018). Sexually transmitted infections among Rohingya refugees in Bangladesh. *The Lancet HIV, 5*(7), Article e342. https://doi.org/10.1016/s2352-3018(18)30140-1

Hossain, M., & Dawson, A. (2022). A systematic review of sexual and reproductive health needs, experiences, access to services, and interventions among the Rohingya and the afghan refugee women of reproductive age in Asia. *WHO South-East Asia Journal of Public Health, 11*(1), 42. https://doi.org/10.4103/who-seajph.who-seajph_144_21

Huda, M. N., Hossain, S. Z., Mohsin, M., Azim, S., Rahman, M., Ferdous, A., & Hossain, M. A. (2022). Exploring knowledge and practices regarding menstrual hygiene management among Bihari women in the Geneva camp in Bangladesh. *Women Midwives and Midwifery, 2*(1), 84–97. https://doi.org/10.36749/wmm.2.1.84-97.2022

*Improving healthcare for refugees in India—India*. (2018, March 18). ReliefWeb. https://reliefweb.int/report/india/improving-healthcare-refugees-india

IRC. (2022, June 27). *Why refugee women want contraception*. The IRC. https://www.rescue.org/article/why-refugee-women-want-contraception

Islam, A., Mozumder, T., Rahman, T., Shatil, T., & Siddique, A. (2024, April 25). *Healing in crisis: Investing in women's mental health and child development in refugee camps has huge benefits*. VoxDev. Retrieved August 3, 2024, from https://voxdev.org/topic/health/healing-crisis-investing-womens-mental-health-and-child-development-refugee-camps-has#:~:text=Rohingya%20refugees%20in%20Bangladesh&text=Over%2080%25%20of%20Rohingya%20women,country%20(Fortify%20Rights%202020

Jean, K. (2020, July 20). Knowledge as a tool for empowerment for Rohingya refugee women and girls. *UNICEF*. Retrieved August 4, 2024, from https://www.unicef.org/rosa/stories/knowledge-tool-empowerment-rohingya-refugee-women-and-girls

Kamdar, B. (2021, June 15). Poor access to safe abortions is killing South Asian Women. *The Diplomat*. https://thediplomat.com/2021/06/poor-access-to-safe-abortions-is-killing-south-asian-women/#:~:text=A%20recent%20study%20by%20the,58%20percent%20to%2090%20percent

Khan, M. N., & Khanam, S. J. (2023). Women's participation in childbearing decision-making and its effects on short-interval births in Rohingya refugee camps of Bangladesh. *The Lancet Regional Health—Southeast Asia, 15*, Article 100250. https://doi.org/10.1016/j.lansea.2023.100250

Kruglinski, J. (2023, December 4). Malnutrition: Baby Nur's story. *UNICEF*. Retrieved August 4, 2024, from https://www.unicef.org/bangladesh/en/stories/malnutrition-baby-nurs-story

Kumari, S. (2012). Burmese refugee women in India: Victims and agents of empowerment. *Peace Prints: South Asian Journal of Peacebuilding, 4*(1), 1–16. https://wiscomp.org/peaceprints/4-1/4.1.5.pdf

Kumari, S. (n.d.). Burmese refugee women in India: Victims and agents of empowerment. *Peace Prints: South Asian Journal of Peacebuilding, 4*(1). https://wiscomp.org/peaceprints/4-1/4.1.5.pdf

Mahat, P. (2023, September 18). *UNICEF calls for more investment as South Asia remains a global epicentre for undernourished and anaemic adolescent girls and women*. UNICEF. Retrieved August 3, 2024, from https://www.unicef.org/rosa/press-releases/unicef-calls-more-investment-south-asia-remains-global-epicentre-undernourished-and

Majumdar, S. (2023, October 9). *Rohingya refugee volunteers combat stresses of camp life with mental health support*. UNHCR. Retrieved August 4, 2024, from https://www.unhcr.org/news/stories/rohingya-refugee-volunteers-combat-stresses-camp-life-mental-health-support

Makhanu, S. K. K., & Waswa, G. (2018). BIOSAN Latrine for Refugee Camps. *ResearchGate*. https://www.researchgate.net/publication/324081535_BIOSAN_LATRINE_FOR_REFUGEE_CAMPS/link/5abcd666a6fdcccda656c7f3/download?_tp=eyJjb250ZXh0Ijp7ImZpcnN0UGFnZSI6InB1YmxpY2F0aW9uIiwicGFnZSI6InB1YmxpY2F0aW9uIn19

*Maldive Islands—Migrants & Refugees Section*. (2023, April 3). Migrants & Refugees Section. https://migrants-refugees.va/country-profile/maldive-islands/#:~:text=In%202021%2C%20there%20were%20182%2C666,the%20remaining%2089%25%20were%20men

Manchanda, R. (2004). Gender conflict and displacement: Contesting "infantilisation" of forced migrant women. *Economic and Political Weekly, 39*(37), 4179–4186. http://www.jstor.org/stable/4415535

Meganathan, M., & Rizvi, D. (2023). Empowering Afghan refugees through medical camps in Pakistan. *IPPF*. Retrieved October 25, 2025, from https://eseaor.ippf.org/stories/empowering-afghan-refugees-through-medical-camps-pakistan

Midwifery programme tackles Afghanistan's high maternal and infant mortality rates. (2023, October 25). *UNHCR*. https://www.unhcr.org/news/midwifery-programme-tackles-afghanistan-s-high-maternal-and-infant-mortality-rates

*Migration data in Southern Asia*. (n.d.). Migration Data Portal. https://www.migrationdataportal.org/regional-data-overview/southern-asia#:~:text=By%20the%20end%20of%202019,neighbouring%20their%20countries%20of%20origin

Nagesh, N., Ip, C. H. L., Li, J., Fan, H. S. L., Chai, H. S., Fan, Y., Wong, J. Y., Fong, D. Y., & Lok, K. Y. W. (2023). Exploring South Asian women's perspectives and experiences of maternity care services: A qualitative evidence synthesis. *Women and Birth*. https://doi.org/10.1016/j.wombi.2023.12.002

Nair, R. (1997). Refugee protection in South Asia. *Journal of International Affairs, 51*(1), 201–220. https://www.jstor.org/stable/24357479

Nepal/Bhutan: Refugee Women Face Abuses. (2020, October 28). *Human Rights Watch*. https://www.hrw.org/news/2003/09/25/nepal/bhutan-refugee-women-face-abuses

Oishi, N., & The Center for Comparative Immigration Studies. (2002). *Gender and migration: An integrative approach* (Working Paper 49). https://ccis.ucsd.edu/_files/wp49.pdf

Pandit, K., Hasan, M. J., Islam, T., & Rakib, T. M. (2022). Constraints and current practices of menstrual hygiene among Rohingya adolescent girls. *Heliyon, 8*(5), Article e09465. https://doi.org/10.1016/j.heliyon.2022.e09465

Pessar, P. R., & Mahler, S. J. (2003). Transnational migration: Bringing gender in. *International Migration Review, 37*(3), 812–846. https://doi.org/10.1111/j.1747-7379.2003.tb00159.x

*Population of Southern Asia (2024)—Worldometer*. (n.d.). https://www.worldometers.info/world-population/southern-asia-population/#:~:text=The%20current%20population%20of%20Southern,of%20the%20total%20world%20population

Raja, A. (2016, June). Sakhi set to export 12 low-cost sanitary pad machines to Jordan refugee camps. *Indian Express*. Retrieved August 4, 2024, from https://indianexpress.com/article/india/india-news-india/sakhi-set-to-export-12-low-cost-sanitary-pad-machines-to-jordan-refugee-camps-2878320/

*Refugee population by country or territory of asylum for South Asia*. (2024, July 2). FRED | St. Louis Fed. https://fred.stlouisfed.org/graph/?g=1s4FG

San Suu Kyi, A. (n.d.). *Gendering refugee crisis in South Asia—The case of Rohingya refugee women*. http://www.mcrg.ac.in/RLS_Migration_2019/FULL_PAPERS_2019/MODULE_E_Sreetapa_Chakrabarty.pdf

Selim, F., & English, J. (2022, April 21). *Child immunization programme reaches Rohingya refugee children on Bhasan Char Island*. UNICEF. Retrieved August 4, 2024, from https://www.unicef.org/press-releases/child-immunization-programme-reaches-rohingya-refugee-children-bhasan-char-island

*South Asia—Population, Female—2024 Data 2025 Forecast 1960–2023 Historical*. (n.d.). Trading Economics. https://tradingeconomics.com/south-asia/population-female-wb-data.html#:~:text=Population%2C%20female%20in%20South%20Asia,compiled%20from%20officially%20recognized%20sources

*South Asian Association for Regional Cooperation and United Nations call for commitment to support millions of pregnant girls and young mothers in South Asia*. (2024, July 12). https://www.who.int/southeastasia/news/detail/12-07-2024-south-asian-association-for-regional-cooperation-and-united-nations-call-for-commitment-to-support--millions-of-pregnant-girls-and-young-mothers-in-south-asia

Stauffer, W. M., Kaiser, R., Painter, J., Weinberg, M., Berman, S., & Mamo, B. (2012). Sexually transmitted infections in newly arrived refugees: Is routine screening for Neisseria gonorrheae and Chlamydia trachomatis infection indicated? *American Journal of Tropical Medicine and Hygiene, 86*(2), 292–295. https://doi.org/10.4269/ajtmh.2012.11-0527

*Strategic Health Information | UNHCR India*. (n.d.). UNHCR India. https://www.unhcr.org/in/what-we-do/safeguard-human-rights/public-health/strategic-health-information

*The 1951 Refugee Convention | UNHCR India*. (n.d.). UNHCR India. https://www.unhcr.org/in/about-unhcr/who-we-are/1951-refugee-convention

Ussher, J. M., Perz, J., Metusela, C., Hawkey, A. J., Morrow, M., Narchal, R., & Estoesta, J. (2017). Negotiating discourses of shame, secrecy, and silence: Migrant and refugee women's experiences of sexual embodiment. *Archives of Sexual Behavior, 46*(7), 1901–1921. https://doi.org/10.1007/s10508-016-0898-9

Waghmare, H., Ahamed Mondal, N., & Prasad, R. D. (2022). Determinants of nutritional status among women in South Asian countries: A cross-sectional study. *Demography India, 51*(2), 100–110. https://iasp.ac.in/uploads/journal/006-1688886074.pdf

Wylie, H. (2023, March 7). *Malnutrition in mothers soars by 25 per cent in crisis-hit countries, putting women and newborn babies at risk*. UNICEF. Retrieved August 3, 2024, from https://www.unicef.org/rosa/press-releases/malnutrition-mothers-soars-25-cent-crisis-hit-countries-putting-women-and-newborn

Yeo, S., Park, Y., McClelland, D. J., Ehiri, J., Ernst, K., Magrath, P., & Alaofè, H. (2023). A scoping review of maternal health among resettled refugee women in the United States. *Frontiers in Public Health, 11*. https://doi.org/10.3389/fpubh.2023.1157098

# Chapter 6
# COVID-19's Impact on Sexual and Gender-Based Violence in Rohingya Refugee Communities in Bangladesh: Health Sector Response

**Jannatul Ferdous**

**Abstract** The Cox's Bazar camp in Bangladesh did not house a Rohingya refugee group before the catastrophic COVID-19 pandemic. The public wellness initiatives that were initiated in response to the epidemic have been partially blamed for the rise in recorded cases of sexual and gender-based violence (SGBV). Furthermore, the COVID-19 limits imposed by the Bangladeshi government affected the provision of comprehensive care for victims of sexual assault. The purpose of this study was to better understand SGBV among Bangladeshi Rohingya survivors and the resources that are accessible to them. Healthcare providers encountered challenges throughout the pandemic that made it more difficult to provide necessary services, such as camp access, early funding denials for SGBV programmes, problems with telemedicine and communication, worries about anonymity, and pressure from donors. This chapter examines gender-based violence (GBV) in Myanmar from various perspectives and emphasises the impact of the COVID-19 pandemic on the health and welfare of Rohingya women. The Bangladeshi government did not prioritise comprehensive SGBV assistance, complicating support for Rohingya survivors. Although the research primarily focuses on Rohingya migration, its findings apply to similar political, social, and humanitarian contexts, particularly in the global south. Government regulations hindered providing accessible and comprehensive SGBV care and services. Bangladesh's experience balancing the needs of homeless populations with COVID-19 containment efforts offers valuable insights for monitoring service delivery during pandemics and epidemics in humanitarian settings. Developing strategies to lower the incidence of illness and provide complete support to SGBV victims remains a top priority.

**Keywords** Covid-19 · Refugee · Gender-based violence · Health

---

J. Ferdous (✉)
Department of Public Administration, Comilla University, Cumilla, Bangladesh
e-mail: jannat.lata@yahoo.com



P. Chouhan et al. (eds.), *Women's Health Dynamics in South Asia*, Asian Perspectives on Public Health, https://doi.org/10.1007/978-981-95-2321-4_6

## 6.1 Introduction

The Rohingya women who have migrated illustrate the worst humanitarian crisis the world has ever seen (Jannat et al., 2023). Marginalised groups are more likely to experience violence, exploitation, or neglect during emergencies or crises; sadly, gender identities frequently contribute to these awful, abhorrent, and cruel outcomes (Kirby, 2015). Those already dealing with humanitarian crises have been hit particularly hard by the COVID-19 pandemic, which has disrupted the lives of millions. Movement limitations have made it challenging for people residing in densely populated regions, such as refugee camps, to exercise social distancing, obtain the assistance they require, and take preventative measures to stop the COVID-19 virus from spreading. Accommodations in Cox's Bazar, Bangladesh, were home to 855,000 Rohingya refugees in March 2020, when the outbreak started. And they have been greatly affected by these difficulties (Chowdhury et al., 2022). Human rights violations, such as violence against women, have devastating effects on victims, their communities, and nations worldwide (Vyas et al., 2023). Many female victims of gender-based violence (GBV) are afraid to speak out about the abuse they suffered or seek help after the fact because of societal and cultural norms that discourage such behaviour (Benjamin & Fancy, 1998). In response to a pressing humanitarian crisis, the UN General Assembly established Sustainable Development Goal 5.2, which is to end violence against women and girls worldwide (UN, 2024). Onyango et al. (2019) noted that SGBV and IPV rose during the pandemic in several countries, and this trend is consistent with a history of public health crises that have raised the risk of SGBV. Many people were worried that the COVID-19 confinements and other social exclusion practices would increase the prevalence of SGBV as a means of controlling the virus (UNFPA, 2020).

As to Dey et al. (2020), the initial indication of SARS-CoV-2-related sickness in Bangladesh was documented on March 8, 2020. As a precaution against the spreading of the coronavirus, the authorities of Bangladesh issued a statewide stay-at-home order in late March 2020. They locked down the Cox's Bazar district, limiting movement both within and outside the surrounding refugee camps and suppliers of essential services (Hossain, 2020). The Office of the Refugee Relief and Repatriation Commissioner (RRRC) issued an order on March 23, 2020, stating that all non-essential services in the camps were to be halted. The order further said that groups primarily aim to provide medical care and supply food, water, and hygiene should not engage in other activities. Rumours have it that they're also attempting to restrict the movement of vehicles and people into and out of the camps (Chowdhury et al., 2022).

The lockdowns prevented many humanitarian relief providers from reaching the refugee settlements in Cox's Bazar, as Spoerri et al. (2020) reported. During the lockdown era, not all parts of complete SGBV services were considered significant (Chowdhury et al., 2022). Due to mobility constraints, SGBV did not have easy access to essential humanitarian resources like as healthcare, economic opportunities, and support networks (UNFPA, 2015). The number of cases of sexual and gender-based violence (SGBV) in the camps has increased since the COVID-19 outbreak began, according to organisations that focus on this issue. This increase is caused by a combination of variables, including stress, overcrowding in confined spaces, demands associated with the pandemic, and trauma in general (UNFPA, 2015). This is in line with the results showing that containment measures intensified domestic violence and sexual assault against women in Bangladeshi refugee camps and the country as a whole and that people were more worried about their safety (Guglielmi et al., 2020; Palit et al., 2022). Women and girls in Bangladesh and the Rohingya people who have experienced or survived abuse, trafficking, child marriage, or other forms of gender-based violence can use these services. Unfortunately, the safe spaces facilities have either temporarily closed or ceased to operate in their prior capacity due to the nationwide lockdown and suspension of "non-essential" services. These programmes, usually operated out of multipurpose facilities or areas designated particularly for women and girls, adopt a multisectoral approach that provides access to a range of services for survivors of SGBV in the camps. A case worker assists survivors in obtaining medical treatment, psychological assistance, safety nets, and legal representation in these settings (Jean & Miks, 2020a, 2020b). Understanding the root causes of Rohingya women's gender-based violence is a crucial focus of this chapter. Additionally, this chapter will address the impact of their experiences in the Bangladeshi refugee camps, especially regarding the ongoing global COVID-19 pandemic.

### *6.1.1 Rohingya Crisis and Violence Against Rohingya Women*

According to Ware and Laoutides (2018), the Muslim minority of northern Myanmar's Rakhine state (previously Arakan) is usually referred to as the Rohingya. According to historical records, the Rohingya people lived in Arakan for about a thousand years. While dealing with the Rohingya, the Burmese government acknowledged them and their choice of ethnic designation on multiple occasions throughout the 1950s (Priddy et al., 2022). Among Myanmar's 135 recognised ethnic groups, the Rohingya were omitted from the 1982 Burma Citizenship Law's official roster. Due to discriminatory citizenship laws that do not adhere to international standards, a large population of Myanmar does not possess citizenship (Arraiza & Vonk, 2017; Kyaw, 2017). The Rohingya people have endured displacement, oppression, and the present-day dangers of refugee camps spread throughout Bangladesh because they are not citizens of the country they were born (Ahmed, 2010; Mohsin, 2020). In particular, since August 2017, the Tatmadaw, the Myanmar Army, has tortured and murdered thousands of Rohingyas. Approximately one million Rohingyas have been forced to move to adjacent Bangladesh as a result of this (Farzana, 2015; Yasmin & Akther, 2020). People often say that this Muslim group in Myanmar is "the greatest oppressed minority in the world" because they believe they have been genocide victims (Human Rights Council, 2017). As they flee from Myanmar into Bangladesh, the Rohingya have been the object of scorn and stereotypes (Zawacki, 2012). Given that they were de-naturalised in 1982 (Cheung, 2012), being unable to reside in Myanmar legally signifies that they are considered to be in an "illegal" position, which has further isolated them and placed them at risk of cultural and structural forms of violence (Zawacki, 2012). After being forcibly removed from their homeland by the military dictatorship in Myanmar, the ethnic minority now faces a period of uncertain transition and instability brought about by prejudice, brutality, and tyranny (Goodman & Mahmood, 2019).

Discriminatory laws play a significant role, as Rohingya refugees are denied legal status in Bangladesh, restricting their ability to seek formal justice for sexual and gender-based violence. The absence of comprehensive legal protections leaves many survivors without recourse, reinforcing cycles of impunity. Bangladesh's current laws and regulations outline equality and nondiscrimination. However, insufficient attention is paid to GBVH-related difficulties in the workplace (Yasmin, 2020). Bangladesh does not currently have laws that forbid or protect against discrimination based on gender, sexual orientation, caste, religion, or other identification markers. The National Human Rights Commission created a draft anti-discrimination bill in 2013 that forbids discrimination against any person or group on various grounds, including caste, religion, sexual orientation, age, disability, pregnancy, marital status, place of birth, sex (male, female, or third gender), custom, culture, occupation, and religion. The draft is under legislative scrutiny and has not yet garnered significant support for enactment (Yasmin, 2020).

Unfortunately, it is not uncommon for women to be victims of violence in times of war (Kreft, 2020). If we want to make sense of this complex GBV situation, we need to know what violence is (Priddy et al., 2022). More than half of Bangladesh's Rohingya population consists of women, and in the neighbourhoods around the camps, one out of six households is headed by a single mother (Sang, 2018). The vast majority of them have first-hand experience with or knowledge of gender-based violence in Myanmar (UN WOMEN, 2018). As they flee ethnic conflict in Myanmar for safety in Bangladesh, they take with them some cultural characteristics of that violence. As it stands, many Rohingya women in refugee camps are still dealing with the aftereffects of gender-based violence. Patriarchy is deeply ingrained in Rohingya culture, with women traditionally expected to stay at home and raise children (Akhter & Kusakabe, 2014; Ullah, 2011). The situation has become more complex due to the COVID-19 worldwide pandemic. Many social services that were previously accessible in the camps have been cut down to reduce the dangers of the virus spreading (Sullivan, 2020). The general health of Rohingya women is greatly affected by this crippling condition.

### 6.1.2 Impacts of COVID-19 Pandemic on GBV

Men and women are affected differently by any significant public health catastrophe. Since testing has proven to be difficult, the COVID-19 epidemic has made life in the camps for Rohingya people more difficult (Akter et al., 2021). Physical separation from the Rohingya camps is practically impossible due to their dense population (Kamal et al., 2020). Those who were displaced and relocated to countries with low or medium incomes have been hit the worst by the pandemic. Bangladeshi Rohingyas are not an exception. There are two official camps and thirty-two unregistered camps housing over a million Rohingyas (Ullah & Chattoraj, 2018). Girls and women comprise most of the Rohingya population (52%) (Kumar et al., 2022). Government travel restrictions make it harder for women, especially those who are pregnant or trying to conceive, to get the sexual and reproductive wellness treatments they need. The absence of clean water, proper sanitation, and hygiene practices puts refugee camp residents at high risk of contracting a variety of infectious diseases, including dengue fever, TB, and diarrhoea (COVID-19) (Tahir et al., 2021). Because of their unique developmental stage, adolescent refugees are more likely to experience internalising problems and symptoms of post-trauma than boys (Derluyn & Broekaert, 2007). Because of this, they are more likely to suffer from anxiety and PTSD.

In the early months of the COVID-19 pandemic, women's clinics and safe spaces received less attention, while food supplies and emergency medical attention were limited to specific areas of the campsites (Ullah & Ferdous, 2022; Ullah et al., 2020). Furthermore, most women have chosen to stay indoors because they fear contracting the viral disease (v et al., 2021). COVID-19 has exacerbated GBV in all of its manifestations and social stigma, which could seriously impair women's and girls' ability to navigate the constrained social norms that mold their lives (Nasar et al., 2023). Rohingya women still needed their husbands' permission to get essentials like soap and masks, and 61% of them needed it to get related to sexuality, reproduction, and maternal health services (such as treatment centres and isolation) even though they had symptoms similar to COVID-19 (ISCG, 2020). The total number of camp authorities has been reduced, and few help centres exist. As a result, there has been an alarming increase in domestic violence, sexual assault, polygamy, underage marriage, people trafficking, and brutality against female sex workers (Jean & Miks, 2020a, 2020b).

Under these circumstances, the fear of disease causes increased stress in the camps, making safety a more pressing concern. A profound pandemic-related fear has broken out among Rohingya refugees because of safety concerns and inadequate funding (Ahmed et al., 2021). Thankfully, a few Rohingya volunteers in health clinics, disseminating vital information about the virus and fostering confidence in the community (Akter et al., 2021). The World Health Organisation (WHO) has trained about 1400 volunteer refugees to look for symptoms of sickness, dispel rumours, and advise on the value of testing. Even when the transmission of a worldwide epidemic illness is low-scale, a high-scale epidemic can develop among refugees (Truelove et al., 2020). When responding to a public health emergency, such as a pandemic, it is imperative to prioritise the health of the host community and the refugees. Failure to do so could lead to unimaginable losses. Priddy et al. (2022) suggest that relationships, collaborations, and engagements may be crucial in reducing risk. According to Akter et al., (2021a, 2021b), even though there have been numerous complaints of spousal abuse and prejudice against women and girls as a result of the COVID-19 pandemic and the lockdown that followed, they are hoping that the Women Friendly Spaces and Women Leading Centers would provide a bridge to sunshine.

To sum up, it is advised that interventions incorporating decentralised psychosocial activities be planned and that women and girls be more actively involved in their empowerment. This means that women who remain at home can lend a hand around the house to other people who have been unable to make it to the centres. Second, males need to be made aware of the significance of preventing child marriage, dowries, intimate partner violence, and gender-based violence and carefully preparing for case management to safeguard women and girls from all types of violence.

Depending on an individual's age, gender, and other intersecting factors like marital status, gender-based violence in the Rohingya community varies significantly. Married teenage girls and Rohingya women claim that intimate relationship abuse is the most common kind of gender-based violence. However, men, adolescent boys, and unmarried females do not perceive this as a direct threat. Men and boys brought up the fact that individuals outside of the Rohingya group perpetrate gender-based violence, but by women and girls, it was ignored entirely. There was widespread alarm over the worsening security situation in the camps and reports of community violence from respondents across all demographics (Guglielmi et al., 2022). Toma et al. (2018) examined health sector coordination from 2017 to 2019, paying particular attention to the HSSAG and Health Sector Working Groups' (HSWG) successes and failures. Epidemiology, case management, sexual and reproductive health, community health, and public health were covered by these subgroups. Early in the reaction, essential service criteria were set for primary healthcare, a crucial first step that made it possible to standardise services according to critical needs. Likewise, the foundation for using this significant health workforce was the establishment of community health outreach standards. Innovative strategies were implemented for infectious disease responses to varicella and acute watery diarrhoea using cross-sectoral partnerships. Improvements in treatment for abortion, family planning, competent delivery attendants, and assistance for gender-based violence were highlighted after the crisis's initial prioritisation of reproductive and sexual health services. Although mental health treatments have been better made available through community-based initiatives, primary healthcare facilities still do not have enough psychiatrists to incorporate mental health programming adequately.

Violence between spouses has become more common in areas surrounding Rohingya camps (Toulemonde, 2020), notwithstanding the health hazards associated with the COVID-19 epidemic (Ferdous & Ullah, 2022b). Remarkably, every Rohingya woman is at risk of gender-based violence, irrespective of their age, marital status, or the social status of their household (Parray et al., 2022). However, these elements work in concert with other components, including geography, literacy level, ease of access to resources, and mobility, to determine an individual's susceptibility to gender-based violence (Karin, 2020). Due to cultural norms, Rohingya adolescent girls face severe limitations on their movement, which poses a significant obstacle to their utilisation of GBV services, including reporting (Guglielmi et al., 2021; Karin, 2020). According to Guglielmi et al. (2022), GBV sub-sector partners, the most vulnerable Rohingya community members, receive the GBV response. Even though many Rohingya and camp-level officials might disagree, partners feel that their presence is felt and that the community is aware of the variety of private services they provide to victims of gender-based violence. Underreporting of gender-based violence has been identified as a severe problem that affects the response to GBV and may even further marginalise vulnerable community members. Partners also stated that, in contrast to determining who is left behind by programming, the normalisation of violence is a more urgent concern. Partners thought that rather than being an abuse that has to be reported to the authorities, many Rohingya women and girls view severe discipline as a means of teaching and showing love.

There are several reasons why the Rohingya refugees have suffered. The health of migrants is a vital topic that needs to be addressed because a substantial number of them are female and teenagers. Separation from male breadwinners (husbands or fathers) puts Rohingya women and children in an already precarious position; COVID-19 has only made matters worse (Tay et al., 2018). Here, we take a look at the three main areas where the mental, sexual, and reproductive health effects of the COVID-19 pandemic on Rohingya refugee girls and women were felt, as well as the relevant variables (Kumar et al., 2022). According to Banerjee (2019), the Rohingya camps serve as a breeding ground for COVID-19 infections due to the cramped living conditions of the women and children living in temporary shelters with poor sanitation. The statewide lockdown has limited resources from the government and outside organisations, which has hindered healthcare provision. This will immediately affect the severe consequences of COVID-19 and the clinical challenges of other disorders. The lack of diagnostic and treatment options in rural areas significantly contributes to the suffering of adult women with chronic illnesses, such as chronic liver disease (CLD) and chronic kidney disease (CKD) (Kumar et al., 2022).

A concerning number of Rohingya people suffer from chronic ailments, including diabetes and hypertension, nevertheless, which is believed to be exacerbated by high-risk factors such as smoking, use of nicotine-free cigarettes, indoor air pollution, and other similar issues (WHO-SEAR, 2018). After the outbreak, things are probably going to get worse. While some studies indicated a decline in child marriages among the Rohingya population after the initial epidemic lockdown, this trend is likely to reverse itself in the coming years (Guglielmi et al., 2020). The closure of some youth programming and children services during the epidemic has resulted in increased difficulty for the Rohingya refugees in Bangladesh to access aid (Kumar et al., 2022). Premature birth, postpartum fistulas, and mental illnesses, including depression and PTSD, are more common among women and girls, while STDs and other obstetrical complications are more common among them (Kumar et al., 2022). Pandemic-related anxiety and worry haven't subsided. In response to Rohingya women's desperate needs, a few safe spaces for women have gradually begun to appear. Despite COVID-19, community volunteers are working extremely hard to maintain these sites. During this period, women can be informed that some spots are still available by doing home check-ins and spreading the word (Priddy et al., 2022). Kumar, among others, in the year 2022, we investigate the effects of COVID-19 on the health and socioeconomic standing of Bangladeshi Rohingya women and teenagers. Over 63% of Rohingya adolescent females experienced food deprivation as a result of the restrictions. A protein deficit resulted from respondents cutting back on meal frequency, according to the vast majority of respondents (87%) to the survey. Since arriving in Bangladesh, they have had restricted access to healthcare and educational resources. Things have gotten worse because of the pandemic. Girls are more susceptible to pregnancy, early marriage, sexual and gender-based abuse, and dropping out of school. The Jannat group, 2023 Ensuring Rohingya refugees' safe and improved sexual and reproductive health is undoubtedly one of the social policy's implied responsibilities, along with satisfying societal demands, education, health, migration, poverty, and other critical global variables. In addition to guaranteeing better health, simple access to SRH care products, and security from harm or judgement, social policy should focus on safeguarding and prioritising SRH.

### *6.1.3 Breaking the Cycle of Violence*

It will take a lot of work to resolve the Rohingya situation. We must recognise that numerous actors, sectors, and agencies must work together to prevent and respond to GBV. This includes providing health care, psychosocial assistance, safety, and emergency security. Similar circumstances exist for more than one million Rohingya in Bangladesh. According to Priddy et al. (2022), the government of Bangladesh is collaborating with numerous international and domestic humanitarian organisations to offer life-saving help to the Rohingya. According to Akhter and Kusakabe (2014), the Rohingya people are at risk on both sides of the border due to their unlawful status in Myanmar and the fact that they are not considered refugees in Bangladesh. More action from the governments of Myanmar and Bangladesh, as well as international development partners, and the active engagement of male and female Rohingya members in the Rohingya camps in Bangladesh and Myanmar, are necessary to reduce gender-based violence against Rohingya women significantly (Tanabe et al., 2019). There may be projects with a longer time horizon among them. There are both immediate and long-term ways to address the issue of Rohingya women experiencing violence in the refugee camps of Bangladesh during the epidemic.

Information regarding domestic violence services in the camps should be made known to Rohingya women. The difficulty of conveying both information and risk during COVID-19 is already high. Various national and international organisations supported hundreds of welcoming places for Rohingya girls, women, and teenagers before the COVID-19 pandemic. Priddy et al. (2022) noted that these services have been severely reduced or nonexistent due to the pandemic in the past few months.

Humanitarian organisations should wisely focus on educating and supporting parents, especially women beneficiaries, to serve as community agents for risk communication. This can be effectively achieved by implementing a block-centred strategy, considering the refugee camps are divided into numerous blocks. To guarantee that women and girls in the Rohingya area receive the assistance they require, this community engagement plan must be sensitive to gender issues (Priddy et al., 2022). In a typical improvised room constructed from bamboo sticks and tarps, four or five Rohingya people—including children—sleep. When it rains, the plastic sheets or papers people lie on become muddy floors (Islam & Nuzhath, 2018). The government should equitably provide food and other necessities to safeguard marginalised communities from discrimination and abuse. Humanitarian organisations must expand their service offerings to include psychosocial assistance and teleconsultation to meet women's and youth's unique requirements (Kumar et al., 2022).

Because of the congestion and close quarters, Rohingya women are more likely to be victims of illnesses, fires, and other types of gender-based abuse in the camps (ISCG & UNHCR, 2019). The refugee camps' inadequate layout often makes cases of sexual violence outside the home even more common. Here, ladies are griping about how unsafe it is, especially at night, due to the absence of proper lighting and restroom door locks (WHO, 2020). According to Sang (2018), the Rohingya camps have found that gender-separate restrooms work. The Kara Tepe camp in Greece, which houses about a thousand displaced individuals, is not the first to implement the practice of separating restrooms in refugee camps (Priddy et al., 2022). Returning the Rohingya people to Myanmar in a dignified and safe manner is of the utmost importance. A more impartial evaluation of the feasibility of repatriation, including Rohingya and independent observers like the UN, is necessary (Landgren, 1998). A viable and long-term remedy to the Rohingya crisis is being considered by the Bangladeshi government and the international community: repatriation. Because of this, the Rohingya people could stop the fighting and thoroughly exercise their human rights (Priddy et al., 2022).

Giving women the tools they need to enter local job markets is an effective way to reduce violence against women (Kumar et al., 2022). Domestic violence and exploitation are more likely to occur when one partner is economically dependent on the other. To improve quality of life and work prospects, providing all young adolescents and women with diverse, high-quality education or vocational training would be beneficial. To help the Rohingya people escape the suffering caused by the COVID-19 pandemic, the government of Bangladesh, along with international organisations and world leaders, must act swiftly to repatriate them to their home country.

## 6.2 Applying the Capability Approach to Address Sexual and Gender-Based Violence in Rohingya Refugee Camps During COVID-19

The capacity Approach, developed by Amartya Sen and Martha Nussbaum, holds that practice and policy must be evaluated in terms of freedom to utilise one's assets and not in terms of one's assets or access to them (e.g., wealth, earnings, social institutions) (Abadeer, 2015; Nussbaum, 2012; Sen, 1994). This Approach can serve as a critical lens through which sexual and gender-based violence (SGBV) and its impact on Rohingya refugee women in Bangladesh, specifically during the pandemic period of COVID-19, can be analysed. In terms of this Approach, real empowerment is not a matter of legal protection but a matter of extending freedom, options, and capabilities for a life with dignity (Kimhur, 2020; Robeyns, 2005; Vizard et al., 2011). Women and girls who have reached Bangladesh, sometimes alone with their children, face additional obstacles, such as abuse, lack of security, and restricted freedom of movement or voice and opportunity to contribute to society (Oxfam, 2022). These factors make them more susceptible to exploitation, forced marriages, and domestic violence (Goodman & Mahmood, 2019). The pandemic further exacerbated these issues by disrupting essential GBV response services, including safe shelters, legal aid, and psychosocial support, leaving survivors with even fewer options to seek help (Chowdhury et al., 2022; Smith, 2021). Deeply entrenched patriarchal norms continue to limit women's ability to make decisions about their safety and well-being (Rahman et al., 2024). The capability approach highlights the urgent need for policy interventions that go beyond emergency relief—ensuring that health and legal systems in refugee camps not only respond to violence but actively work to expand women's agency, access to education, and economic participation. By framing SGBV through the lens of capabilities, we can move towards transformative solutions that enhance women's autonomy and resilience, even in crisis settings.

## 6.3 Further Research Direction

The main focus of future study should be the effectiveness of volunteer-based programmes and modified programming, as well as the long-term effects of COVID-19 on SGBV support services in refugee camps. It will be essential to look into how government regulations affect how services are provided and strategies for enhancing privacy and communication in telehealth. Research comparing comparable humanitarian situations may yield important lessons for creating resilient, flexible SGBV support systems during pandemics and other emergencies.

**Declarations**

**Conclusion** It is impossible to find answers to the horrifying Rohingya predicament due to its immense complexity. We need to act quickly in response to the dire effects of COVID-19 on the health and welfare of Rohingya women and adolescents. The wide-ranging psychological and societal impacts of COVID-19 suggest that a concerted effort may be required to adequately protect these vulnerable groups (Kumar et al., 2022). Instead of simplifying the problem, this study aims to raise awareness about a critical aspect of the Rohingya crisis on a national and international level, encourage active engagement, and provide potential clarity. The search for knowledge, action, and ultimate peace is far from over. Investigations into the causes of the Rohingya people's forced migration and catastrophic displacement are continuing and may take new turns at any time.

Conversely, this challenge presents an excellent chance for additional investigation into creative and durable remedies. The public is now more aware of the issue, and a solution analysis has emerged from the evaluation and collection of data regarding the gender struggle and the culture of violence. In addition, with the increasing worries about studies on gender-based violence, marriage between kids, gender-equal relationships in families, and the consequences of teen pregnancies in the long run, homeschooling should be allowed again for children. Community engagement between refugees from Myanmar, their host communities, and the government should be enhanced through joint efforts by national and international partners to ensure the safest, most thorough response for those in need.

This study investigates the impact of COVID-19 on sexual and gender-based violence (SGBV) in Rohingya refugee communities in Bangladesh, focusing on health sector responses. No conflicts of interest; ethical guidelines were strictly followed.

## References

Abadeer, A. S. Z. (2015). The capability approach and gender discrimination. In *Palgrave Macmillan US eBooks* (pp. 71–83). https://doi.org/10.1057/9781137395283_4

Ahmed, S., Simmons, W. P., Chowdhury, R., & Huq, S. (2021). The sustainability–peace nexus in crisis contexts: How the Rohingya escaped the ethnic violence in Myanmar, but are trapped into environmental challenges in Bangladesh. *Sustainability Science, 16*, 1201–1213.

Ahmed, I. (2010). *The plight of the stateless Rohingya*. The University Press Limited.

Akter, S., Dhar, T. K., Rahman, A. I. A., & Uddin, M. K. (2021a). Investigating the resilience of refugee camps to COVID-19: A case of Rohingya settlements in Bangladesh. *Journal of Migration and Health, 4*, Article 100052.

Akter, F., Ahmad, N., Jaohari, N. A. S. B. & Rahman, A. R. A. (2021). During COVID-19, Rohingya women are facing challenges due to lockdown affects their psychosocial condition in refugee camps in Cox's bazar. International Webinar Community Development in Southeast Asia 2021 (IWCDSA2021).

Akhter, S., & Kusakabe, K. (2014). Gender-based violence among documented Rohingya refugees in Bangladesh. *Indian Journal of Gender Studies, 21*(2), 225–246.

Arraiza, J. M., & Vonk, O. (2017). *Report on citizenship law: Myanmar*. European University Institute.

Banerjee, S. (2019). The Rohingya crisis: A health situation analysis of refugee camps in Bangladesh.

Bean, T. M., Eurelings-Bontekoe, E., & Spinhoven, P. (2007). Course and predictors of mental health of unaccompanied refugee minors in the Netherlands: One year follow-up. *Social Science & Medicine, 64*(6), 1204–1215.

Benjamin, J. A., & Fancy, K. (1998). *The gender dimensions of internal displacement: Concept paper and annotated bibliography*. Office of Emergency Programmes, UNICEF.

Cheung, S. (2012). Migration control and the solutions impasse in South and Southeast Asia: Implications from the Rohingya experience. *Journal of Refugee Studies, 25*(1), 50–70.

Chowdhury, S. A., McHale, T., Green, L., Mishori, R., Pan, C., & Fredricks, I. (2022). Health professionals' perspectives on the impact of COVID-19 on sexual and gender-based violence (SGBV) and SGBV services in Rohingya refugee communities in Bangladesh. *BMC Health Services Research, 22*(1), 743.

Dey, S. K., Rahman, M. M., Siddiqi, U. R., & Howlader, A. (2020). Exploring epidemiological behavior of novel coronavirus (COVID-19) outbreak in Bangladesh. *SN Comprehensive Clinical Medicine, 2*(10), 1724–1732.

Derluyn, I., & Broekaert, E. (2007). Different perspectives on emotional and behavioural problems in unaccompanied refugee children and adolescents. *Ethnicity and Health, 12*(2), 141–162.

Farzana, K. F. (2015). Boundaries in shaping the Rohingya identity and the shifting context of borderland politics. *Studies in Ethnicity and Nationalism, 15*(2), 292–314.

Ferdous, J., & Ullah, A. A. (2022a). The COVID-19 pandemic: The price Bangladesh pays. *Thammasat Review of Economic and Social Policy, 8*(2), 89–112.

Ferdous, J., & Ullah, A. K. M. (2022b). COVID-19 and the migrant population: The resilience of South Asians. *International Journal of Asia-Pacific Studies, 18*(2).

Goodman, A., & Mahmood, I. (2019). The Rohingya refugee crisis of Bangladesh: Gender based violence and the humanitarian response. *Open Journal of Political Science, 9*(3), 490–501.

Guglielmi, S., Seager, J., Mitu, K., Baird, S., & Jones, N. (2020). Exploring the impacts of COVID-19 on Rohingya adolescents in Cox's Bazar: A mixed-methods study. *Journal of Migration and Health, 1*, Article 100031.

Guglielmi, S., Mitu, K., & Seager, J. (2021). 'I just keep quiet': Addressing the challenges of married Rohingya girls and creating opportunities for change. *The European Journal of Development Research, 33*(5), 1232–1251.

Guglielmi, S., Mitu, K., Jones, N., Ala Uddin, M., & Seager, J. (2022). *Gender-based violence. What is working in prevention, response and mitigation across Rohingya refugee camps, Cox's Bazar, Bangladesh* (Report). Gender and Adolescence: Global Evidence, London.

Human Rights Council. (2017). Human Rights Council opens special session on the situation of human rights of the Rohingya and other minorities in Rakhine State in Myanmar.

Human Rights Council. (2022). Report of the Special Rapporteur on the situation of human rights in Myanmar, Thomas H. Andrews. Agenda item 4: Human rights situations that require the Council's attention, reference A/HRC/49/76.

ISCG, I. & UNHCR. (2019). 2019 Joint Response Plan for Rohingya Humanitarian Crisis (January-December).

Jannat, S., Sifat, R. I., & Khisa, M. (2023). Sexual and reproductive health conditions of women: Insights from Rohingya refugee women in Bangladesh. *Sexuality Research and Social Policy, 20*, 855–868.

Jean, K., & Miks, J. (2020). *Preventing a silent crisis for Rohingya women and girls during COVID-19 pandemic.* UNICEF. https://www.unicef.org/coronavirus/preventing-silent-crisis-rohingya-women-and-girls-during-covid-19-pandemic. Accessed on 9 July 2023.

Hossain, I. (2020, April 08). Cox's Bazar put under lockdown. *Dhaka Tribune*. https://www.dhakatribune.com/bangladesh/health/206251/cox's-Bazar-put-under-lockdown. Accessed on 10 April 2024.

Inter-Sector Coordination Group. (2020). *In the shadows of the pandemic: The gendered impact of COVID-19 on Rohingya and host communities.* https://reliefweb.int/attachments/9c6df541-20ef-32ca-b6e7-cad2e557b699/advocacy_brief_in_the_shadows_of_the_pandemic_the_gendered_impact_of_covid-19_on_rohingya_and_host_communities.pdf

Islam, M. M., & Nuzhath, T. (2018). Health risks of Rohingya refugee population in Bangladesh: A call for global attention. *Journal of Global Health, 8*(2).

Jean, K., & Miks, J. (2020). Preventing a silent crisis for Rohingya women and girls during COVID-19 pandemic. *UNICEF [Internet], 29.*

Karin, S. (2020). Status of Rohingya in refugee camps of Bangladesh: A review study. *Open Access Library Journal, 7*(09), 1.

Kamal, A. H. M., Huda, M., Dell, C., Hossain, S. Z., & Ahmed, S. S. (2020). Translational strategies to control and prevent spread of COVID-19 in the Rohiynga refugee camps in Bangladesh. *Global Biosecurity, 1*(4), 1–10.

Kreft, A. K. (2020). Civil society perspectives on sexual violence in conflict: Patriarchy and war strategy in Colombia. *International Affairs, 96*(2), 457–478.

Kimhur, B. (2020). How to apply the capability Approach to housing Policy? Concepts, Theories and challenges. *Housing Theory and Society, 37*(3), 257–277. https://doi.org/10.1080/14036096.2019.1706630

Kirby, P. (2015). Ending sexual violence in conflict: The Preventing Sexual Violence Initiative and its critics. *International Affairs, 91*(3), 457–472.

Kumar, B., Pinky, S. D., Pulock, O. S., Kamal, R. S., & Aziz, R. (2022). COVID-19 and the Rohingya refugees in Bangladesh: Socioeconomic and health impacts on women and adolescents. *International Journal of Asia Pacific Studies, 18*(2), 179–199.

Kyaw, N. N. (2017). Unpacking the presumed statelessness of Rohingyas. *Journal of Immigrant & Refugee Studies, 15*(3), 269–286.

Landgren, K. (1998). The future of refugee protection: Four challenges. *Journal of Refugee Studies, 11*(4), 416–432.

Mohsin, A. (2020). Caught between the nation and the state: Voices of Rohingya refugee women in Bangladesh. *Asian Journal of Comparative Politics, 5*(2), 144–157.

Nasar, S., Nadim, A. S. M., Raz, S., Jabbar, A., Hossain, M. R., Aktar, B.,... & Rashid, S. F. (2023). Livelihood challenges of single female household heads in the Rohingya and host communities in Cox's Bazar, Bangladesh during the COVID-19 pandemic. *BMC Public Health, 23*(1), 2084.

Nussbaum, M. C. (2012). The capabilities approach and animal entitlements. In *Oxford University Press eBooks* (pp. 228–252). https://doi.org/10.1093/oxfordhb/9780195371963.013.0009

Onyango, M. A., Resnick, K., Davis, A., & Shah, R. R. (2019). Gender-based violence among adolescent girls and young women: a neglected consequence of the West African Ebola outbreak. In *Pregnant in the time of Ebola: Women and their children in the 2013–2015 West African epidemic* (pp. 121–132).

Oxfam. (2022, May 25). *Breaking barriers for Rohingya refugee women | Oxfam International.* Oxfam International. Retrieved January 29, 2025, from https://www.oxfam.org/en/breaking-barriers-rohingya-refugee-women

Palit, S., Yang, H., Li, J., Khan, M. A. S., & Hasan, M. J. (2022). The impact of the COVID-19 pandemic on the mental health of Rohingya refugees with pre-existing health problems in Bangladesh. *Conflict and Health, 16*(1), 10.

Parray, A. A., Hossain, M. R., Sultana, R., Aktar, B., & Rashid, S. F. (2022). "Younger women had more access to COVID-19 information": An intersectional analysis of factors influencing women and girls' access to COVID-19 information in Rohingya and host communities in Bangladesh. *PLOS Global Public Health, 2*(12), Article e0000459.

Priddy, G., Doman, Z., Berry, E., & Ahmed, S. (2022). Gender-based violence in a complex humanitarian context: Unpacking the human sufferings among stateless Rohingya women. *Ethnicities, 22*(2), 215–232.

Rahman, A., Strong, J., Mondal, P. P., Maynard, A., Haque, T., Moore, A. M., &Afsana, K. (2024). Perceptions and attitudes of Rohingya community stakeholders to pregnancy termination services: a qualitative study in camps of Cox's Bazar, Bangladesh. *Conflict and Health, 18*(1). https://doi.org/10.1186/s13031-024-00574-9

Robeyns, I. (2005). The Capability Approach: A theoretical survey. *Journal of Human Development, 6*(1), 93–117. https://doi.org/10.1080/146498805200034266

Sang, D. (2018). *One year on: time to put women and girls at the heart of the Rohingya response.* Oxfam GB.

Sen, A. K. (1994). Well-being, capability and public policy. *GiornaleDegliEconomisti E Annali Di Economia, Nuova Serie, Anno 53, 7/9*, 333–347. https://www.jstor.org/stable/23247762

Smith, M. D. (2021, March 22). *Protection risks during COVID-19 in the Rohingya refugee response*. Frontline Negotiations. Retrieved January 29, 2025, from https://frontline-negotiations.org/blog/protection-risks-during-covid-19-negotiating-safe-access-to-gender-based-violence-services-in-the-rohingya-refugee-response-in-coxs-bazar-bangladesh/

Spoerri, M., Ullah, Y., & Nwangwu, N. C. (2020). The Rohingya and COVID-19: Towards an inclusive and sustainable policy response. *Independent Diplomat*.

Sullivan, M. (2020). COVID-19 has arrived in Rohingya refugee camps and aid workers fear the worst.

Tanabe, M., Greer, A., Leigh, J., Modi, P., Davis, W. W., Mhote, P. P., … & Parmar, P. (2019). An exploration of gender-based violence in eastern Myanmar in the context of political transition: findings from a qualitative sexual and reproductive health assessment. *Sexual and Reproductive Health Matters, 27*(2), 112–125.

Tahir, A. R. M., Ee, X. W., Rashid, A. A., Yahaya, A. Y. B., & Devaraj, N. K. (2021). The proportion of infectious disease cases, its associated factors, and the appropriateness of antimicrobial prescription among Rohingya refugee pediatric patients in IMARET mobile clinics. *Journal of Immigrant and Minority Health, 23*(6), 1159–1169.

Tay, A. K., Islam, R., Riley, A., Welton-Mitchell, C., Duchesne, B., Waters, V. & Ventevogel, P. (2018). *Culture, context and mental health of Rohingya refugees: A review for staff in mental health and psychosocial support programmes for Rohingya refugees*. Geneva: United Nations High Commissioner for Refugees (UNHCR).

Toma, I., Chowdhury, M., Laiju, M., Gora, N., & Padamada, N. (2018). *Rohingya refugee response gender analysis: Recognizing and responding to gender inequalities*.

Toulemonde, M. (2020). COVID-19 outbreak: Cox's Bazaar rapid gender analysis. *Inter Sector Coordination Group, UN Women, CARE, and Oxfam, 17*.

Truelove, S., Abrahim, O., Altare, C., Lauer, S. A., Grantz, K. H., Azman, A. S., & Spiegel, P. (2020). The potential impact of COVID-19 in refugee camps in Bangladesh and beyond: A modeling study. *PLoS Medicine, 17*(6), e1003144. https://doi.org/10.1371/journal.pmed.1003144

United Nations (UN). (2024). *Goal 5: Achieve gender equality and empower all women and girls*. https://www.un.org/sustainabledevelopment/gender-equality/. Accessed on 11 June 2024.

United Nations Population Fund (UNFPA). (2015). *Minimum standards for prevention and response to gender-based violence in emergencies*. https://www.unfpa.org/sites/default/files/pub-pdf/GBVIE.Minimum.Standards.Publication.FINAL_.ENG_.pdf. Accessed on 10 March 2024.

United Nations Population Fund (UNFPA). (2020). *Gender equality and addressing gender-based violence (GBV) and coronavirus disease (COVID-19) prevention, protection and response*. https://www.unfpa.org/resources/gender-equality-and-addressing-gender-based-violence-gbv-and-coronavirus-disease-covid-19. Accessed on 11 June 2024.

UN Women. (2018). Gender brief on Rohingya refugee crisis response in Bangladesh. *UN Women—Asia-Pacific*.

Ullah, A. A. (2011). Rohingya refugees to Bangladesh: Historical exclusions and contemporary marginalization. *Journal of Immigrant & Refugee Studies, 9*(2), 139–161.

Ullah, A. A., Hossain, M. A., & Chattoraj, D. (2020). Covid-19 and Rohingya refugee camps in Bangladesh. *Intellectual Discourse, 28*(2), 793–806.

Ullah, A. A., & Chattoraj, D. (2018). Roots of discrimination against Rohingya minorities: Society, ethnicity and international relations. *Intellectual Discourse, 26*(2), 541–565.

Ullah, A. A., & Ferdous, J. (2022). *The Post-pandemic World and the global politics*. Springer.

Vizard, P., Fukuda-Parr, S., & Elson, D. (2011). Introduction: The capability approach and human rights. *Journal of Human Development and Capabilities, 12*(1), 1–22. https://doi.org/10.1080/19452829.2010.541728

Vyas, S., Jansen, H. A., Gardner, J., Tuladhar, S., Hammond, K., & Diemer, K. (2023). An analysis of changes in the prevalence and patterns of intimate partner violence against women in seven Asian countries. *BMC Women's Health, 23*(1), 399.

Ware, A., & Laoutides, C. (2018). *Myanmar's' Rohingya'conflict*. Oxford University Press.
World Health Organization. (2020). *Global progress report on water, sanitation and hygiene in health care facilities: Fundamentals first*.
WHO-SEAR. (2018, May 7). *Bangladesh: Rohingya refugee crisis 2017–2018*. Public health situation analysis.
Yasmin, L., & Akther, S. (2020). The locals and the Rohingyas: Trapped with an uncertain future. *Asian Journal of Comparative Politics, 5*(2), 104–120.
Yasmin, T. (2020). *Overview of laws, policies and practices on gender-based violence and harassment in the world of work in Bangladesh*. International Labour Organization.
Zawacki, B. (2012). Defining Myanmar's Rohingya problem. *The Human Rights Brief, 20*, 18.

# Chapter 7
# Social Status of Women in the *Khap* Panchayat Belt, Northern India: Bane or Boon?

**Ravita Yadav, Mukesh Kumar, and Bishwajeet Besra**

**Abstract** *Khap Panchayats* are the caste councils which are found in northern India and are mostly prominent among upper castes, especially the *Jat* caste (an agrarian caste in northern India). Unity, honor, community, and brotherhood are the base of these traditional councils. The primary objective is to examine the impact of *Khap Panchayats* on women's rights and empowerment in the *Khap Panchayat* belt of Northern India, evaluating both the restrictive and potentially empowering aspects of these traditional bodies. The study focuses on understanding women's participation in *Khap Panchayats*, their roles, and the social norms enforced by these traditional bodies. The chapter employs the mixed method approach (quantitative as well as qualitative), involving field observations and interviews with community members and local leaders in rural Haryana. Findings reveal that women are largely excluded from decision-making processes in *Khap Panchayats*, with their involvement limited to peripheral roles. Patriarchal values are deeply entrenched, manifesting in restrictions on women's autonomy and public participation. However, there are isolated instances where *Khaps* have contributed to empowering and ensuring women's safety, indicating a potential for positive change. Addressing the gender disparity in *Khap Panchayats* is crucial for enhancing women's social status in rural Haryana. Promoting women's active participation in decision-making processes can lead to broader societal benefits, including improved health outcomes and greater empowerment. The study calls for inclusive reforms to traditional governance systems to achieve gender equality and social progress.

**Keywords** Khap Panchayats · Women's Empowerment · Gender Equality · Patriarchy · Traditional Governance · Rural Haryana

R. Yadav (✉) · M. Kumar · B. Besra
Department of Migration and Urban Studies, International Institute for Population Sciences, Mumbai, Maharashtra, India
e-mail: ravita240495@gmail.com

 
P. Chouhan et al. (eds.), *Women's Health Dynamics in South Asia*, Asian Perspectives on Public Health, https://doi.org/10.1007/978-981-95-2321-4_7

## 7.1 Introduction

The traditional social institution known as a *KhapPanchayat* is mostly prevalent in the northern Indian states of Rajasthan, Uttar Pradesh, and Haryana. In North India, the caste *Jat* is the foundation stone of the Khap Panchayat. By using the concept of *bhaichara* (brotherhood), the *Khaps* can establish dominance over the entire village, group of villages, or clan. *Khap* is a type of traditional caste panchayat, which maintains the four pillars of rural life: *aikya* (unity), *izzat* (honor), *biradari* (community), and *bhaichara* (brotherhood) (Chowdhry, 2007). In the past, the purpose of *Khap Panchayats* was to uphold social order, settle disputes, and enforce local traditions and standards (Chowdhry, 2007). The *Khap Panchayat* is a hierarchical organization headed by a '*Pardhan*' or '*Chaudhary*' who oversees meetings and drives the decision-making process. These councils have a great deal of social power, and society respects their decisions, which are frequently founded on customary law in resolving land disputes, marriages, and other social conflicts as one of the *Khap Panchayat's* main functions. It has been argued that their customs, especially about women's autonomy and inter-caste marriages, violate individual rights and uphold regressive norms (Kaur, 2010). Such a customary practice is not unique in India alone. It is an ancient practice found among societies worldwide in one form or another. In the *Pashtoon* society of Afghanistan and Pakistan, it is called *Jirga* (Carter & Connor, 1989; Faqir & Atta, 2013; Wardak, 2003; Zaman et al., 2018); in Bangladesh, it is called *Shalishi* (Riaz, 2005). This institution is similar in many respects to the institutions of *Lekgotla* in Southern Africa (Rammala, 2021); and *Mediation Committees* in China (Clark, 1989; Li, 1979). The names of the traditional panchayats found in various parts of the Indian subcontinent vary; some examples are *Khap* in Haryana and Uttar Pradesh, *Pal* among the *Meos* of Haryana and Rajasthan (Hussain, 2022), *Manjhi Pargainait* in Santhal, *Hatu, Parha* among the Oraon and Munda tribes of Jharkhand (Hussain, 2022; Singh, 2008), *Peddala panchayat* in Begatha tribes in Eastern Ghats (Rajpramukh & Palkumar, 2005), *Kula, caste panchayats* in the East and West Godavari districts of Andhra Pradesh (Ramesh, 2021), *Katta Panchayats* in Tamil Nadu (Tulsyan, 2022). In the Indian subcontinent, local informal justice systems of this kind have long served as the foundation for the administration of rural justice (Khan & Sharma, 1982). Despite going by many names, they all have the same approach i.e., informal and regional. *Khaps*are is a type of customary panchayat based on caste and is common throughout rural Northern India, which is the subject of the current study.

The village is the first level of organization within a *Khap Panchayat*, and this panchayat is completely different from the democratic village panchayat which is based on the legitimate and fair election of the head and is, therefore, a constitutional body. On the other hand, the decisions made by traditional bodies frequently defy human rights and established legal norms, operating beyond the purview of the constitution (Sharma, 2011). The role that these bodies play in upholding patriarchal standards that are detrimental to women's rights has been extensively documented. Research indicates that these organizations promulgate directives that curtail the liberty of women, which have a detrimental effect on women's rights and self-governance (Vaisey & Miles, 2017). These bodies impede women's participation in public life and economic endeavors, perpetuating outdated gender norms and impeding women's empowerment and advancement. The fact that attempts to question these unconstitutional practices have frequently encountered opposition suggests how deeply ingrained these patriarchal systems are (Menon, 2012). *Khap Panchayat*-specific literature emphasizes their dual social roles. They are recognized as substantial barriers to women's rights and gender equality even if they are recognized as defenders of custom and social order (Chowdhry, 2007). *Khap Panchayats* are found to enforce moral codes that limit women's freedom of movement, options for marriage, and engagement in public life, all of which serve to further marginalize and oppress them (Kaur, 2010). Another noteworthy position is opposition to dowries and exorbitant wedding costs. Notwithstanding these encouraging developments, there is still controversy in the reports of media, around the influence of *Khap Panchayats* on women's rights and empowerment, with wide differences in opinions and results (Yadav, 2024). These practices perpetuate cycles of discrimination and violence against women.

Women's health and use of healthcare are severely harmed by the absence of their rights, autonomy, and empowerment. When women are deprived of their rights and autonomy, they often face significant barriers to accessing healthcare services. This can lead to poor health outcomes, including higher rates of maternal mortality, malnutrition, and chronic illnesses (Sen & Ostlin, 2011). Empowerment is closely linked to women's ability to make decisions about their health and seek medical care when needed. Without empowerment, women may be unable to negotiate safe sex practices, resulting in higher rates of sexually transmitted infections and unintended pregnancies (UNFPA, 2014). Furthermore, women's development is critical to achieving better health outcomes because it increases their access to and affordability of healthcare services through education and economic independence. Research suggests that women who feel empowered are more likely to make use of healthcare services, make sure their kids get immunizations, and have healthier lives (WHO, 2019). As a result, depriving women of their rights and empowering them not only impedes their personal growth but also negatively impacts their general health and welfare. The existing literature shows that unconstitutional local governance often suppresses women's rights, autonomy, empowerment, and overall development, negatively affecting their health and well-being. Although *Khap Panchayats* are long-practiced unconstitutional assemblies that predominantly interfere in several decisions affecting residents, including female residents, there is a lack of existing literature that portrays the social status and health of women in the *Khap* environment in India. Therefore, this chapter aims to present the scenario of women's social status in the *Khap Panchayat* region. The social status of women is intricately linked with their health, making this chapter significant for drawing further research on the linkage between women's social status and health based on the present findings.

## 7.2 Materials and Methods

From the sampling point of view, the focus was on the hotspots of *Khap* activities in Haryana, There are four districts where most of the *Khap*s are based: *Rohtak, Jind, Sonipat*, and *Jhajjar* in the state. Among the four districts, *Jhajjar* and *Rohtak* districts are predominated by the *Jat* population, and *Khaps* are the most common in *Jats* as compared to any other castes. Therefore, the study has been conducted in the two most active *Khap*s, *Gulia Khap* of *Jhajjar*district and *Maham Chaubisi Khap* of *Rohtak* district in Haryana.

The study has been built mainly based on primary data collected by using structured and semi-structured schedules and guidelines in two phases and has been carried out using Kobo Toolbox software. In the first phase of fieldwork (qualitative phase), open-ended questions in the interview schedule (guidelines) cover the fundamental details about the individuals and households (Fig. 7.1). One Focused-Group Discussion (FGD) from each district was conducted. The FGD's guidelines compromise the meaning of 'honor' from individuals' points of view, various spaces that construct caste and patriarchy, the age at marriage for girls, the impact of *Khaps* on the lives of women and people from other castes, etc. The study identified leaders of *Khaps,* elected village panchayats, NGO activities, college professors, school teachers, and administrative officials, women participants as lead observers, media persons, and police officials as key-informants and interviewed them with the help of key-informant guidelines (Table 7.1). Different methods used for the qualitative analysis are as follows: Case study Method, Narrative Model, Grounded Theory Approach, Phenomenological Method, Ethnographic Model, FGD, Word Cloud, Mind Map.

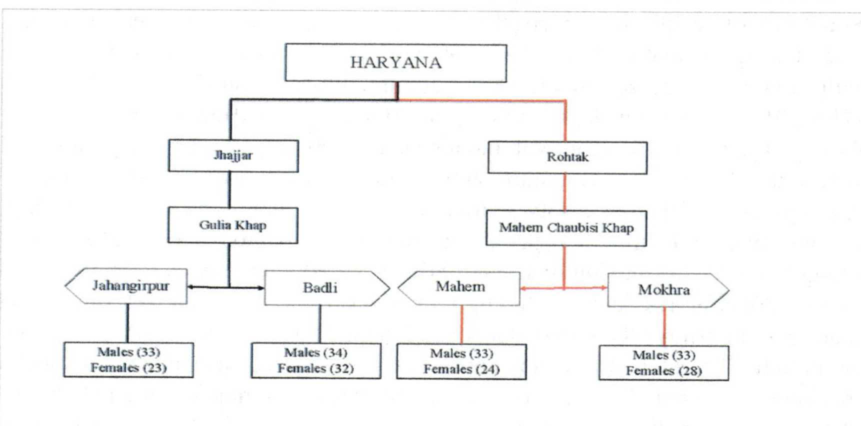


**Fig. 7.1** Schematic flow of sample selection

**Table 7.1** Qualitative phase data collection tools

| S. No | Qualitative tools used | Key stakeholders | No. of interviews |
|---|---|---|---|
| 1 | In-depth Interviews | | 16 |
| 2 | Key- Informants Interview | *Khap*leaders and members (2), *Khap*supporters (2), Teachers / Professors (2), Social workers (2), *Dalits* (2), Affected people (2), Older people (2), Educated university students (2) | 16 |
| 3 | Case Studies | 3 Case studies per district | 6 |
| 4 | Focus Group Discussion | One FGD per district (Men) | 2 |

*Source* Prepared by Researcher

The qualitative data was collected using the PAPI (Pen and Paper Interview) method and audio-visual aid. Software such as NVivo, Atlas ti, and Microsoft Office were used to analyze the data.

Even after selecting the district and village, it was impossible to interview each and every individual of the village in the second phase of data collection (Quantitative phase), the selection of the 240 individual units of the survey was done by purposive sampling. Comprehensive data collection is accomplished by utilizing a structured questionnaire in the second phase. Stata version 15.0 and MS Excel were used for the data wrangling, analysis, and visualization of the quantitative data analysis. A bivariate analysis was conducted. An array of $2 \times 2$ tabulations was presented. In order to test for unadjusted associations, these tables were supplemented with a Chi-square p-value.

The total fieldwork was stretched over six months in two phases; the first phase of fieldwork was carried out in the months of June, July, and August of 2022, and the second phase was carried out in the months of October and November 2022. Along with collected field data from both male and female members of different age groups (Table 7.2), the study also uses the secondary data collected from various government reports, newspaper reports and clippings, relevant articles, and various empirical studies conducted by NGOs and social workers.

### 7.2.1 *Structure of* Khap *and Women's Participation*

The Panchayati Raj Act of 1992 is now in effect in India. Three tiers serve as the foundation for this amendment. Under this arrangement, elected representatives must have a 33.0% female reserve. Panchayats are referred to as gram panchayats at the village level, *Panchayat samiti* at the block level, and *Zila Parishads* at the district level. Although the Panchayati Raj Act reserves certain seats for women, women actually do not participate in panchayats very much. Numerous studies have also

**Table 7.2** Percentage distribution of the respondent's background characteristics, 2022

| Background Characteristics | | Frequency |
|---|---|---|
| Gender | Male | 55.4 |
| | Female | 44.6 |
| Age group (in years) | 18–35 | 43.7 |
| | 36–50 | 26.3 |
| | Above 50 | 30 |
| Marital status | Married | 54.2 |
| | Unmarried | 37.9 |
| | Separated | 0.8 |
| | Widowed | 7.1 |
| Educational status (years of schooling) | Below 10 years | 33.5 |
| | 11–14 | 31.7 |
| | Above 15 | 35.8 |
| Social group | Jats | 33.3 |
| | Non Jats* | 35 |
| | Non Jats SC | 31.7 |
| Occupation | Agricultural Owner Cultivator | 32.5 |
| | Tenant Cultivator | 10.4 |
| | Agricultural labourer | 13.3 |
| | Government Services | 4.2 |
| | Self-employed/Private Job | 7.9 |
| | Student | 32.1 |
| Land profile | Landless | 16.3 |
| | 0–3 | 29.6 |
| | 4–6 | 8.8 |
| | 7–9 | 10.8 |
| | Above 9 | 34.5 |
| | Total Sample | 240 |

Non *Jat** refers to non *Jats* who are in OBC and General category.
*Source* Field Survey July–Nov, 2022.

shown that when women are elected as representatives, their husbands or relatives use their authority. However, we can state that the current situation is evolving.

During one of the meetings of *Gulia Khap* Panchayat in village *Jahangirpur, Jhajjar*, which was attended by the researcher, it was observed that there was absolutely no participation of women. No women were seen in the meeting, only two women were seen that too outside the *Chabutra*, in a room, for preparing tea and food, even though they were not allowed to serve. The males were only serving the

**Table 7.3** Women's place in the structure of social *Panchayats*

| Hierarchy of Social *Panchayat* | *Gulia Khap* in *Jhajjar* District | | *Maham Khap* in *Rohtak* District | |
|---|---|---|---|---|
| | Men | Women | Men | Women |
| Village level *Pardhan* | ✔ | ✖ | ✔ | ✖ |
| *Gawand* level *Pardhan* | ✔ | ✖ | ✔ | ✖ |
| *Tappa* Level *Pardhan* | ✔ | ✖ | ✔ | ✖ |
| *Khap*Panchayat *Pardhan* | ✔ | ✖ | ✔ | ✖ |
| *Sarvkhap* Panchayat *Pardhan* | ✔ | ✖ | ✔ | ✖ |

*Source* Field Survey July–Nov, 2022

snacks and other eatable items, all this brings out the fact that women have absolutely no place in these panchayats.

The absence of women in every *Khap Panchayat* observed during fieldwork in the research area is highlighted in Table 7.3. It clearly shows the total dominance of men in the composition of Haryana's *Khap* panchayats. Villagers in Haryana's *Khap* region say that women are not allowed to join '*chaupals*,' where men gather to make decisions for different wrongdoings. Women have never been permitted in *Panchayats*, which are overwhelmingly male settings. Men were observed playing cards and bubbling *huqqah*, particularly in Haryana's *Khap* belt. Women in the community were required to cover their faces and heads in front of male *chaupal* members if they were passing by.

## 7.3 Results

### *7.3.1 Women's Perception on Khap Participation*

The information regarding women's current participation and opinion on women's participation in *Khaps* is shown in Fig. 7.2. Regarding women's involvement, a small percentage of respondents—13.0% of the sample as a whole—said that women participate occasionally, while a sizable majority—81.0%—said that women do not participate, and 6.0% responded DK (Fig. 7.2a). In terms of views on women's involvement, the data shows that a sizable percentage of study participants—66.0% of the sample—said they are in favor of women taking part. On the other hand, 9.0% of participants said they did not want any participation from women. Moreover, a significant portion of participants (25%) chose DK as a response (Fig. 7.2b).

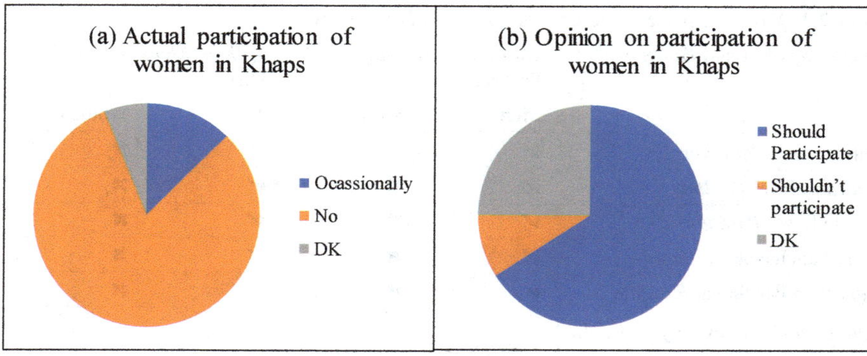


**Fig. 7.2** Women's perception on the participation of women in *Khap Panchayats*, 2022. **a.** Actual participation of women in Khaps. **b.** Opinion on participation of women in Khaps. Non *Jat** refers to non *Jats* who are in OBC and General category; DK refers to Don't Know. *Source* Field Survey July–Nov, 2022

### 7.3.2 Authority of Khap to Establish Laws Pertaining to Women's Issues

This section explores the capacity of *Khap Panchayats* to establish laws specifically concerning women's issues. It aims to shed light on how these traditional bodies shape and regulate the legal aspects affecting women's lives in Haryana, reflecting their significant role in local governance. The authority of *Khap* to establish laws concerning women's issues saw 22.5% of respondents expressing disagreement, 55.0% showing agreement, and 22.5% responding DK (Fig. 7.3). Gender analysis reveals that female respondents showed higher agreement (56.1%) compared to males (54.2%). Among different age groups, younger respondents (18–35) exhibited the highest agreement rate at 60.0%, whereas the elder age group (50+) had the highest disagreement rate at 34.7% (Fig. 3). Looking at social groups, *Jats* had the highest agreement rate at 78.8%, while the highest disagreement rate was among Non *Jats** (36.9%) and the highest DK rate was among Non *Jat* SC at 34.2%. Regarding education, respondents with 0–10 years of education showed lower agreement (39.7%) compared to those with 11–14 years (55.3%) and 15+ years (68.6%).

### 7.3.3 Does Khap Panchayat Try to Impose Patriarchy in Society?

According to Fig. 7.4, more than half of respondents responded that society is forced to conform the patriarchy by *Khap* panchayats (60%). Of the respondents, 16.7% said that *Khap* decisions do not attempt to impose patriarchy and 23.3% provide DK response (Fig. 7.4). If we talk about the same context but with different background

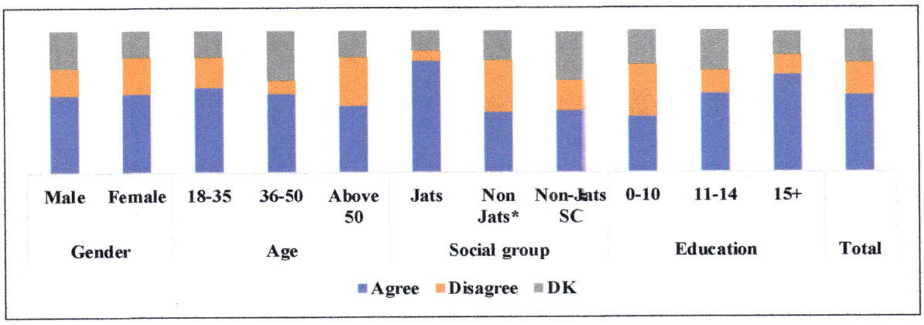


**Fig. 7.3** Respondent's perception on the authority of *Khap* to establish laws pertaining to women's issues. Non *Jat** refers to non *Jats* who are in OBC and General category; DK refers to Don't Know. *Source* Field Survey July–Nov, 2022

**Fig. 7.4** Respondent's perception on *Khap Panchayat* try to impose patriarchy in Society (Overall), Haryana, India, 2022 ($n = 240$). *Source* Field Survey July–Nov, 2022; DK refers to Don't Know

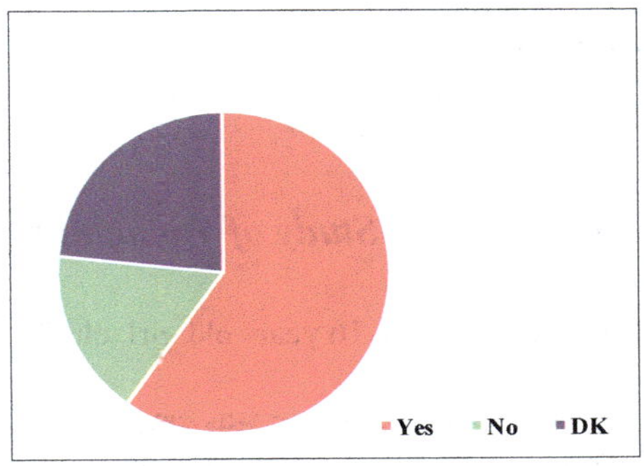


characteristics, such as gender, age, education, and social group, the results are shown in the following figure (Fig. 7.5).

Among male respondents, 25.5% responded that KP does not impose patriarchy, while among female respondents, 72.0% said that KP imposes patriarchy. Regarding age groups, the majority of respondents aged 18–35 (97.1%) and 36–50 (50.8%) answered that KPs impose patriarchy, while a significant proportion of those above age 50 (40.2%) was against this notion (Fig. 7.5). In terms of social groups, Non *Jat* SCs had the highest agreement rate (68.4%) regarding KPs imposing patriarchy, followed by Non *Jats** (64.3%) and Jats (47.5%). Education-wise, respondents with 0–10 years and 11–14 years of education had a higher proportion (37.2% and 14.5%, respectively) who replied that *Khaps* do not impose patriarchy compared to those with 15+ years of education (0%).

> It is not only because of Khaps but the very structure of our society, where questions are being raised on the speech of women. Since the Vedic period, the status of women was lower than that of men, with the passage of time some people have changed but in reality, Khaps are old and their working method is also old in which women have not yet got the status equal to men. The man is the leader of the society and he is the leader of the home also. Khaps are also hindering this further. (KII, Female Professor [38])

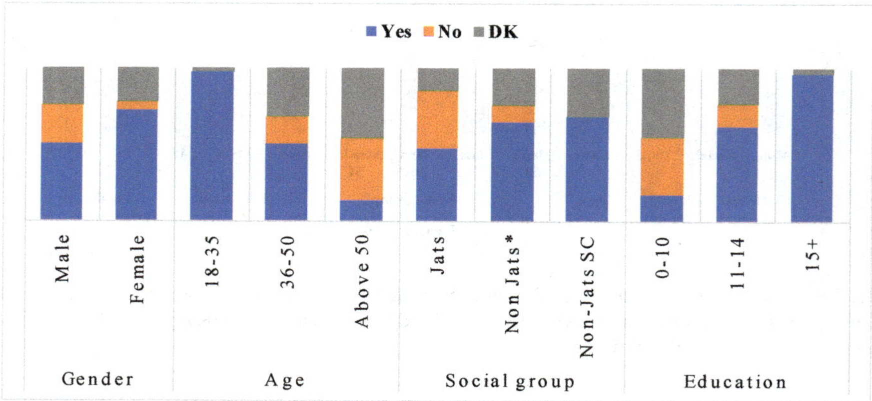


**Fig. 7.5** Respondent's perception on *Khap Panchayat* try to impose patriarchy in society (in %). Non *Jat** refers to non *Jats* who are in OBC and General category; DK refers to Don't Know. *Source* Field Survey July–Nov, 2022

## *7.3.4 A Case Study of Women in* Khap *Region*

**Case Study**: Riya, 16 years old girl, eloped from school. According to the principal of her school.

One day Riya's phone was caught in the class, and I told his family, his family kept an eye on her for a few days and did not send her to school for two weeks. After two weeks she started coming to school, after that, she started to come to school and one day her father called me and said that the girl has not come home from school. His family members started pointing out the mistakes of the school. You tell me what is the fault of the school if the girl does not go home after getting off the school bus. At that time the image of the school is brought into disrepute. For a few days, her family kept frowning that we helped their daughter to elope and threatened that they would close the school forever. After two to three days, they came to know about the girl, the boy ran away, with whom she eloped. Now her family is marrying her. It may be seen as wrong that she is marrying at 16 years only that too with a middle-aged man, but what could the parents think, what would they do if she ran away again? Her parents lost the respect due to her death at the school. By the way, she was not paying attention to her education, in such a way, she did not become a collector by studying, but it affected other girls too. Parents are afraid of educating their daughters so that they do not become the reason for disreputation in the society. Riya's family did the right thing by marrying her for the sake of their *izzat*.

### 7.3.5 Women's Restriction in Khap Belts

> The job of earning money at home is of men and the job of taking care of the house is of women because women are the honor of the house. (FGD 1)
>
> In a village where no tradition has been established, if a girl marries of her own free will, then all the people in the village are associated with their respect. (FGD 2)
>
> The turban is not just a piece of cloth, it is a symbol of honor for our elders. (FGD 2)
>
> It is better if your daughter gets married and reaches home at the right age and time. (FGD 2)
>
> Did we give birth to our daughter just to see this day? Is our daughter so educated that she will now impart knowledge to her parents? (FGD 1)
>
> These women have destroyed the entire culture by dancing on Instagram and Tik-Tok. (FGD 1)
>
> Respect is so double-faced, only women are robbed of respect, no Chaudhary or Pradhan of this society is robbed. (Female, 34)
>
> A young girl should leave her home at the right time, for her parents, this will equal to take bathe in Ganga, otherwise there is fear of running away from home, hence she should get married at the age of 18 years, she will do the rest of her education at her in-law's house. (Khap Leader, 54)
>
> The rule of Khap Panchayats, their grandeur, their dominance is only on the poor people, the khaps do not even open their mouth in front of wealthy people and officials. What laws and what justice do these Khap Panchayat talk about? (NGO worker, female, 46)

From the above case study, KIIs and FGDs glimpses, we can say that the agrarian society of rural Haryana in *Khap* region restricted the women for the honor of the family.

### 7.3.6 Contribution of Khaps to Women Empowerment

Respondents were asked about the role of *Khap Panchayats* in women empowerment. They were aware of the '*Beti bachao, Beti padhao*' campaign and recognized its success. Haryana recorded a sex ratio at birth of 922, in the first six months of 2020 (Haryana Department of Health; DTE, 2023). This indicates a strong emphasis on education and support for sports in the community. Additionally, there is a clear stance against dowry and over-expenditure, as well as a call for stricter rules to prevent these practices.

Figure 7.6 presents a pie chart that illustrates the respondents' opinions on whether *Khap Panchayats* contribute to women's empowerment. The responses are divided into three categories: Yes, No, and Don't Know (DK). A significant portion of respondents, 64%, believe that *Khap Panchayats* do contribute to women's empowerment (Fig. 7.6).

Additionally, 18% of respondents feel that *Khap Panchayats* do not contribute to women's empowerment. On the other hand, 64% of respondents believe that *Khap*

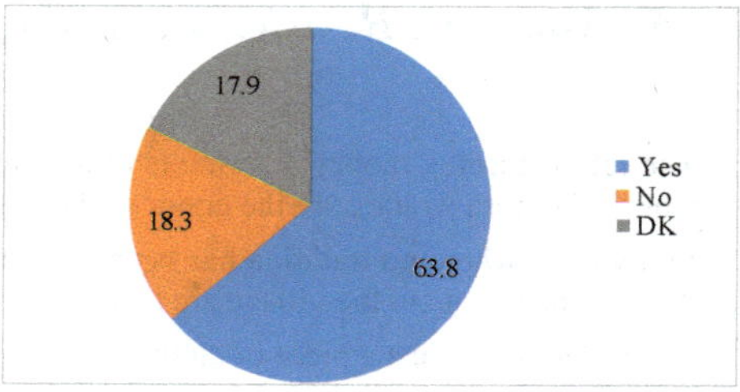


**Fig. 7.6** Respondent's perception of the contribution of *Khaps* to women empowerment

*Panchayats* contribute to women's empowerment. Another 18% of respondents are unsure or do not know whether these *panchayats* contribute to women's empowerment. This distribution shows a varied perception *of Khap Panchayats'* role in empowering women, with a plurality believing in a positive contribution, while a significant portion remains unsure (Fig. 7.7). If we look at the same context but with different background characteristics, the following figure helps us to understand the picture.

Figure 7.7 provides insights into how men and women view *Khap's* authority differently.

Among males, 71.4% whereas among females, 54.2% think that *Khaps* contribute to women's empowerment. The following two tables (Table 7.4 and Table 7.5) show the distribution of males and females who think that *Khaps* play a positive role in empowering women according to their social group and educational status.

Non *Jat** refers to non *Jats* who are in OBC and General category.

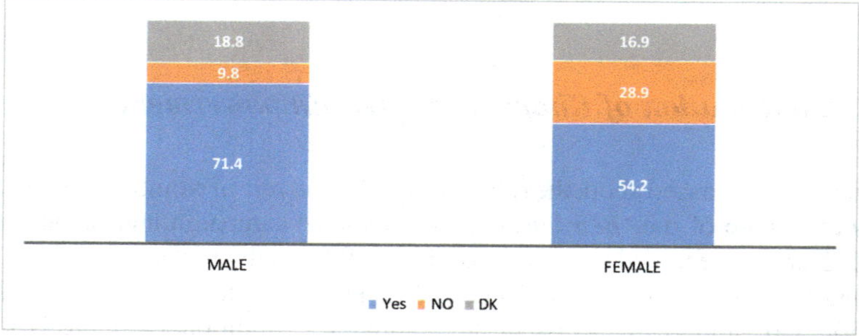


**Fig. 7.7** Respondent's perception on contribution of *Khaps* in women empowerment by gender. *Source* Field Survey July–Nov, 2022; DK refers to Don't Know

**Table 7.4** Respondent's perception on the contribution of *Khaps* in women empowerment by gender and social group

| Social group | Male | Female |
|---|---|---|
| *Jat* | 36.8 | 24.3 |
| Non-*Jat** | 24.1 | 16.8 |
| Non-*Jat* SC | 10.5 | 13.1 |

**Table 7.5** Respondent's perception on contribution of *Khaps* in women empowerment by gender and educational status

| Education (years of schooling) | Male | Female |
|---|---|---|
| 0–10 | 27.1 | 24.3 |
| 11–14 | 29.3 | 11.2 |
| 15 + | 15.0 | 18.7 |

*Source* Field Survey July–Nov, 2022

*Source* Field Survey July–Nov, 2022.

Among the *Jat* males, 36.8% think that *Khaps* contribute to women empowerment, whereas only 24.3% of the females from the same category have the same opinion. Secondly, only 16.8% of females from Non *Jat* (who are in OBC and General category) as compared to 24.1% of Non *Jats* males have the opinion that *Khaps* play a positive role in women empowerment. The same flow is shown in the Non *Jat* SC category, more males are in favor of *Khaps* as compared to females.

In terms of education, 27.1% of males having less than 10 years of schooling percept that the *Khaps* are favoring women empowerment while for the same years of schooling the percentage of females is quite low (24.3%) whereas males with more than 15 years of education only 15.0%, whereas 18.7% of females having same category of educational status have the opinion that *Khaps* are working for empowering the women.

Some of the glimpses from the qualitative data also support the above results which are as follows:

> Khaps have done a lot of work in the direction of women moving ahead in society, promoted their education, and helped them to move ahead by locking at their interest in sports. But still, there is a need for improvement in many places, one of them is the entry of women in the cave. (Gulia Khap Member [38, Private Job])

### 7.3.7 *Khaps and Women's Property Rights: Tradition vs. Modernity*

The right to property is a fundamental aspect of human rights and socioeconomic development. Article 300A of the Indian Constitution guarantees the right to property, stating, 'No person shall be deprived of his property save by authority of law.' This constitutional provision ensures that every citizen, irrespective of gender, has the right to acquire, hold, and dispose of property. In India, women are subordinate to men in all spheres of family life, across all castes and social strata. Because men possess tenancies and own and manage most land, women are dependent on men. Other than in cases where there is no male ancestry, customs assist daughters in not inheriting land. When a parent passes away, it is unfair that a woman does not inherit his/her belongings. It is false to claim that women receive a dowry, or their portion of patrimony, when they marry (Davar, 1999). However, the practical enforcement of these rights often clashes with traditional and patriarchal structures, particularly in rural areas governed by *Khap Panchayats*. This section is to shed light on the perception of the respondents of the study on the property rights status of women in *Khap*-dominated regions. The respondents' perceptions of property rights for women in the *Khap* region reveal that a majority, comprising 63.0%, believe women have no property rights. Meanwhile, 31.0% perceive that women have limited property rights, and a minority of 6.0% believe that women have equal property rights (Fig. 7.8).

> If I take my father's land, then I also have to give it to my sister-in-law, and after marriage, the girl's house will change, so what will I do with that land? (Jahangirpur village [62, Female, Head of the family])

There is a notable gender disparity in the perception of property rights for women shown in Fig. 7.9, with female respondents (81.3%) more likely to perceive no property rights compared to male respondents (48.9%).

There are significant variations in the perception of property rights for women across different social groups, with Non *Jats** being more likely to perceive limited

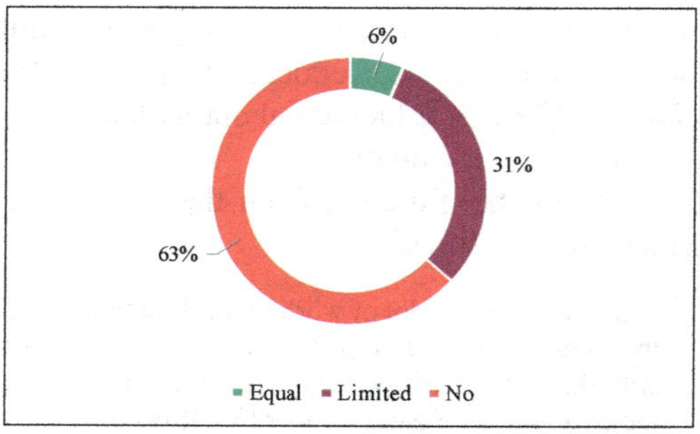


**Fig. 7.8** Respondent's perception on the property right status of women

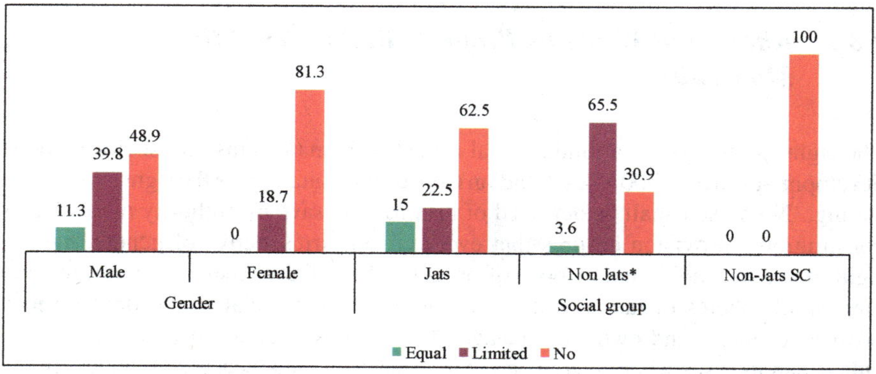


**Fig. 7.9** Respondent's perception on the property right status of women. Non *Jat** refers to non *Jats* who are in OBC and General category

property rights compared to *Jats*. Among Non *Jat* SC, no one responded to property rights for women as equal or limited, and 100.0% answered no property rights for women. Among *Jats*, 15% perceive property rights for women as equal, 22.5% perceive them as limited, and 62.5% perceive no property rights for women. Among Non *Jats**, 3.6% perceive property rights for women as equal, 65.5% perceive them as limited, and 30.9% perceive no property rights for women.

Overall, the majority of respondents perceive no property rights for women in the *Khap* region, with notable variations across gender and caste.

> The son has the right on the father's property, a lot is given to the daughter in the form of dowry at the time of marriage and after that even on festivals, a little bit is given to her throughout her life? (Maham Village [42, Female, Housewife])

### 7.3.8 *Khap Restrictions on Women in Public*

In many regions of North India, women's participation in public life has long been severely restricted by *Khap Panchayats* or traditional village councils. Rigid gender norms are reinforced by these limitations, which frequently determine how women behave, dress, and interact with males outside of their homes. These laws severely restrict the freedoms and opportunities available to women, impacting their ability to access social services, work, and education. *Khap* decrees have a pervasive influence that hampers women's socioeconomic development and promotes gender inequality in certain places. This section examines the different public restrictions put in place by *Khaps*.

Figure 7.10 indicates varying opinions regarding the banning of mobile phones for girls and women in public. When the survey asks whether the use of mobile phones is banned for girls and women in public, it is inquiring about whether there are any restrictions or prohibitions on using mobile phones in open spaces such as streets, parks, markets, public transportation, and other communal areas where people gather or move about freely (Fig. 7.10).

The overall result shows that 68.0% of respondents responded that there is nothing such as a ban, while 22.0% expressed that yes the use of mobile in public areas is banned, and 10.0% responded DK.

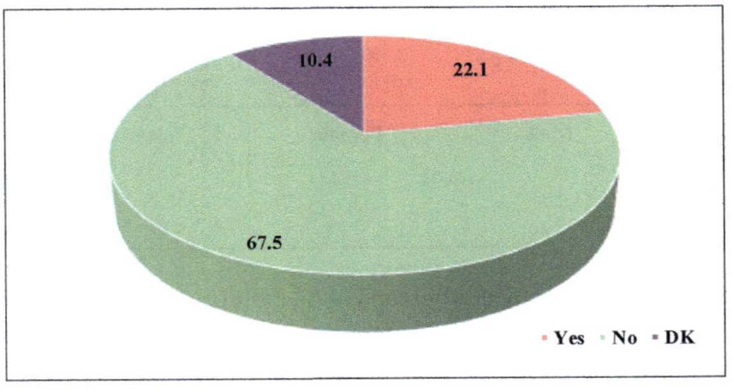


**Fig. 7.10** Respondent's perception on mobile use restrictions in public for women. DK refers to Don't Know

Among male respondents, the majority (80.4%) replied that there is no such ban, whereas 15.8% reported about the ban, and 3.8% responded DK. Conversely, among female respondents, a smaller percentage (51.4%) replied that there is no ban on the usage of mobile in public places, while 29.9% replied that yes there is, as shown in Fig. 7.11.

Across different social groups, Non *Jat** had the highest percentage of respondents who answered that there is no such ban (73.8%), followed by Non *Jats*SCs (71.1%) and *Jats* (57.5%).

> Some khap panchayats ban women from using phones. But we consider mobile phones a means of development for women, we consider them a means of communication and connection in today's times. But they should also take care that they are not used for wrong purposes. (Maham Khap Member [38, Male, Government Servant])

Responses about the imposition of a dress code for girls and women in public places reveal that 29.0 percent of the sample believes that *Khaps* do not impose any dress code (Fig. 7.12). Conversely, approximately half of the respondents feel that girls and women should dress decently in public, hence supporting the restrictions imposed by *Khaps.*

A significant gender disparity in perspectives on dress code restrictions is evident in Fig. 7.13, with 45.9% of males acknowledging the existence of such restrictions for girls and women in public, compared to 57.0% of females (Fig. 7.13).

> The decision to ban jeans and mobiles in Meerut was a decision of one locality, it was linked to a conspiracy that it is a terrorist decision, a Taliban decision, what does it mean? (Maham Khap Member [50, Male, Agriculturist])

This section presents a word cloud generated from the qualitative data collected for the study. A word cloud is a visual representation of text data, where the size and

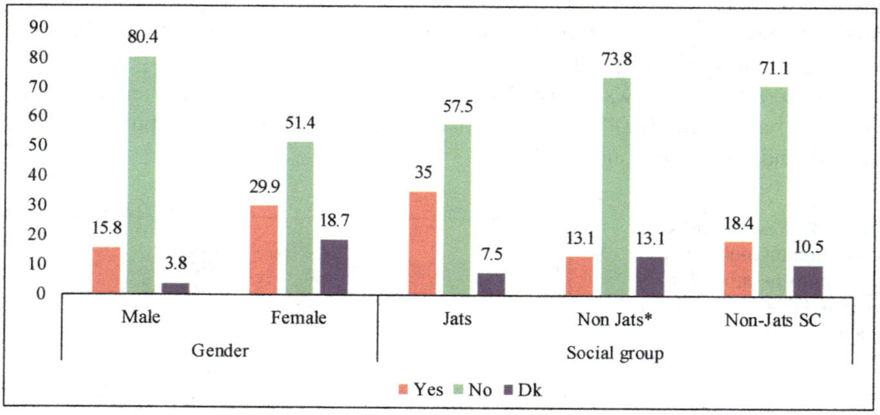


**Fig. 7.11** Respondent's perception on mobile use restrictions in public for women. Non *Jat** refers to non *Jats* who are in OBC and General category; DK refers to Don't Know. *Source* Field Survey July–Nov, 2022

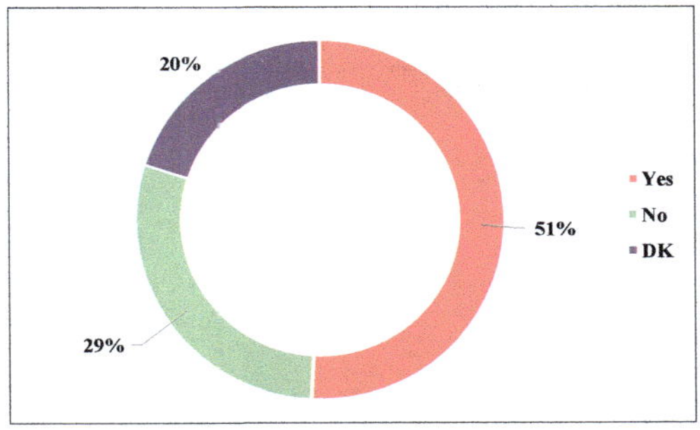


**Fig. 7.12** Respondent's Perception on Dress/ *Parda* restrictions in public for women. DK refers to Don't Know. *Source* Field Survey July–Nov, 2022

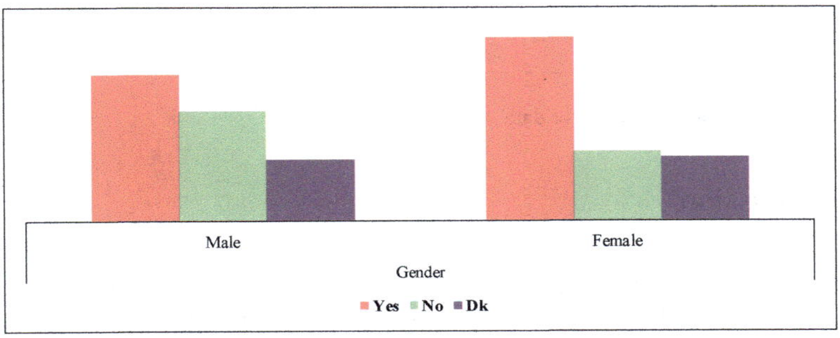


**Fig. 7.13** Respondent's perception on dress/ *Parda* restrictions in public for women. DK refers to Don't Know. *Source* Field Survey July–Nov, 2022

font of each word indicate its frequency or importance. This visual highlights the prominent themes and concepts discussed in the field and supports the goal of the study, which is to clarify the ways in which gender, caste, and traditional governance continue to shape the rural society structure and change it over time.

The study's word cloud, which was produced using qualitative data, effectively captures the complex interactions that exist in rural Haryana between caste dynamics (*Jats* and gotra), traditional government (*Khaps*), and gender roles (male and female). It draws attention to the extent to which these factors are woven into the community's social fabric and affect every facet of life, including marital customs, property ownership, and societal status.

The frequent mention results in the predominance of words such as *Panchayat,* tradition, honor, *pagdi*, male, social, land, women, *parda*, caste, etc. which underscores the influence of long-standing cultural practices on the daily lives and social structures within the rural society of Haryana (Fig. 7.14).

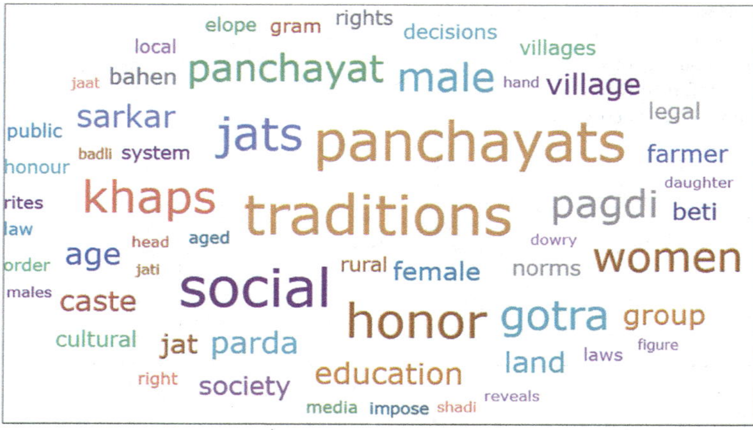


**Fig. 7.14** Word cloud of qualitative data

## 7.4 Discussion

This study delves into the intricate dynamics of caste, gender, and the role of *Khap Panchayats* in rural Haryana, focusing on how these traditional bodies influence the social status of women. As we all know, the progress of a community is measured by the progress of its women. Despite this, women in many parts of the world, including India, continue to face significant challenges due to the prevailing patriarchal structure that subordinates them to men. This patriarchal structure is deeply ingrained in the cultural and social fabric of rural Haryana, where women's roles are often confined to the domestic sphere. The Panchayati Raj Act of 1992, which mandates a 33% reservation for women in local governance, has not significantly altered women's participation in *Khap Panchayats*. Observations from the field, reveal that women are entirely absent from decision-making processes. They are relegated to peripheral roles, such as preparing food, with no involvement in the actual meetings or discussions. This exclusion is starkly evident in the hierarchical structure of social panchayats, where all leadership positions at various levels are occupied exclusively by men (Datta, 2023). The study highlights the mixed impact of *Khap Panchayats* on women's rights and empowerment. On one hand, these bodies uphold deeply patriarchal values, restricting women's autonomy and participation in public life. For instance, a significant majority of the respondents believe that women should not participate in *Khap Panchayats*, reflecting entrenched gender biases. Women are often excluded from decision-making processes, and relegated to peripheral roles like preparing food for meetings rather than participating in them (Chowdhry, 2007). The *Khaps* wield significant influence over the community, enforcing norms related to marriage, property rights, and social conduct (Kaur, 2010). The study also cites instances of *Khap Panchayats* dictating dress codes and restricting women's use of mobile phones in public. Such measures are intended to control women's behavior and maintain the community's honor but result in significant constraints on women's freedom and rights (Menon, 2012). Their responsibilities often include resolving disputes within the community, but they are particularly notorious for their rulings on issues related to honor, particularly concerning women's conduct and marriages (Kaur, 2010).

However, it is essential to acknowledge that the influence of *Khaps* is not uniformly negative. Some respondents noted that *Khaps* can contribute to women's empowerment by promoting social harmony and resolving disputes that might otherwise escalate. For example, in certain cases, Caste Councils have intervened to ensure women's safety and well-being within the community (Basu, 2018). These instances, though less common, indicate that the potential for positive change exists if *Khaps* can be reformed to include women's voices and perspectives (Jayaram, 1979). The topic includes a poignant case study of Riya, a 16-year-old girl who eloped, highlighting the severe social consequences of challenging traditional norms (Rahaman et al., 2022a, 2022b). Her family's decision to marry her off to a much older man, despite her youth, reflects the community's prioritization of family honor over individual rights and well-being (Rahaman et al., 2022a, 2022b). Focus group discussions further illuminate how deeply ingrained the concepts of honor and tradition are in the community, affecting women's autonomy and opportunities. The restriction of women's rights and autonomy by *Khap Panchayats* has profound negative implications for their health and healthcare utilization. Moreover, the study underscores the importance of women's development in achieving broader health and societal outcomes. Research suggests that women who feel empowered are more likely to access healthcare services, ensure their children are immunized, and lead healthier lives overall (WHO, 2019). Therefore, depriving women of their rights and empowerment not only impedes their personal growth but also negatively impacts their general health and welfare (Sharma et al., 2020).

Women make up around half of a society's human resources. The advancement of civilization depends on individual contributions. Women have traditionally been portrayed as weak, repressed, and excluded from decision-making processes in the majority of the world's nations. The underlying reason for this problem is the prevailing patriarchal society structure, which holds that men are superior to women and have greater control over resources, opinions, and ideologies. In our multifaceted society, women occupy a multitude of positions. There are significant differences in women's status across the Indian subcontinent based on a variety of factors, including occupation, property rights, caste, religion, class, cultural background, etc. Each of these components plays an important part in figuring out where they fall within various categories. Social stratification, tradition, and culture of Indian society are affecting women's status. Women ignore all knowledge inhibition and subordination which is responsible for increasing discrimination and pain (Mazumdar, 2001). The study supports, that patriarchy is one of the consequences of *Khap*by both theoretical analysis and empirical evidence. The social, cultural, and legal influence of *Khap Panchayats* plays a significant role in sustaining patriarchal norms in rural Haryana. They are seen as upholders of '*izzat*' (honor) and maintain a deep-rooted cultural emphasis on honor and control over women's sexuality and mobility (Rahaman &

Das, 2024). Three Key Challenges for Women in the *Khap Panchayat* Belt: First, women in the *Khap Panchayat* belt face severe restrictions on their autonomy and mobility. Traditional norms enforced by these councils often limit women's freedom to make personal decisions, participate in public life, or even move freely outside their homes. This lack of autonomy hinders their ability to pursue education, employment, and personal growth. Second, women are largely excluded from decision-making processes within *Khap Panchayats*. These councils are dominated by male elders who make decisions affecting the entire community, including women, without their input. This exclusion perpetuates gender inequality and prevents women from advocating for their rights and interests. Third, the patriarchal norms upheld by *Khap Panchayats* contribute to poor health outcomes for women. Restrictions on women's behavior and social stigma associated with violating community norms deter women from seeking timely medical care. Additionally, practices like honor killings and punishment for perceived moral transgressions pose significant safety risks to women.

Balancing respect for traditional institutions with promoting gender equality and women's rights is a challenge. To address the challenges faced by women in the *Khap Panchayat* belt, the following policy recommendations are proposed: First, the media plays a crucial role in reporting *Khap* excesses, which has gained attention from various stakeholders like the judiciary, political class, and academia. It is important for the media to maintain objectivity in their reporting and provide a balanced view of the situation. By highlighting the positive aspects of *Khap Panchayats* alongside their shortcomings, the media can contribute to a better understanding of the issues at hand. Ultimately, a collaborative effort involving all stakeholders is crucial for bringing about positive social change in the *Khap* belt. The media must be mindful of their influence and responsibility in shaping public perception and promoting constructive dialogue. Second, implement and enforce legal reforms that protect women's rights and ensure their inclusion in decision-making processes. Laws should be strengthened to prohibit discriminatory practices by *Khap Panchayats* and to safeguard women's autonomy and freedom. Third, invest in educational and vocational training programs specifically targeted at women in these regions. Providing women with access to education and economic opportunities can empower them to challenge traditional norms and improve their social and economic status. Fourth, conduct community engagement and awareness programs to challenge patriarchal norms and promote gender equality. These programs should involve both men and women and aim to shift societal attitudes toward women's rights and empowerment. Fifth, improve access to healthcare services for women in rural areas, including reproductive health services. Mobile health clinics and community health workers can play a crucial role in ensuring that women receive timely medical care without facing social stigma or restrictions.

### 7.4.1 Limitations and Strengths of the Chapter

The current study has various limitations concerning both conceptual and physical factors. Some of the limitations of the study are as follows: The first is the time constraints for studying a topic in an area that is vast. When talking about the *Khap* panchayats, the *Jats* being studied are extremely antagonistic. Many of them are aware that outsiders propagate bad news about their esteemed institutions. The leaders of the *Khap* panchayats are afraid to disclose precise data since the panchayats are involved in various such activities which are not correct, legally. Due to the immense influence of these caste panchayats, the *Pardhans* and other members hesitate to give an accurate image. The weaker segments of society, such as those from lower castes, are afraid of the *Khap* leaders and are reluctant to give accurate information. As every *Khap* has different rules regarding some issues, the results can't be generalized completely. Since women in society are not permitted to communicate with outsiders on their own, the researcher also was not allowed to interact directly with the females during the fieldwork. It appears that the information provided by their male counterparts on their behalf is manipulated and biased. Due to the higher non-response rate among women, equal representation was not possible. The topic of the murders committed by the *Khap* panchayats is quite sensitive, and people hesitate to discuss it. Despite these drawbacks, the researcher has built a rapport with the community and organized the gathering of reliable data. The acquired data has also been cross-checked by the researcher using a variety of methods.

## 7.5 Conclusion

In conclusion, the study provides a nuanced understanding of the role of *Khap Panchayats* in shaping the social status of women in rural Haryana. While these traditional bodies continue to enforce patriarchal norms that limit women's autonomy, there are indications of their potential to contribute positively to women's empowerment if inclusive reforms are implemented. Addressing the gender disparity in *Khap Panchayats* and promoting women's active participation in decision-making processes are crucial steps toward achieving gender equality and enhancing the social status of women in this region. This aligns with the need for structural reforms in traditional governance systems to promote gender equality.

## References

Basu, S. (2018). Gender and Law. *Critical Themes in Indian Sociology, 282.*

Carter, L., & Connor, K. (1989). *A preliminary investigation of contemporary Afghan councils.* ACBAR.

Chowdhry, P. (2007). Contentious marriages, eloping couples: Gender, caste, and patriarchy in Northern India. *(No Title)*.

Clark, J. P. (1989). Conflict management outside the courtrooms of China. In *Social control in the People's Republic of China* (pp. 57–69).

Datta, P. K. (2023). Gender quota and women's participation in rural local bodies in India: The context, constraints and consequences. *Indian Journal of Public Administration, 69*(4), 832–844.

Davar, B. V. (1999). Indian psychoanalysis, patriarchy and Hinduism. *Anthropology & Medicine, 6*(2), 173–193.

Faqir, K., & Atta, M. A. (2013). Jirga: A conflict resolution institution in Pukhtoon society. *Gomal University Journal of Research, 29*(1).

Hussain, A. (2022). *Negotiating the question of caste, Islam and Indian Muslims: Caste elements among Meos of Mewat*.

Jayaram, N. (1979). Higher education, inequality and social change in India. *Sociological Bulletin, 28*(1–2), 46–58.

Kaur, R. (2010). Khap panchayats, sex ratio and female agency. *Economic and Political Weekly*, 14–16.

Khan, M. Z., & Sharma, K. (1982). Profile of a Nyaya panchayat.

Li, V. H. (1979). Law without lawyers: A comparative view of law in China and the United States. *Philosophy East and West, 29*(2).

Mazumdar, V. (2001). Whose past, whose history, whose tradition?: Indigenizing women's studies in India. *Asian Journal of Women's Studies, 7*(1), 133–153.

Menon, N. (2012). *Seeing like a feminist*. Penguin UK.

Ministry of Women and Child Development. (2020). *Beti Bachao Beti Padhao: Compendium of Best Practices*. Government of India.

Rahaman, M., & Das, K. C. (2024). Differentials in self-reported health status and healthcare utilization among homeless women during the antenatal period in urban settings: Does migration status matter? *Journal of Migration and Health*, 100246.

Rahaman, M., Roy, A., Kapasia, N., & Chouhan, P. (2022a). Spousal violence in India: Does risk of spousal violence higher among polygynous unions? *Cogent Social Sciences, 8*(1), 2103945.

Rahaman, M., Sen, S., Rana, M. J., & Ghosh, S. (2022b). Is consanguineous marriage related to spousal violence in India? Evidence from the National Family Health Survey, 2015–16. *Journal of Biosocial Science, 54*(6), 959–974.

Rajpramukh, K. E., & Palkumar, P. D. S. (2005). Livelihood challenges and strategies: The Valmikis of Eastern Ghats. *The Anthropologist, 7*(2), 153–160.

Ramesh, T. (2021). Problems and prospects of Gutti Koyas: A case study of Gutti Koyas of West Godavari District, Andhra Pradesh. *Asian Journal of Multidisciplinary Research and Review, 3*(6), 100–110.

Rammala, M. N. R. (2021). Lekgotla and idiomatic expressions in traditional dispute resolution: The case of Makapanstad, North West Province, South Africa. *International Journal of African Renaissance Studies, 16*(1), 220–241.

Riaz, A. (2005). Traditional institutions as tools of political Islam in Bangladesh. *Journal of Asian and African Studies, 40*(3), 171–196.

Sen, G., & Ostlin, P. (2011). *Gender inequity in health*. World Health Organizations.

Sharma, K. (2011). Unheard voices: Honour killings in India. *International Journal of Criminal Justice Sciences, 6*(1–2), 83–97.

Sharma, S., Mehra, D., Akhtar, F., & Mehra, S. (2020). Evaluation of a community-based intervention for health and economic empowerment of marginalized women in India. *BMC Public Health, 20*, 1–16.

Singh, P. K. (2008). Traditional self governance system and its existential realities in Jharkhand. *The Oriental Anthropologist, 8*(1–2), 221–241.

Tulsyan, A. (2022). *The issue of the dogged Khap Panchayats in India*. Available at SSRN 4018757.

UNFPA. (2014). *State of world population 2014: The power of 1.8 billion*. United Nations Population Fund.

Vaisey, S., & Miles, A. (2017). What you can—And can't—Do with three-wave panel data. *Sociological Methods & Research, 46*(1), 44–67.

Wardak, A. (2003). *Jirga—A traditional mechanism of conflict resolution in Afghanistan* (pp. 1–20). University of Glamorgan, Centre for Criminology.

WHO. (2019). *Women's empowerment and gender equality: The need for action and the role of health systems.* World Health Organization.

Yadav, R., Dakua, T., & Das, K. C. (2024). Khap panchayats in India: An analysis from media and movies. *Indian Journal of Social Studies and Humanities, 1*(18), 69–83.

Zaman, L., Khan, Q., & Naz, A. (2018). Critical discourse analysis: Jirga and its Survival in Pakistan. *Pakistan Journal of Criminology, 10*(3), 29–40.

# Part III
# Sexual, Reproductive, and Maternal Health

# Chapter 8
# The Human Right to Late-Stage Abortion in India: A Legislative and Judicial Analysis of the Medical Termination of Pregnancy (Amendment) Act, 2021

**Adam Dubin and Shreya Srivastava**

**Abstract** This chapter reviews the judgments of the Indian Supreme Court and several High Courts since the coming into effect of the 2021 Amendment to the Medical Termination of Pregnancy (MTP) Act, 1971, to analyze how Indian courts have addressed the issue of late-stage abortion (after 24 weeks). The chapter finds that while many courts have upheld the spirit of the law, the judicialization of abortion has led to divergent approaches which have created an emerging line of case law in which abortion rights have not been upheld. In particular, the chapter also finds that some courts have improvised judicial doctrines to prevent late-stage abortions and have failed to consider international legal obligations. From the secondary data that the authors have relied on for exploring the reasons for abortions and impact the lack of safe and legal abortions have, the decision of courts to deny abortions is not conducive to the health and welfare of women. Ultimately, the chapter concludes that a new modification is necessary to the MTP to ensure that courts adhere to constitutional and international laws that uphold women´s personal autonomy and choice to terminate their pregnancies. In addition, there is a need to expedite the setting up of medical boards and sensitization of doctors.

**Keywords** Reproductive rights · India · Abortion · Late stage abortion · MTP (Amendment) Act, 2021

---

A. Dubin (✉)
Faculty of Law, Universidad Pontificia Comillas, Madrid, Spain
e-mail: Adubin@comillas.edu

S. Srivastava
Institute of Law, Nirma University, Ahmedabad, India
e-mail: shreya.srivastava@nirmauni.ac.in

 
P. Chouhan et al. (eds.), *Women's Health Dynamics in South Asia*, Asian Perspectives on Public Health, https://doi.org/10.1007/978-981-95-2321-4_8

## 8.1 Introduction

In 2021, the Parliament of India amended the 1971 Medical Termination of Pregnancy Act, 1971 (hereinafter, the MTP Act, 1971) to allow abortion up to 24 weeks, with the possibility of accessing abortion later in pregnancy (referred to here as ALP, also sometimes referred to as late-stage abortion) for certain category of women under limited circumstances with the approval of the Courts. This change came in response to the need to broaden the scope of safe and legal abortions in a country where thousands of women die each year from unsafe terminations of pregnancy.

This chapter asserts that ALP, while not specifically referenced in international human rights law, has nonetheless evolved into a human right that must be guaranteed at least in certain instances. The MTP Amendment allows women the right to terminate their pregnancies after 20 weeks but up to 24 weeks with the permission of medical boards. Any termination beyond that period can only be done with the final approval of the high courts of Indian states. This has since produced several important cases in which the courts have had to determine whether women can abort legally after 24 weeks.

This judicialization of abortion access in India has resulted in many cases granting women the right to terminate their pregnancies at these later stages, upholding the spirit of the MTP Amendment, 2021. However, the courts in India have in other cases denied the plea of abortion of some women. Despite the obligations under the Constitution of India and also the international human rights law, leaving this decision to the discretion of the courts leads to the denial of reproductive rights justice, potentially threatening reproductive access in a country with high rates of maternal mortality, especially among poor women.

This chapter analyzes how Indian high courts have applied the 2021 Amendment. It finds that while much of the case law produced since the Amendment went into effect meets fundamental rights obligations, other cases are in contravention of women´s rights and put at risk the maternal health of poor women, in particular. This chapter begins by discussing abortion access worldwide and then asserts that ALP is a human right, before discussing the precarious state of maternal health and abortion rights in India. Afterwards, the chapter moves into an analysis of the courts´ jurisprudence since the 2021 Amendment, analyzing both the tendencies in upholding the Amendment along with ways in which judicializing abortion rights has led to violations of women´s rights. The chapter concludes that to remedy this problem, the Government of India should once again amend the MTP to insert language that binds the courts to certain constitutional and international rights principles, thereby removing the discretion left to judges in deciding on abortion rights access. Further, training and sensitization of registered medical practitioners and setting up of medical boards will strengthen the procedure for termination of pregnancy.

### 8.1.1 Abortion Worldwide

Most countries around the world statutorily recognize some degree of abortion rights, though access to a safe and legal abortion is still elusive for millions of women, especially poor women. According to a report by the United Nations Population Fund (UNFP), the global abortion rate is approximately 39 per 1,000 pregnant women (UNFPA, 2022). Seventy-three million abortions worldwide take place annually. 29% of all pregnancies and 61% of unintended pregnancies globally end in abortion. The WHO (2024) reported that approximately 45% of all abortions globally take place under unsafe conditions, a public health crisis leading to the hospitalization of millions of women and costing governments upwards of 550 million USD and individual households nearly 1 billion USD in post-abortion treatment costs (UNFPA, 2022: 11).

From 2003 to 2012, between 4% and 13% of maternal deaths were due to unsafe abortions, according to the WHO, though they estimate that this figure is probably underreported (WHO, 2024). Most unsafe abortions occur in Asia, especially in the regions of central and South Asia. According to the WHO, nearly 75% of all abortions were unsafe in Latin America and Africa. Approximately half of the abortions conducted were also deemed to be "least safe" in Africa (2024).

The reasons why abortion access may be limited go beyond just restrictive laws, though this does play a prominent role. In many countries, geographic isolation from reproductive health services, poverty, lack of know-how, family pressures, and patriarchy, in addition to untrained and ideologically opposed medical staff, often working in highly underfunded health care systems, can make abortion access difficult, if not impossible, for millions of women.

This inaccessibility of safe abortions, it goes without saying, has direct and tragic effects on the life and health of women. As noted above, tens of thousands of women continue to die each year from unsafe abortions, and many more suffer life-altering health complications, from punctures of internal organs to sepsis and other infections. Families lose mothers and breadwinners, and even where women do survive, they are often incapacitated, unable to work, and shunned by society.

Access to safe and legal abortions, on the other hand, not only provides for better health outcomes, but studies suggest also increases socio-economic productivity and gender equality. For example, legal and accessible abortion has a positive impact on female educational attainment and labor market participation. Comparatively, restrictive laws lead to poverty among women and their dependency on public assistance (Van Der Meulen Rodgers et al, 2021). In addition, restrictive laws also create higher healthcare expenditures for governments and individuals. In the Philippines, for example, medical procedures to fix incomplete abortions cost the Government nearly 8 million USD in 2021 (Ray, 2024).

Access to safe and legal abortion throughout the entirety of a pregnancy is an issue that also has implications beyond health and well-being. Allowing women to make decisions about their own bodies, irrespective of mores, traditions, and patriarchy, ensures that women are bearers of their rights and can exert full control over their bodies and personal autonomy. This not only saves lives and protects their right to health but also contributes to greater socio-economic development, the advancement of gender equality, and progress toward the Sustainable Development Goals, particularly Goal 3.1 to reduce maternal mortality.

### *8.1.2 Toward a Recognition of ALP in International Human Rights Law*

Abortion, a human right, is not a single right but an amalgamation of international rights that have evolved over time to strengthen and affirm women´s rights to terminate their pregnancies. Human rights apply from the time of birth to the time of death but do not regulate the rights of the unborn.

What was once conceived largely in the context of population control, especially in the developing world, the right to abortion has increasingly become understood as a right that gives women control and autonomy over their bodies. Decisional and bodily autonomy are at the center of this right, however, international law leaves a margin to states to regulate abortion access outside several prescribed grounds. This is allowed to the extent the measures regulating voluntary terminations of pregnancy do not lead to the violation of the right to life of a pregnant person. Other rights mentioned under the Covenant can also not be violated in the garb of these regulations. In other words, while abortion, including ALP, is guaranteed in international law under certain circumstances, it is not an absolute right.

The right to abortion is a right protected under international, regional, and domestic frameworks. This includes recognition by all three regional human rights systems that safe and legal abortion, at least under certain circumstances, must be guaranteed. It is worth noting that despite the challenges of guaranteeing access to safe and legal abortions across Africa, the *Protocol to the African Charter on Human and Peoples' Rights on the Rights of Women in Africa* codifies abortion as a human right, making it the only human rights treaty to specifically recognize abortion.

The basis of this right stems from Article 12 of the 1979 United Nations Convention on the Elimination of Discrimination Against Women, under which the State Parties are under an obligation to provide access to health care services. This also includes the commitments related to family planning (CEDAW, 1979). However, over time, other UN Conventions and human rights bodies have also recognized this right, which when not protected can also trigger a violation of other rights, including privacy, health, liberty, and the prohibition against torture rights.

The language of CEDAW is notably absent from a specific recognition of abortion rights. This was due, in part, to the Clinton Administration´s attempt to seek more "abortion-neutral" terminology to appease opponents of abortion (Venter, 2012: 455). On a broader level, however, the language of the document itself sought to find common ground among nations and avoid alienating countries opposed to recognizing abortion rights, particularly since at that time abortion rights were not as prominently part of the international women´s rights agenda.

Between the time of drafting CEDAW until its final version, there was an important substantive change made to Article 12 that strengthened women´s autonomy to make decisions over their bodies. In a 1974 draft version of CEDAW by the United Nations Working Group to the Commission on the Status of Women, then Article 10 sought to guarantee only "information to family planning." However, the final version of health rights, which eventually became Article 12, recognizes a more actionable right to "access to health care services, including those related to family planning." This shift in language creates a responsibility on the state to respect, protect, and fulfill access to family planning services—not only information—while also recognizing women as the bearer of the right of access.

This empowerment of women over their own bodies was also reflected in the outcome of the UNFP International Conference on Population and Development, which in its 1994 Program of Action recognized unsafe abortions "as a global priority" toward protecting women´s health (Erdman, 2023: 1119). It put women more squarely in their center of reproductive and sexual rights, and, as noted by one scholar, there was a shift by the global community, and instead of prioritizing State interests in the sphere of reproductive rights, the focus shifted to the rights of women (Pillai, 2024).

Recognizing that abortion rights discourse was increasingly evolving toward greater recognition of reproductive rights and greater decisional autonomy, the U.S. Government engaged in a failed attempt to halt the elevation of abortion into the global rights agenda during the negotiations leading up to the1995 Beijing Declaration and Platform for Action. It sought to insert a reservation stating that the Platform does not create any new human rights, including the right to abortion (Pietilä, 2007: 101).

Instead, the final Declaration explicitly recognized the threat unsafe abortions pose to women and their right to control their own sexual and reproductive health, without any limitation on gestational periods. The Declaration reflected overwhelming evidence on the number of women dying from unsafe abortions and how the passage of restrictive abortion laws contributes to increases in maternal health deaths (Haddad & Nour, 2009).

With continuing high levels of maternal mortality due to unsafe abortions, especially among poor women in developing countries, CEDAW took its first steps through the publication of General Recommendation 24 of 1999 (para. 31c) on Women and Health to call on states to amend legislation that criminalises abortions and make the right of abortion more accessible.

An important turning point came in 2005 through *K.L. v. Peru* (2003) in which the U.N. Human Rights Committee, in a case involving a 17 year old girl who was carrying a fetus with severe fetal abnormalities, was denied access to an abortion. The Human Rights Committee found for the applicant, holding that such restrictions on abortion amount to an interference in her private life under Article 17 of the ICCPR. In addition, the Committee also found that forcing a woman to carry a fetus to term is also a violation of Article 7 prohibition against torture. This case represents an important shift in abortion rights by placing the question of abortion into the sphere of the female´s private life and arguably extending the right without gestational limits when Article 7 is triggered.

From this point on, the United Nations embarked on what can be described as a fairly rapid evolution toward recognizing the personal autonomy of women to make decisions over their own bodies. In response to a Communication by three NGOs to CEDAW against the Philippines filed in 2008 (and ruled in 2015) for promoting natural family planning at the expense of women´s sexual and reproductive rights, CEDAW called on the Philippines to legalize abortion in certain cases, prevent unsafe abortions, and guarantee post-abortion health care. The Committee reinforced the concept of private life, noting that by failing to provide abortion access, the state will deprive women of their autonomy over a right that is fundamental (CEDAW, 2015:12).

In two separate cases in 2016 and 2017, respectively, the United Nations Human Rights Committee ruled that not being able to terminate a non-viable pregnancy and having to travel abroad, amounts to a violation of the right against cruel and unusual treatment, and also constitutes a violation of privacy and non-discrimination rights. Importantly, with respect to the question of non-access constituting a violation of the prohibition against cruel and unusual punishment, the Committee (Mellet, 2016: para. 7.6) seems to suggest more explicitly that abortion regulations cannot be applied where a woman undergoes severe physical or mental suffering. According to the General Comment No. 20 of the Human Rights Committee, Article 7 of the ICCPR, does not leave room for limitation or justification for invocation of extenuating circumstances to excuse a transgression of Article 7.

From 2016 onward, a series of general comments and recommendations reflected the growing consensus on abortion as a human right. The Committee of the International Covenant on Economic, Social and Culture Rights released General Comment 22 (2016) on the Right to Sexual and Reproductive Health, which further anchored access to safe and legal abortion as a right by obligating states to respect, protect, and fulfill the right and noting that ideological opposition to the right cannot be a barrier to access. The General Comment requires states to provide legal recognition for the right to abortion, noting that states must guarantee women's access to safe abortions. This should also include post-treatment care. Training of health care providers is a must if the former are to be ensured (CESCR, 2016: para. 22). Importantly, the General Comment also recognizes the bodily and decisional autonomy of women, explicitly referring to women's autonomy over their reproductive and sexual health (CESCR, 2016: para. 28). In addition, CEDAW General Recommendation 35 recognized that the denial or delay of safe abortions, or the forced continuation of pregnancy, may amount to torture, and Human Rights Committee in a 2018 General Comment 36 (para. 8) reinforced the Recommendation on providing safe and legal access to abortion facility especially when the woman is in substantial pain or there is a threat to her life.

While the right to safe and legal abortion has evolved considerably in the last twenty years, uncertainties remain, particularly as international law has sought to balance the right of women with the sovereignty of states to put in place certain restrictions to regulate the voluntary termination of pregnancy. The right guarantees access to safe and legal abortion in cases of rape, incest, threat to life, or substantial physical or mental suffering, but beyond that, states have a margin to adopt laws aimed at regulating abortion.

In cases where abortions are sought during later stages of pregnancy, states can likely place gestational certain limits on abortions but only where doing so would not violate the guarantees provided in international law on sexual and reproductive health. Nor can such restrictions lead to violations of other fundamental rights, such as life or prohibitions against torture.

### 8.1.3 Abortion Access in India

Between 2015 and 2019, there were 48,500,000 documented pregnancies, 16 million of which ended in abortion (Guttmacher). A 2015 study published in The Lancet estimates that the abortion rate in India among women aged 15 to 49 years old is 47 per 1,000 pregnancies and that only 22% of abortions were legal, i.e., they were obtained safely through registered medical practitioners and hospitals; 73% of abortions were medication abortions that did not take place within medical facilities, likely making them illegal; 5% were abortions outside of health facilities using non-medical methods, also likely making them illegal. In total, the article estimates that nearly 1 million unsafe abortions took place in 2015 (Singh et al., 2018).

For millions of women around India, access to a safe abortion continues to be elusive. 10% of maternal health deaths in India occurred because of unsafe abortions, according to report by Chandra et al. (2021). In Concluding Observations to India in 2014, the CEDAW Committee raised concerns about the lack of safe abortion and post-abortion care in response to many civil society reports highlighting the scarce access for millions of women. The CEDAW Committee (2014: 31b) urged India to create an infrastructural framework to ensure access to high-quality and safe abortion services, as well as for the management of complications that arise due to unsafe abortions.

The report by Chandra et al. (2021) highlights the challenges faced by millions of Indian women in obtaining abortions, including stigma and patriarchy, poverty, difficulty accessing the public health care system, as well as spatial geographies that disproportionately affect rural women. Some doctors, including those at large public hospitals, have expressed their ideological opposition to abortion, making it difficult for poor women, who cannot afford to go to private hospitals, to terminate their pregnancies. In addition, Dalit women frequently experience caste-based discrimination by doctors, and the poor generally often find themselves confronting high medical fees, making abortion access difficult (Rao, 2023).

There is also an unfilled need among pregnant women in India to access abortion services after the 24-week gestational limit expires. This is due to several factors, such as the late diagnosis of fetal abnormalities, women not attending their first antenatal screening until the fourth or fifth month of pregnancy, and sexual assault survivors not revealing their pregnancies until they are visibly pregnant (Chandra et al., 2021:52). However, women seeking abortions after 24 weeks often find themselves struggling to access safe and legal abortions, even though the MTP Amendment 2021 permits it under certain exceptions. The report by Chandra et al. (2021) found that many doctors refuse to consider abortions after the gestational limit, believing incorrectly that abortions are prohibited after 24 weeks. The United Nations and WHO have condemned the use of judicial and medical board authorization in India because it denies women the right to an abortion forces women to submit to medical examinations and other processes that by their very nature deny women autonomy over their own bodies (OHCHR, 2014).

Overall, while the right to abortion is recognized in India and provides for a regulatory framework that has benefited millions of women and has helped to improve safeguards for a safe abortion, thousands more continue to abort in unsafe and illegal conditions. The difficulties for many women to access a safe and legal abortion throughout their pregnancies has created a perilous situation, especially for the poor, lower caste, and geographically isolated, who are often forced to either carry the fetus to term against their will or undergo potentially life-threatening unsafe abortions.

### 8.1.4 ALP Access in India

The history of abortion laws in India has been stringent until the passing of the Medical Termination of Pregnancy Act, 1971. The law and policy debate is rooted in the ethical argument of taking human life. As a result, inducing an abortion is a criminal offense in India, unless it is done to save the life of the pregnant woman. This led to an increase in illegal abortions, but they were related to high mortality rates as they were being conducted in unsanitary conditions and by unqualified persons. As a significant matter of public health, the Shantilal Shah Committee (hereinafter the Shah Committee) was appointed in 1964 to study the question of rationalization of abortion in India. The Shah Committee report also found that mostly married women were seeking abortions, and therefore, had no reason to enshroud their pregnancy (Shah, 1964, 39).

The Shah Committee recognized that abortion has legal, social, economic, moral, medical, and religious aspects. However, the looming presence of illegal abortions leading to high maternal morbidity, wastage of medical skill and resources, as well as the commitment of the State toward family planning led to the determination of the question on the necessity of legal abortions in the country by broadening of the right of legal abortion for women. It became a significant question of public health.

Considering the causes necessitating abortions, the Shah Committee recommended the need for liberalizing abortion laws in India. The earlier restrictive application of the law that allowed abortions only in case of medical grounds was suggested to be amended by including humanitarian as well as eugenic grounds. Thus, India fell in that group of countries which allowed abortions under a broad range of circumstances, thereby acknowledging the actual and foreseeable environment of a woman as well as taking into account her socio-economic factors (Deo, Pg. 283).

The recommendations of the Shah Committee were incorporated in the Medical Termination of Pregnancy Act, 1971 (hereinafter the MTP Act, 1971). The intent of the Act is to protect the health of a pregnant person and facilitate safe, hygienic, and legal abortions. Termination of pregnancy was legal during the first twelve weeks if continuation of the pregnancy involved a threat to the mother's life would be gravely injurious to her health, both physical as well as mental; or, if the child, if born, would suffer from serious abnormalities (MTP Act, 1971, Section 3). The law presumed injury to the mental health of the woman if the pregnancy was caused by rape, or, in the case of a married woman, pregnancy occurred as a result of failure of any contraceptive process. Thus, by delineating the limits of termination of pregnancy, compelling state interest in the protection of life has also been ensured.

Termination of pregnancy falls within the inviolable privacy of an individual, which is a postulate of human dignity. It fosters the inviolability of the body and the mind of an individual (*Justice K.S. Puttaswamy* v. *UoI*). In 2009, the Supreme Court in the case of *Suchita Srivastava & Anr.* v *Chandigarh Administration* (2009) has also explicitly stated that under Article 21 of the Constitution of India, reproductive choices can be exercised by a woman as it ensures a life of dignity. Thus, the "personal liberty of a woman includes not only the right to procreate, but also to abstain from procreation" (*Suchita Srivastava*, 2009, Para 10). Since this choice is based on a woman's reproductive autonomy and bodily autonomy, abortion rights have been embedded within the human rights framework. Between the choice of the woman and the life of the fetus, some decisions have even stated that the right of a woman cannot be overshadowed by placing the right of the unborn fetus on a higher pedestal (*High Court on its own motion* v *State of Maharashtra*, para 20).

International treaties of human rights and covenants which are ratified by India are also binding on the State if they expound on fundamental rights. ICCPR, ICESR, and CEDAW require State parties to provide for the sexual and reproductive health of their people. The statutory right under the MTP Act, 1971 echoes this commitment. Access to legal and safe abortion is not only about the reproductive freedom of women, but also of their agency. Thus, it has been interpreted to endow a pregnant person with decisional and bodily autonomy, both facets of personal liberty, thereby, empowering a woman to choose the course of her life.

### 8.1.5 The 2021 Amendment

The earlier limited gestational period led to the filing of several writs and in the constitutional courts of India. More than 100 writs were filed in the various High Courts and 26 petitions were filed in the Supreme Court during 2017–2018 seeking to terminate pregnancy beyond the gestational period on grounds of fetal abnormalities and conception due to rape (Deo, Pg. 283). Moreover, there has been the advancement of medical technology which allows the determination of fetal anomalies in 20th and 21st weeks of pregnancy.

Against this backdrop, the MTP (Amendment) Bill 2021 was introduced in the Parliament and was passed on 25th March 2021. The Bill was formulated after consultation with all possible stakeholders, relevant ministries and Ethics Committee of Experts formed by the ministry of Health and Family Welfare. Now, pregnancies can be terminated until twenty weeks on the advice of one registered medical practitioner and until twenty-four weeks in case of a special category of women. This group is more vulnerable to social stigma, or, may not be able to continue the pregnancy due to their actual or reasonably foreseeable environment and social or economic circumstances. According to Rule 3B of the MTP (Amendment) Rules, 2021, it includes survivors of the offense of rape, sexual assault, or incest; minors; widows or women whose marital status has altered during the pregnancy (such as the cases of divorce); women who suffer mental and physical disabilities; and pregnant women in humanitarian settings such as war, natural disasters, or any other situation that may be considered to be an emergency; or, where the fetus suffers from malformations that are incompatible with life.

A landmark case where the new rules and amended law was discussed extensively by the Supreme Court is *X* v *Principal Secretary, Health and Family Welfare Department, Government of NCT of Delhi & Anr.* (2023) (hereinafter, *X* v *NCT case*). Societies often exercise control over women's bodies legally as well as socially. Reproduction itself is both biological as well as political. In India, this was also observed in the unamended MTP Act, 1971 wherein only a married woman could use the law for the termination of pregnancy that occurred due to the failure of contraceptive, whereas an unmarried woman could not according to Section 3(2)(b) of the MTP Act, 1971. Since the unamended MTP Act, 1971 prominently discussed rights of married women, an unmarried woman had no option but to take recourse to unsafe and illegal abortion. Allowing abortion for an unmarried girl due to social stigma was recognized in the Shantilal Shah Committee Report.

The *X* v *NCT case* upholds the progressive nature of the amended MTP Act, 1971. The petitioner was an unmarried woman who had become pregnant in a consensual relationship. She wanted to terminate her pregnancy as her partner did not want to marry her. The context of her immediate and foreseeable circumstances was the social stigma and harassment of single parents and no source of livelihood. Since her case did not fall into any of the categories mentioned in Rule 3B of the MTP (Amendment) Rules, 2021, the High Court of Delhi rejected her petition.

However, the Supreme Court undertook the interpretation of this statute in the widest possible manner. It reinforced that the scheme of the MTP Act, 1971 does not distinguish between married and unmarried women, thereby interpreting the law beyond the patriarchal principles of what constitutes "permissible sex"*(X* v. *NCT*, Para 127). It held that the said rule is applicable when women are abandoned by their "family or partner." Thus, it broadened the scope of application of this provision considering the beneficial purpose that this statute serves and dissociated this right from the institution of marriage.

### 8.1.6 Analysis of the Trajectory of Court Decisions in ALPs After the 2021 Amendment

Generally, courts have had regard to the pregnant woman's psychological status, sociocultural and economic conditions while passing a favorable order for the termination of pregnancy. In analyzing many of the cases since the MTP Amendment 2021 went into effect, the approaches of the Indian courts can be grouped to demonstrate how the courts have dealt with this complicated issue. From this analysis, certain conclusions can be extrapolated which highlight the tendencies of the Indian courts in applying this amendment since it went into effect.

One of the identifiable considerations by the court is the woman's actual or reasonable foreseeable circumstances to adjudicate such cases. In doing so, the opinion of the pregnant person has to be given primacy (*A* v *State of* Maharashtra, 2024). For instance, in *XYZ v Dean of B.J. Govt. Medical College and Sassoon Hospital through the Professor, HoD and* Ors. (2021), the High Court of Bombay allowed the termination of pregnancy at the gestational period of 26 weeks on the firm choice of the petitioner. Though the pregnancy was a result of a consensual relationship, and the fetus had no abnormalities, the psychological impact of bearing the child and the lower income status of the woman were determinative factors.

Pregnancy resultant from acts of sexual assault and rape are a category of cases where the law presumes grave mental injury to the pregnant mother, and, as such, the courts have generally approached this question in a way that aligns with the international law of human rights. Denying the woman termination of the pregnancy, even though it could be beyond the statutory gestational limit, would amount to forcing motherhood upon her and at the same time denying her the human right and fundamental right to live with dignity. In an aggravated case where the woman was raped and also found HIV positive, the Supreme Court opined that the failure of the medical authorities to act on time upon receiving the consent of the woman for termination of the pregnancy not only amounted to a violation of her human rights but also amounted to torture. As a result, the Supreme Court not only observed that it was the duty of the State to act in an effective and expeditious manner to protect her life and liberty by allowing the termination, but also that she was eligible for grant of compensation under the public law (Z v *State of Bihar*, 2018).

Where the case is of sexual assault of minor girls, the courts have also been forthcoming in allowing termination of pregnancies even beyond the statutory limit. The sole and only consideration for the courts in such cases becomes the safety and welfare of the minor, as demonstrated through case law. Women's bodies at such tender ages are not equipped to physically and mentally handle pregnancies. If a girl is forced to carry the pregnancy to term, childbirth will lead to severe damage to her body and in some cases may even be fatal for her. Even if she successfully delivers the child, the trauma of such young, forced motherhood is unimaginable. In some of these cases, courts have also been conscious of the intersectionalities of caste and gender. Thus, in *X* v *Union of India represented by Secretary & Ors.* (2024), where a 16-year-old Dalit girl was raped and became pregnant, the Kerala

High Court allowed the termination of her pregnancy at 28 weeks because the court was aware that the exclusion and ostracization of the victim from the community, even though she was very young, was probable (*X* v. *Union of India* 2024: para 9).

Another identifiable and important aspect of the courts´ jurisprudence has been a notable emphasis on safeguarding the right of reproductive choice and the comprehensive health of women, especially in cases of rape and sexual assault. Courts have laid down guidelines for the effective functioning of agencies set up under the MTP Act, 1971. In *X* v *State of Karnataka* (2023), the Court stated that immediately upon registration of a sexual offence under Protection of Children from Sexual Offences Act, 2012 or rape under the Indian Penal Code, 1870 (now Bhartiya Nyay Sanhita, 2023), a medical examination of the victim should be conducted and if she is found to be pregnant, she and her family members must be apprised of the legal process of termination of pregnancy. She should also be given counseling in a language which is known to her. The High Court of Delhi has stated that at the time of medical examination, mandatory tests for determination of pregnancy should be carried out and if the victim desires to terminate her pregnancy, she should be immediately produced before the Medical Board. All the necessary documentation should be expeditiously prepared so that when the case comes before the court, it does not waste any more time. The lack of medical boards was a significant hurdle observed by the Court, and accordingly, it ordered the State government to ensure that all government hospitals in the district have proper MTP centers and the medical boards should be mandatorily constituted at these hospitals (*Minor R* v. *State*, 2023).

### 8.1.7 Omission of International Law and the Misuse of Judicial Doctrines: The Arbitrary Denial of Abortion Rights at Late Stages of Pregnancy in Indian Case Law Following the 2021 Amendment

Despite substantial case law by Indian courts recognizing abortion rights after the 24-week limit, there is also a line of cases denying late-stage abortion access, in contravention of women´s fundamental rights. The decisions denying abortions at late stages often fail to consider Indian law and international obligations and, more so, tend to hide behind improvised judicial doctrines that ultimately infringe on the rights of women seeking to terminate their pregnancies.

The use of courts in determining abortion access reinforces the concerns of the United Nations and reproductive rights activists that the judicialization of abortion rights risks putting ideological beliefs over the health and personal autonomy of the female, as well as avoiding the obligations provided for under international human rights law. The overturning of *Roe v Wade* (1973) in the United States and the ensuing back and forth at state court levels is a case in point that reinforces the tenuous nature of abortion rights protection when courts are asked to decide on the matter.

Article 51 of the Constitution of India specifically recognizes the State's responsibility to promote and foster respect for international law and obligation arising from the signing or ratification of treaties by India. The Protection of Human Rights Act, 1993, domesticates international human rights law into the Indian legal framework. As discussed earlier, international human rights law recognizes under certain circumstances the right of women to terminate their pregnancies, including ALP. Furthermore, as discussed previously, the Indian Supreme Court has explicitly recognized the binding nature of human rights law on Indian courts when deciding on the issue of reproductive rights, noting that, "treaties and covenants ratified by India are binding on the State if they have secure and promote the fundamental rights guaranteed by the Constitution of India" (Para 124, in its decision X v. NCT Delhi case). This should be interpreted to mean that where Indian courts are faced with a question of termination of pregnancy, particularly where the life of the mother is at risk or the mother alleges mental suffering, courts should interpret domestic law in light of the guarantees found in international law.

Furthermore, even where the Indian courts may not necessarily identify an exact justification for the termination of pregnancy at later stages under the MTP Amendment, courts in India have margin and judicial coverage for prioritizing the personal autonomy or other fundamental rights of women. This is known as the doctrine of complete justice enshrined in Article 142 of the Constitution of India. According to *State v. Kalyan Singh* (2017: para 22), under the said provision of the Constitution, the Supreme Court has the obligation to do complete justice to the parties before it. In doing so, the Court may relax the law applicable to the parties, or, may even exempt the parties from the rigor of the law. However, this exercise should not lead to a miscarriage of justice and must be undertaken based on the facts and circumstances of each case.

Supported by international human rights law, the Courts could seek a broad interpretation of the MTP Amendment on grounds of personal autonomy and health, particularly in consideration of the difficult circumstances brought in front of courts by poor women petitioners who might otherwise resort to seeking an illegal abortion. Furthermore, considering the extremely high rate of maternal mortality resulting from non-abortion access in India, complete justice is an important doctrine to invoke under these circumstances, with the broader goal of protecting maternal health across India.

In the case of *X v. Union of India* (2023: para. 25), a poor woman failed to realize she was pregnant until approximately 24 weeks. She had previously sought permission at this point in her pregnancy but was denied under the MTP Amendment 2021. By the time this case arrived at the Supreme Court, she was almost 27 weeks pregnant. She argued for permission to terminate based on her postpartum depression and mental condition, and because her husband is the only wage earner in the family and due to the large number of dependents. Nevertheless, the Court in this case refuses to invoke complete justice, noting that, it "may not be attracted in every case." Instead, the court grounds its decision in the likely viability of the fetus and rejects, without very much consideration, the application of complete justice to this case.

A judgment under the complete justice doctrine read in the context of *Kalyan Singh*, would suggest that the Court could likely justify the granting of termination rights for this woman. This is because the complete justice doctrine places a duty on the court to seek justice if doing so would achieve the protection of fundamental rights under Indian constitutional law and international human rights law. *Kalyan Singh* (2017) allows for the relaxation of laws if, by doing so, the court would achieve the protection of rights. In addition, a broader, wide-ranging justice would also be achieved by providing a legal basis for the thousands of women in India each year who are forced to abort through back-alley providers.

In a similar judgment, the High Court of Bombay in *X.Y.Z v Union of India* (2024) denies a woman the right to terminate her late-stage pregnancy at nearly 27 weeks. The woman alleges that she suffers from poor mental and physical conditions and that her financial condition is poor because she is the sole breadwinner and has multiple dependents. In considering the medical reports of the doctors involved, including the psychiatrist who finds that she is fit to carry the fetus to term, the court denies the request.

It does so on grounds of what seems to be an ad hoc philosophy of "judicial conscience," prioritizing the potential life of the fetus over the rights of the mother and raising concerns over feticide, or what one scholar refers to as "the phantasm of feticide" (Tibrewala, 2024). The Court, while recognizing the extreme hardship of the woman and her right to personal autonomy, ultimately overcomes such consideration through a conscientious objector argument and raises the possibility of a current of "pro feotus" jurisprudence (Tibrewala, 2024).

Once again, the court fails to consider international human rights law, which would justify a reliance on Article 142 to ensure complete justice toward the protection of fundamental rights and to mitigate the anguish and burden the court recognizes this woman will have to bear. This conscientious objection approach takes the place of what should be a rights-centered analysis, in which woman´s rights are prioritized over the personal objections of the judges. International law on abortion rights specifically recognizes that conscientious objection should not be an obstacle to protecting women´s abortion rights. While this normally applies in the context of hospitals and medical facilities, the same is true of a court setting, where decisions must be decided on the merits and not based on personal bias.

Both examples demonstrate an overarching concern, as discussed previously, that the courts are not positioned to make decisions about when women should be able to terminate their pregnancies. And while many of the opinions of the Indian courts have properly upheld the spirit of the MTP and its Amendment 2021, there are also cases—and there will certainly be more—where weak judicial reasoning and personal opposition stand in the way of doing complete justice for the thousands of poor women who are required to carry to term their pregnancies, a right strongly grounded in international human rights law. And while the courts in both cases have advocated for adoption as the alternative to abortion, that carries with it tremendous suffering and hardship for women and should not be used by courts as the "go-to" option to justify the denial of abortion rights.

## 8.2 Conclusion

Looking ahead, the MTP Act should again undergo a modification to incorporate language that references the obligation of judges to interpret cases in accordance with international human rights law and the complete justice doctrine. By doing so, women seeking access to abortion at later stages would be less subject to the whims of arbitrary decision-making by judges. Courts would have less margin to rule through personal conviction and instead be required to act toward the fulfillment of justice found in accordance with Indian constitutional and international human rights principles.

Although abortion generates tremendous discord between advocates and opponents, including within the judicial system, the reality of maternal health in India needs to be at the center of judicial decision-making. The reality is that thousands of women, most of whom live in extreme poverty, lose their lives each year because of an inability to access safe, affordable, and legal abortions. The courts therefore cannot be a barrier toward protecting the health, lives, and fundamental rights of women seeking to terminate their pregnancies.

In addition to the alignment of the role of courts in the backdrop of the human and fundamental right of health, delays and complexities that arise due to the registered medical practitioners and medical boards should also be looked into. Registered medical practitioners should not fear criminal prosecution if they are acting in good faith. They must use the least invasive and modern practices for inducing abortions. This can be ensured through training and sensitization programs that should be spearheaded by the medical fraternity and advocates having medico-legal expertise. State governments should also expedite the process of setting up medical boards in every district, in consonance with the law and judicial orders, so that no time is lost first in their constitution and later in their decision-making.

By strengthening the language of the MTP Act to incorporate references to international law and the complete justice doctrine, setting up of medical boards and sensitization of registered medical practitioners, the Government would reaffirm its commitment to abortion rights and continue to improve maternal mortality outcomes across India.

## References

### *Cases*

CEDAW, General Recommendation No. 24: Article 12 (Women and Health), adopted in 1999.

CEDAW. (2015). Summary of the inquiry concerning the Philippines under article 8 of the Optional Protocol to the Convention on the Elimination of All Forms of Discrimination against Women. United Nations.

CEDAW. 2014. Concluding observations on the combined fourth and fifth periodic reports of India. CEDAW/C/IND/CO/4–5. United Nations.

CESCR. General Comment No. 22 on the Right to Sexual and Reproductive Health: Article 12 (Right of everyone to the enjoyment of the highest attainable standard of physical and mental health), adopted in 2016.

Convention on the Elimination of All Forms of Discrimination against Women (CEDAW). adopted 18 December 1979, 1249 U.N.T.S. 13, entered into force 3 September 1981.

Chandra, A., et al. (2021). Legal Barriers to Accessing Safe Abortion Services in India: A Fact-Finding Study [online]. Center for Reproductive Rights. https://reproductiverights.org/wp-content/uploads/2021/08/Legal-Barriers-to-Accessing-Safe-Abortion-Services-in-India_Final-for-upload.pdf. Accessed July 8, 2024.

Deo, S. (2020, March 17). *Lok Sabha, Third Session.* Parliament of India, Lok Sabha Digital Library. https://eparlib.nic.in/bitstream/123456789/794800/1/lsd_17_03_17-03-2020.pdf#search=abortion. Accessed July 10, 2024.

Erdman, J. N. (2023). The WHO abortion care guideline: Law and policy—Past, present, and future. *International Journal of Gynecology and Obstetrics, 162*(3), 1119–1124. https://doi.org/10.1002/ijgo.15017

Guttmacher Institute. India: Meeting the Needs for Services. https://www.who.int/news-room/fact-sheets/detail/abortion. Accessed July 4, 2024.

Haddad, L. B., & Nour, N. M. (2009, January 1). Unsafe abortion: unnecessary maternal mortality. PubMed Central (PMC). https://www.ncbi.nlm.nih.gov/pmc/articles/PMC2709326/.

HRC. K.L. v. Peru, CCPR/C/85/D/1153/2003, Communication No. 1153/2003.

Mellet, Amanda Jane v Ireland, Merits, UN Doc CCPR/C/116/D/2324/2013, IHRL 4106 (UNHRC 2016), 31st March 2016, United Nations [UN]; United Nations General Assembly [UNGA]; United Nations Human Rights Council [UNHRC].

Pietilä, H. (2007). The Unfinished Story of Women and the United Nations. UNCTAD/NGLS/2007/1. U.N. Non-Governmental Liaison Service.

Pillai, G. (2024, April 17). *India's push-and-pull on reproductive rights.* Published on Verfassungsblog on Matters Constitutional. https://verfassungsblog.de/indias-push-and-pull-on-reproductive-rights/. Accessed July 1, 2024.

Rao, S. (2023, November 2). Feminists in India laud their abortion rights—but they don't extend to Dalit women. *The Guardian.* https://www.theguardian.com/global-development/2022/aug/03/india-abortion-rights-dalit-women. Accessed July 7, 2024.

Ray, N. (2024, May 13). *In brief: unveiling the realities of laws on abortion in the Philippines.* Center for Reproductive Rights. https://reproductiverights.org/abortion-law-philippines-brief/

Shah. (1964). Ministry of Health and Family Planning, Report of the Committee to Study the Question of Legislation of Abortion.

Singh, S., Shekhar, C., Acharya, R., Moore, A. M., Stillman, M., Pradhan, M. R., Frost, J. J., Sahoo, H., Alagarajan, M., Hussain, R., Sundaram, A., Vlassoff, M., Kalyanwala, S., & Browne, A. (2018). The incidence of abortion and unintended pregnancy in India, 2015. *Global Health/The Lancet. Global Health, 6*(1), e111–e120. https://doi.org/10.1016/s2214-109x(17)30453-9

Tibrewala, M. (2024, January 25). Guest post: The phantasm of 'feticide'—On the Delhi High Court's abortion order in R v. Union of India on Constitutional Law and Philosophy. Accessed July 19, 2024.

UN General Assembly, Convention on the Elimination of All Forms of Discrimination Against Women, United Nations, Treaty Series, vol. 1249, p. 13, 18 December 1979.

UN Office of the High Commissioner for Human Rights (OHCHR), Reproductive Rights are Human Rights: A Handbook for National Human Rights Institutions Published jointly with UNFPA and the Danish Institute for Human Rights, HR/PUB/14/6, 2014. Accessed July 8, 2024.

UNHCR. General Comment No. 35: Article 9 (Liberty and Security of Persons), adopted in 2014.

UNHCR. General Comment No. 36: Article 6 (Right to Life), adopted in 2018.

United Nations Population Fund: UNFPA. (2022). The case for action in the neglected crisis of unintended pregnancy. https://www.unfpa.org/swp2022.

Van Der Meulen Rodgers, Y., Coast, E., Lattof, S. R., Poss, C., & Moore, B. (2021). The macroeconomics of abortion: A scoping review and analysis of the costs and outcomes. *PloSOne, 16*(5), Article e0250692. https://doi.org/10.1371/journal.pone.0250692

Venter, C. M. (2012). *International women's rights, equality, and justice: A context and practice casebook*. Carolina Academic Press.

World Health Organization: WHO. (2024, May 17). Abortion. https://www.who.int/news-room/fact-sheets/detail/abortion.

*A (Mother of X)* v. *State of Maharashtra* 2024 SCC Online SC 835.

*High Court on its Own Motion* v. *State of Maharashtra* (2016) 3 AIR Bom R (Cri) 575).

*Justice K.S. Puttaswamy (Retd.) & Anr.* v *Union of India &Ors.* AIR 2017 SC 4161

*Minor R Thr. Mother H* v. *State (NCT of Delhi)* (2023) 1 HCC (Del) 198.

*State* v. *Kalyan Singh* (2017) 7 SCC 444.

*Suchita Srivastava & Anr.* v. *Chandigarh Administration* (2009) 14 SCR 989.

*X* v *Principal Secretary, Health and Family Welfare Department, Government of NCT of Delhi & Anr* (2023) 9 SCC 433.

X v Union of India 2023 SCC Online SC 1338.

*X* v. State of Karnataka 2023 SCC Online Kar 75.

*X* v. *State of West Bengal* 2023 SCC OnLine Cal 2399.

*X* v. *State of West Bengal* 2023 SCC Online Cal 2609.

*X* v. *UoI represented by Secretary &Ors.* 2024 SCCOnline Ker 2135.

*X* v. *UT of J&K & Others* 2023 SCC Online J&K 197.

*X.Y.Z v Union of India* W.P. No. 8920 of 2024.

*X.Y.Z. v. Dean of B.J. Govt. Medical College and Sassoon Hospital through the Professor, HoD* and Ors W.P. No. 5123 of 2021.

*Z* v. *State of Bihar* (2018) 11 SCC 572.

# Chapter 9
# Empowering Choices: The State of Reproductive Rights for Women in India

**Rahul Jain** and **Kapil Bhati**

**Abstract** Women's reproductive rights primarily emphasize their reproductive choices. The right to women's overall health is reflected in women's rights to reproductive health and sexual freedom including the right to life, liberty, and security of the person; freedom from cruel, inhuman, or degrading treatment; to health care and information; and to be free of all forms of discrimination and coercion in the distribution of resources for health services, as well as their availability and accessibility. Therefore, the chapter frames a comprehensive and in-depth exploration of women's reproductive rights using both primary and secondary data. The key results of the chapter were: Early marriage is positively linked with low education of women. Contraceptive choices among less educated women were limited. Abortion legality awareness is low among women, irrespective of educational background. In conclusion, there is a need to focus on women's education to promote sexual and reproductive health (SRH) rights among Indian women. Concurrently, SRH literacy with a particular focus on abortion subject is need to focus in India.

**Keywords** Autonomy · Equality · Maternal health · Reproductive rights

## 9.1 Introduction

The concept of "reproductive health" was formally introduced by the World Health Organization during the late nineteenth century at the International Conference on Population and Development (ICPD) in Cairo, (Ghebreyesus & Kanem, 2018). Reproductive health encompasses the reproductive psycho-physical and social well-being. For a woman to achieve, maintain, and sustain her reproductive health, her sexual and reproductive rights must be respected, safeguarded, and upheld (World

R. Jain (✉) · K. Bhati
Research Scholar, Bennett University Greater Noida, Greater Noida, India
e-mail: l22solp0023@bennett.edu.in; gjrj239@gmail.com

K. Bhati
e-mail: l23solp0007@bennett.edu.in



P. Chouhan et al. (eds.), *Women's Health Dynamics in South Asia*, Asian Perspectives on Public Health, https://doi.org/10.1007/978-981-95-2321-4_9

Health Organization, 2018). The ICPD firmly established women's reproductive health rights and choices. The Conference affirmed women's right to access information about health options and to utilize services equivalent to those available to men, even if fulfilling such entitlements challenges traditional attitudes. Regarding reproductive freedom, an individual's personal beliefs should not impede their ability to responsibly choose safe and legal family planning methods. Furthermore, these rights to pregnancy and childbearing support a woman's health and the joy of motherhood (Shiva Kumar et al., 2013). Regarding the Indian context of reproductive health, a notable state-level variation in cesarean delivery existed. For instance, Tamil Nadu has the highest average rate of cesarean delivery at 36%, while Bihar reported the lowest rate at 7%. The excerpt focuses on the differences in cesarean delivery across regions and the underlying socio-economic and pregnancy-related factors affecting the differences. Understanding these factors will help in formulating effective policies for mitigating the nationwide uneven distribution of cesarean deliveries (Roy et al., 2021). Furthermore, there is a lack of research on the combination of homelessness, relocation, and maternal well-being, particularly in mega-urban areas. A recent study highlighted a higher prevalence of poor reproductive health among urban homeless in India, predominantly among migrants. The study also added that reproductive health rights and choices are also low among socio-economically marginalized women in India (Rahaman & Das, 2024). Regarding the family planning scenario in India, nearly 51% of women who wanted to postpone childbirth had an unmet need for contraception (UNC). Women's education, their decision-making power, and socio-economic status are some of the significant predictors of UNC in India (Rahaman et al., 2022b). Similarly, the unsafe abortion context highlights that rural women had a higher risk of unsafe abortions than their urban counterparts, which could be linked to the rural–urban gap in socio-cultural, economic, and healthcare accessibility (Rahaman et al., 2023). To overcome the burden of unmet needs for family planning and associated reproductive health vulnerability, a recent study coined that "family planning is indispensable for better health and the Sustainable Development Goals (SDGs) in India". Concurrently, a similar study recommends that there is a need for affordability, coverage, and acceptability of modern reversible contraceptives to ensure the reproductive health rights of Indian women. In addition, the ongoing debate focuses on promoting women's right to bodily autonomy with moral and ethical views on personhood (Shah, 2022). In these backgrounds, addressing the underlying reproductive health issues is crucial to achieving a "better India" (Arya et al., 2001). Based on the above discussion, the present chapter explored that reproductive health rights among women in India have still not been promoted as developed nations furnished them. While the existing literature is substantial in understanding the reproductive health rights (RHRs) in India, no previous study described it comprehensively by framing multi-dimensional segments of the reproductive health of women in India. With this backdrop, the present chapter presents a descriptive critical fabric of reproductive health in India to understand the underlying issues and draw the policy attention. Specifically, the objectives of the present chapter were: (a) to comprehend the significance and notion of reproductive rights. (b) to Review the Status quo of reproductive rights of women in the Indian context.

And (c) assess the relationship between women's autonomy and their control over reproductive rights.

## 9.2 Materials and Methods

### *9.2.1 Research Design*

A cross-sectional survey design was used to investigate how women's autonomy serves as a significant determinant of their control over reproductive rights. Survey research is valuable in this context due to its ability to efficiently gather a large amount of data on the relationship between attitudes and behaviors across various dimensions (Shaughnessy et al., 2011). Gautam Buddha Nagar, Greater Noida, is selected as a study area, purposively.

### *9.2.2 Data Collection Tools*

The primary survey included a total of 100 sampled women of reproductive age between 18 and 45 groups from the Gautam Buddha Nagar district, India. The information was gathered from both primary and secondary sources. Primary data was obtained through in-person face-to-face interviews. To support the study findings, several research articles, reports, periodicals, and books were also reviewed and added in this chapter. To enhance the validity of the present chapter, a structured questionnaire was used during the survey and selected sample using a random sampling technique.

### *9.2.3 Analyses*

Frequency and proportional distribution statistics were used. Specifically, the prevalence of age-specific marriage proportion, prevalence of contraception use, and percentage distribution of SRH awareness are calculated in this chapter to describe the SRH matters.

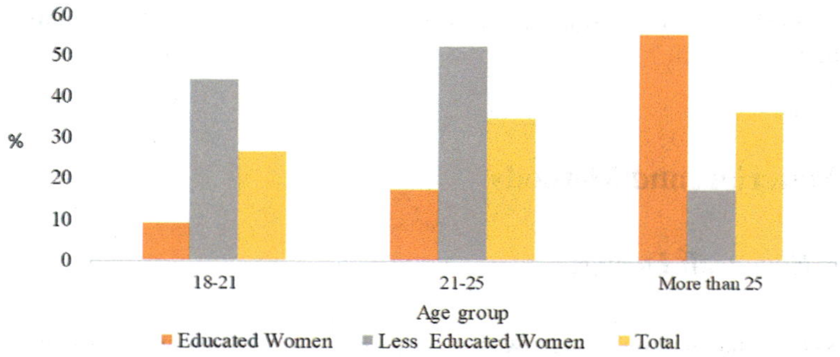


**Fig. 9.1** Age at marriage by education level among sampled women. *Source* Primary Field Survey, 2024

## 9.3 Results

### *9.3.1 Women's Education and Age at Marriage*

Figure 9.1 shows that the prevalence of marriage at early age was higher among less educated women than highly educated women. For example, the level of married women in the age group 18–22 was 44% among less educated women and 9% among highly educated women. Whereas, late-age marriage was found in 55% among educated women, which was 17% among less educated women (Fig. 9.1). A positive relation between education and late-age marriage was observed among the study population.

### *9.3.2 Women's Education and Contraception Choice*

There was substantial variation in patterns in contraception use with women's education (Fig. 9.2). Use of condom use 87% and 68%, among educated women and less educated women, respectively. A similar gap in oral pill (79% and 48%), IUD (40% and 31%), and female sterilization (81% and 57%) use was also found between educated and less educated women. A considerable variation was also observed regarding male sterilization and other contraception.

### *9.3.3 Women's Education and SRH Awareness*

Figure 9.3 reveals variation in SRH awareness among sampled highly educated women. Educated women in the study area exhibited sound knowledge of HIV/AIDS (52%), STIs/RTIs (51%), and contraceptive side effects (62%), with over half

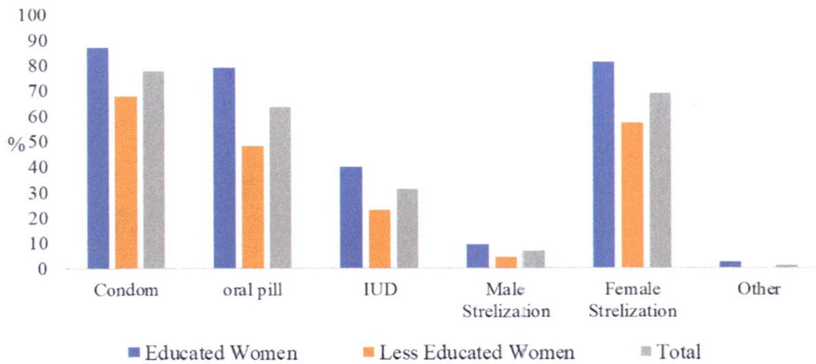


**Fig. 9.2** Contraception choices by women's education among sampled women. *Source* Primary Field Survey, 2024

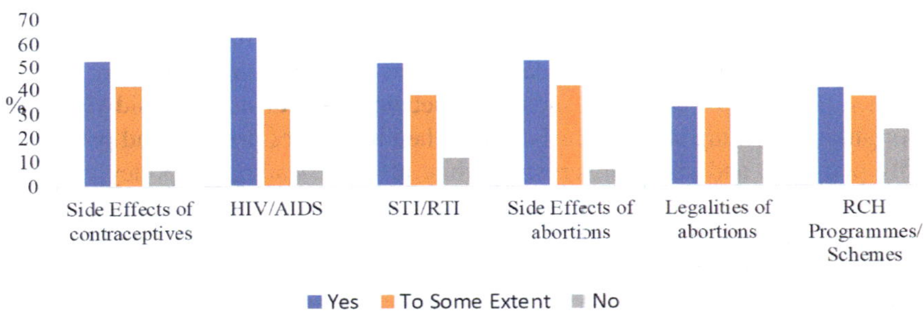


**Fig. 9.3** Sexual and reproductive health awareness among sampled highly educated women. *Source* Primary Field Survey, 2024

being well-informed side effects of abortion. However, they lacked awareness of the legality of induced abortion (32%). Regarding, the RCH programmers, only 40% were aware of the schemes.

In the context of less educated women, the chapter's result shows that only 18% of them were aware of the side effects of contraception (Fig. 9.4). Similar patterns were also observed regarding HIV/AIDS awareness (20%) and side effects of abortion (20%). Related to STI/RTI awareness was only 12% among the less educated women (Fig. 9.4).

### 9.3.4 *Role of Health Care Providers*

Healthcare providers and services are instrumental for a woman to be empowered in reproductive health because she must enjoy access to safe and legal abortions, contraceptives, maternal health, and comprehensive reproductive education (Hoyt

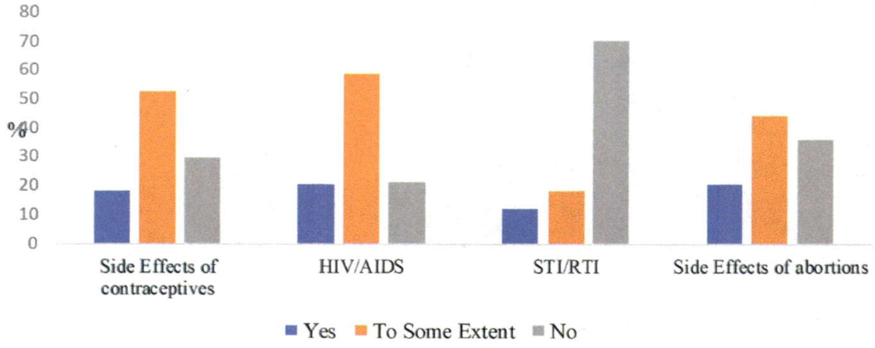


**Fig. 9.4** Sexual and reproductive health awareness among sampled less educated women. *Source* Primary Field Survey, 2024

et al., 2022; Yuan et al., 2019). For women to enjoy their rights fully, in the absence of stigma and bias, an accessible, affordable, and non-discriminating healthcare system is a must. Healthcare providers such as gynecologists, nurses, and midwives are important in providing comprehensive care when it involves prenatal and postnatal, family planning, and abortion services, while also advocating for policy changes and informed consent (Belachew, 2023; Lopes et al., 2022; Mare et al., 2022). Their role extends beyond clinical responsibilities to empower women with knowledge of reproductive health options and rights. Data from prior research has demonstrated that women making their decisions on matters related to contraceptive use tremendously improves reproductive health outcomes, even making them more effective in family planning and using contraceptives (Alspaugh et al., 2021; Håkansson et al., 2018).

The existence and accessibility of modern contraception, legal abortion, maternal and neonatal care, and sexual education create an environment that actively permits a woman to pursue her reproductive rights. Advancements in technology, such as telemedicine and mobile health clinics, will lessen accessibility burdens and further advance rural India concerning better health outcomes. The Indian government has taken up some initiatives, one of which is the Ayushman Bharat scheme, which claims to strengthen primary healthcare and protect the economically vulnerable; however, what is needed is far more, which addresses systemic issues that disrespect the rural healthcare infrastructure. The development of healthcare infrastructure simplifies the intervention process by providing transport facilities from villages to health centers, communication and technology, energy, irrigation, banking, and service facilities concerning economic development and health infrastructure. This will require governmental intervention to bridge the gap between the rural and urban healthcare infrastructure and guarantee an equitable distribution of essential services (Barbieri et al., 2021; Handebo, 2021). The systemic approach to reproductive health will increase value not only for individuals but also for society as a whole in improving maternal and child health outcomes and economic development (Asmamaw, 2024; Howett et al., 2021).

## 9.4 Discussion

The present chapter describes the SRH rights of women in India using micro-level data. To describe the SRH rights, the present chapter included age at marriage, contraception dynamics, and SRH awareness status among women as chapter components. Through the lens of women's education how the status of women's SRH varies is highlighted in the chapter. The present chapter displays that a significant relationship between education and marriage age is crucial for women's reproductive rights and choices. For instance, women with the least amount of education marry at a median age of 17.6 years, while those who have completed more than 11 years of schooling marry at a median age of 23 years. Higher education offers numerous advantages, including longer pursuit of academics, varied job opportunities, improved financial autonomy, and broadened life travel expeditions. Educated women often prioritize their personal and supportive life plans and strategies before considering marriage (Roy & Chouhan, 2021). Where less educated women frequently face early marriage due to limited economic prospects and cultural norms, further negatively affecting their reproductive health and family planning (Roy & Chouhan, 2022). This can significantly impact maternal and child health and educational attainment of future generations and perpetuate cycles of poverty (Ghebreyesus & Kanem, 2018). Promoting educational access for women is crucial to empower them and expand their life choices, thereby enhancing their reproductive rights (Santhya et al., 2010). Targeted interventions such as vocational training and awareness campaigns could support less educated women in delaying marriage if they choose to do so, ultimately contributing to better health and socio-economic outcomes. Early marriages often result in adolescent pregnancies, contributing to millions of cases of maternal illness and death annually, thereby exacerbating poverty (Mbizvo et al., 2023). This issue is particularly prevalent in rural areas. The health issues and fatalities are caused by bleeding and medical complications following unsafe abortions (Kumari et al., 2022). These can range from immediate problems to long-term consequences. Early marriage significantly reduces women's autonomy and control over reproductive health decisions (Preusse et al., 2014). Despite government efforts to improve adolescent well-being and access to contraception, many young wives still choose termination over preventive measures due to cultural taboos surrounding non-procreative intimacy. There is a need for a nuanced understanding of reproductive agency, suggesting that addressing societal stigmas and improving access to safe termination services are crucial for empowering young wives and preventing unintended pregnancies (Bhattacharya, 2019). However, the RCH policy does not provide adequate guidance for young people entering their fertile years, leaving their needs unmet. Schools and colleges are easy entry points to disseminate information on RTIs/STDs, sexual abuse, sexual health, sexual and reproductive rights, contraceptive options, family planning, safe abortion practices as well as gender awareness; but this has not been taken proper care of in the special RCH package launched by the government. In India, sexual education has not yet been incorporated into the school curriculum (Epstein et al., 2023).

The present chapter found that the use of reversible contraception is limited among less educated women. Therefore, the issue related to the skewness of reversible contraception use in India indirectly indicates that the reproductive rights of women in India are limited. In particular, the RCH is more limited to vulnerable women like the homeless (Rahaman & Das, 2024). Therefore, the previous study suggests that there is a need for targeted policy attention to ensure women's family planning methods choices in India. For effective outreach to RCH services, NGOs, self-help groups, voluntary organizations, and the media could be beneficial. Innovative strategies to engage youth and provide vital information on safe sex practices are crucial. The "*Condom Bindaas Bol*" campaign (Eager, 2004). Reproductive and child health policies should focus on ensuring universal access to services, promoting gender equality, respecting all sexual orientations, and protecting women's rights. (Shalev, 2000). A purely medical approach to reproductive rights ignores the realities of inequality and fails to consider issues of choice and lack of independence. Moving forward, policies must account for the diverse human experience and be designed to support the unique circumstances of every individual in the population, which enables personal advancement, regardless of debates about their suitability (Frohmader & Ortoleva, 2014). However, providing and asking for consent and bodily autonomy in general, for individual sexual experiences and decisions, demand respect and permission from all parties involved (Bhattacharya, 2019). Women have the right to autonomy over their reproductive health, including unobstructed access to safe birth control and the authority to make self-directed choices regarding pregnancy (Bagade et al., 2014). This self-determination is crucial for their safety, development, and active involvement in society (Ryan & Deci, 2020). Providing basic reproductive services is essential to prevent maternal mortality and improve health outcomes. (Fleszar et al., 2023) Empowering women leads to better health and educational outcomes for their children, breaking the cycle of deprivation (Nicholson et al., 2023). Upholding their legal rights ensures a just society where they have the same opportunities as men to thrive and contribute to India's progression (Epstein et al., 2023).

The present chapter also found that SRH awareness is also very limited among women, particularly about the legality of abortion care. As a result, 15 million unsafe abortions were reported in India, where 2 million reported accessibility issues of contraception. Additionally, 78% of adolescents with an abortion history reported unsafe performance of the abortion, resulting in 190,000 adolescents without post-abortion treatment (Seth, 2022). Indian state's policy on RHR controlling over individual's SRH rights (Senderowicz & Maloney, 2022). Gender-based violence is treated as a peripheral issue in India's public health system, which views it primarily as a law-and-order problem, despite international guidelines and its significant health consequences (Keith et al., 2022). Consequently, there is a need for safe abortion services in India due to the high rate of unwanted pregnancies and associated maternal deaths (Rahaman et al., 2023). In summary, restricting women's reproductive choices negatively impacts their health, equality, freedom, and quality of life. When safe and legal abortion services are unavailable, women are denied access to critical healthcare like contraception, prenatal care, and safe post-abortion care. The lack of partner support for reproductive agency and equal power is also violated (Ishola et al., 2021). India's commitment to the Family Planning 2030 alliance to expand contraceptive options is a "transformative moment" in advancing women's rights and their ability to self-govern and is expected to increase the use of modern preventive techniques (Yarger et al., 2022). Furthermore, according to the latest NFHS-5 data, only 10% of women in India can independently make decisions about their health, and 11% believe it is acceptable for husbands to use force if a wife refuses to have sex (Tripathi et al., 2023) A substantial proportion of pregnancies in India are unintended, with 49% classified as unplanned. This is exacerbated by non-medical abortions, as 78% of the 15 million abortions occur outside medical facilities (Wallin, 2019). More than 30 million married women of childbearing age lack access to contraception, and around 2 million adolescent girls do not have access to modern contraception. Only a few women receive recommendations for parental checkups. The Indian government has historically focused on controlling population size rather than protecting reproductive rights (Huzaimah et al., 2023). This has resulted in inadequate efforts to ensure universal access to abortion and contraception. Gender-based violence is treated as a law-and-order issue with little impact on women's health (Keith et al., 2022). Non-medical abortions are the leading cause of maternal mortality, with 8 women dying each day, and two-thirds of abortions between 2007 and 2011 classified as unsafe (Wang et al., 2023). The availability of reproductive health services is often constrained by systemic barriers in healthcare systems. For instance, this study reveals that in many regions of the Gautam Buddha district, there is a shortage of trained healthcare providers capable of offering the entire range of reproductive health services, including family planning and the provision of safe abortion care. Political and legal barriers restricting access to these services sharpen the effects of such a shortage, especially in countries where abortion is still criminalized. For instance, in South Africa, despite a supportive legal framework for reproductive rights, many women seeking termination of pregnancy do so outside designated health facilities due to a lack of awareness of their rights and the services available to them (Kaswa & Yogeswaran, 2020). This brings to light a serious gap between policy and practice where even in supportive legal environments, the practical availability of services remains dependent on the needs of women. This study also highlights the neglect of proper women's healthcare and the growing demand for personal autonomy and rights. The present chapter recommends that India should focus on the promotion of women's SRH rights and affordable, accessible, and client-choice-based SRH services to achieve a "healthy India".

## 9.5 Conclusion

The present chapter summary concludes that women's education is an instrument for promoting SRH rights. Findings suggest that the issues of early marriage, lack of contraception choice, and unawareness of SRH matters are considerably high among uneducated or less educated women. Although, the level of education increased significantly in India, the existence of a high proportion of illiterate or less educated women in India attending focus on SRH literacy among them. Among the SRH domains, the awareness regarding abortion legality is found to be considerable, which indicates that there is a need to focus on abortion legality and services campaigns in India.

## References

Arya, S., Menon, N., & Lokaneeta, J. (Eds.). (2001). *Reproductive rights in the Indian context: An introduction*. Saheli Women's Resource Centre.

Asmamaw, D. (2024). Married women decision-making autonomy on contraceptive use in east africa: a multilevel analysis of recent demographic and health survey. *Sage Open, 14*(1). https://doi.org/10.1177/21582440241236567

Alspaugh, A., Reibel, M., & Barroso, J. (2021). "Since i'm a little bit more mature": contraception and the arc of time for women in midlife. *Women S Midlife Health, 7*(1). https://doi.org/10.1186/s40695-021-00062

Bagade, O., Pawar, V., Patel, R., Patel, B., Awasarkar, V., & Diwate, S. (2014). Increasing use of long acting reversible contraception: Safe, reliable, and cost-effective birth control. *World Journal of Pharmacy and Pharmaceutical Sciences, 3*(10), 364–392.

Bhattacharya, S. (2019). Respect for autonomy is the ethical principle associated with enabling patients to make their own healthcare decisions. *Patient Education and Counseling, 102*(9), 1736–1737. https://doi.org/10.1016/j.pec.2019.06.005

Barbieri, M., Herculano, T., Silva, A., Bahamondes, L., Juliato, C., & Surita, F. (2021). Acceptability of ENG-releasing subdermal implants among postpartum Brazilian young women during the covid-19 pandemic. *International Journal of Gynecology & Obstetrics, 154*(1), 106–112. https://doi.org/10.1002/ijgo.13663

Belachew, T. (2023). Married women's decision-making autonomy on modern contraceptive use and its associated factors in high fertile sub-Saharan Africa countries: a multi-level analysis of demographic and health surveys. *Archives of Public Health, 81*(1). https://doi.org/10.1186/s13690-023-01210-3

Eager, P. W. (2004). From population control to reproductive rights: Understanding normative change in global population policy (1965–1994). *Global Society, 18*(2), 145–173. https://doi.org/10.1080/1360082042000207483

Epstein, Y., Ellison, A. M., Echeverría, H., & Abbott, J. K. (2023). Science and the legal rights of nature. *Science, 380*(6646). https://doi.org/10.1126/science.adf4155

Fleszar, L. G., Bryant, A. S., Johnson, C. O., Blacker, B. F., Aravkin, A., Baumann, M., Dwyer-Lindgren, L., Kelly, Y. O., Maass, K., Zheng, P., & Roth, G. A. (2023). Trends in state-level maternal mortality by Racial and Ethnic Group in the United States. *JAMA, 330*(1), 52–61. https://doi.org/10.1001/jama.2023.9043

Frohmader, C., & Ortoleva, S. (2014, July). The sexual and reproductive rights of women and girls with disabilities. In ICPD *International Conference on Population and Development Beyond*.

Ghebreyesus, T. A., & Kanem, N. (2018). Defining sexual and reproductive health and rights for all. *The Lancet, 391*(10140), 2583–2585. https://doi.org/10.1016/s0140-6736(18)30901-2

Hirve, S. S. (2004). Abortion law, policy and services in India: A critical review. *Reproductive Health Matters, 12*(sup24), 114–121. https://doi.org/10.1016/s0968-8080(04)24017-4

Huzaimah, A., Abdillah, M., Laila, N. Q., Tamudin, M., & Astuti, T. M. P. (2023). Disregarding the reproductive rights of women in child marriage in Indonesia. *Samarah: Jurnal Hukum Keluarga Dan Hukum Islam, 7*(2), 1097–1120. https://doi.org/10.22373/sjhk.v7i2.17392

Howett, R., Krogstad, E., Badubi, O., Gertz, A., Bawn, C., Mussa, A., … & Morroni, C. (2021). Experiences of accessing and providing contraceptive implant removal services in Gaborone,

Botswana: A qualitative study among implant users and healthcare providers. *Frontiers in Global Women S Health, 2*. https://doi.org/10.3389/fgwh.2021.684694

Handebo, S. (2021). Informed choice of contraceptive methods among women in Ethiopia: further analysis of the 2016 Ethiopian demographic health survey. *Open Access Journal of Contraception, 12*, 83–91. https://doi.org/10.2147/oajc.s292923

Håkansson, M., Oguttu, M., Gemzell-Danielsson, K., & Makenzius, M. (2018). Human rights versus societal norms: A mixed methods study among healthcare providers on social stigma related to adolescent abortion and contraceptive use in Kisumu, Kenya. *BMJ Global Health, 3*(2), Article e000608. https://doi.org/10.1136/bmjgh-2017-000608

Hoyt, J., Hamon, J., Krishnaratne, S., Houndekon, E., Curry, D., Mbembe, M., ... & Webster, J. (2022). "It was my own decision": The transformational shift that influences a woman's decision to use contraceptives covertly. *BMC Women S Health, 22*(1). https://doi.org/10.1186/s12905-022-01731-z

Ishola, F., Ukah, U. V., & Nandi, A. (2021). Impact of abortion law reforms on women's health services and outcomes: A systematic review protocol. *Systematic Reviews, 10*(1).https://doi.org/10.1186/s13643-021-01739-w

Keith, T., Hyslop, F., & Richmond, R. (2022). A systematic review of interventions to reduce gender-based violence among women and girls in sub-Saharan Africa. *Trauma, Violence, & Abuse, 24*(3), 1443–1464. https://doi.org/10.1177/15248380211068136

Kumari, S., Singh, M., Goswami, S., Gupta, E., Sharma, P., Gupta, V.,... Kishore, J. (2022). Have the relaxations in legislation related to termination of pregnancy made abortions safe in India? A metaanalysis on the prevalence of unsafe abortions among 15–49-year-old females in India. *CHRISMED Journal of Health and Research, 9*.

Kaswa, R., & Yogeswaran, P. (2020). Abortion reforms in South Africa: an overview of the choice on termination of pregnancy act. *South African Family Practice, 62*(1). https://doi.org/10.4102/safp.v62i1.5240

Lopes, S., Constant, D., Fraga, S., & Harries, J. (2022). How women's empowerment influences fertility-related outcomes and contraceptive practices: A cross-sectional study in Mozambique. *Plos Global Public Health, 2*(9), Article e0000670. https://doi.org/10.1371/journal.pgph.0000670

Mare, K., Aychiluhm, S., Tadesse, A., & Abdu, M. (2022). Married women's decision-making autonomy on contraceptive use and its associated factors in Ethiopia: A multilevel analysis of 2016 demographic and health survey. *Sage Open Medicine, 10*. https://doi.org/10.1177/20503121211068719

Mbizvo, M. T., Kasonda, K., Muntalima, N.-C., Rosen, J. G., Inambwae, S., Namukonda, E. S., Mungoni, R., Okpara, N., Phiri, C., Chelwa, N., & Kangale, C. (2023). Comprehensive sexuality education linked to sexual and reproductive health services reduces early and unintended pregnancies among in-school adolescent girls in Zambia. *BMC Public Health, 23*(1). https://doi.org/10.1186/s12889-023-15023-0

Medical Termination of Pregnancy (MTP) Amendment Act § Act 08 of 2021.

Nicholson, S. E., Pasque, P. A., & Sax, L. J. (2023). *Empowering women in higher education and student affairs*. https://doi.org/10.4324/9781003444442

Preusse, C., Gammill, H., Ma, K. K., Li, C. I., McDougall, J., Mahoney, D., & Gadi, V. (2014). PO40 Reproductive health decisions following breast cancer diagnosis. *The Breast, 23*.

Rahaman, M., & Das, K. C. (2024). Differentials in self-reported health status and healthcare utilization among homeless women during the antenatal period in urban settings: Does migration status matter? *Journal of Migration and Health, 10*, Article 100246. https://doi.org/10.1016/j.jmh.2024.100246

Rahaman, M., Rana, M. J., Roy, A., & Chouhan, P. (2022a). Spatial heterogeneity and socio-economic correlates of unmet need for spacing contraception in India: Evidences from National Family Health Survey, 2015–16. *Clinical Epidemiology and Global Health, 15*, 101012. https://doi.org/10.1016/j.cegh.2022.101012

Rahaman, M., Singh, R., Chouhan, P., Roy, A., Ajmer, S., & Rana, M. J. (2022b). Levels, patterns and determinants of using reversible contraceptives for limiting family planning in India: Evidence from National Family Health Survey, 2015–16. *BMC Women's Health, 22*(1). https://doi.org/10.1186/s12905-022-01706-0

Rahaman, M., Roy, A., Chouhan, P., Das, K. C., & Rana, M. J. (2023). Revisiting the predisposing, enabling, and need factors of unsafe abortion in India using the Heckman Probit model. *Journal of Biosocial Science*, 1–21. https://doi.org/10.1017/S002193202300024X

Roy, A., & Chouhan, P. (2021). Girl child marriage in Malda district of West Bengal: Analysis of prevalence and socio-economic factors. *Vulnerable Children and Youth Studies, 16*(4), 293–306.

Roy, A., & Chouhan, P. (2022). Exploring the socioeconomic factors associated with girl child marriage and its impact on pregnancy outcomes: A study from Malda District of West Bengal. *Indian Journal of Community Medicine, 47*(1), 8–11.

Roy, A., Paul, P., Chouhan, P., Rahaman, M., & Kapasia, N. (2021). Geographical variability and factors associated with caesarean section delivery in India: a comparative assessment of Bihar and Tamil Nadu. *BMC Public Health, 21*(1). https://doi.org/10.1186/s12889-021-11750-4

Ryan, R. M., & Deci, E. L. (2020). Intrinsic and extrinsic motivation from a self-determination theory perspective: Definitions, theory, practices, and future directions. *Contemporary Educational Psychology, 61*(1), 1–11. https://doi.org/10.1016/j.cedpsych.2020.101860

Santhya, K. G., Ram, U., Acharya, R., Jejeebhoy, S. J., Ram, F., & Singh, A. (2010). Associations between early marriage and young women's marital and reproductive health outcomes: Evidence from India. *International Perspectives on Sexual and Reproductive Health,* 36(3), 132–139. https://doi.org/10.1363/ipsrh.36.132.10

Senderowicz, L., & Maloney, N. (2022). Supply-side versus demand-side unmet need: Implications for family planning programs. *Population and Development Review, 48*, 689–722. https://doi.org/10.1111/padr.12478

Seth, A. (2022, April 28). Sexual and Reproductive Health Rights (SRHR) in India [Part 1]. *The Times of India.* https://timesofindia.indiatimes.com/blogs/nonpartisan-perspectives/sexual-and-reproductive-healthrights-srhr-in-india-part-1/

Shah, K. H. (2022). Induced abortion across the world and evolution of medical termination of pregnancy law in India: A review. *Journal of South Asian Federation of Obstetrics and Gynaecology, 13*(6), 426–430. https://doi.org/10.5005/jp-journals-10006-1971

Shalev, C. (2000). Rights to sexual and reproductive health: The ICPD and the convention on the elimination of all forms of discrimination against women. *Health and Human Rights, 4*(2), 38. https://doi.org/10.2307/4065196

Shaughnessy, J., Zechmeister, E., & Jeanne, Z. (2011). *Research methods in psychology* (9th ed.). McGraw Hill.

Shaw, A. (2004). Attitudes to genetic diagnosis and to the use of medical technologies in pregnancy: Some British Pakistani perspectives. In M. Unnithan-Kumar (Ed.), *Reproductive agency, medicine, and the state: Cultural transformations in childbearing* (pp. 25–57). Berghahn Books.

Shiva Kumar, A. K., Panda, P., & Ved, R. R. (2013). *Handbook of population and development in India.* Oxford University Press.

Tripathi, S., Pathak, V. K., & Lahariya, C. (2023). Key findings from NFHS-5 India report: Observing trends of health indicators between NFHS-4 and NFHS-5. *Journal of Family Medicine and Primary Care, 12*(9), 1759–1763. https://doi.org/10.4103/jfmpc.jfmpc_377_23

Wallin, A. (2019). *The compatibility of prenatal sex selection with international human rights law: The causes and regulation of non-medical sex selective abortions.*

Wang, S., Rexrode, K., Florio, A. A., Rich-Edwards, J., & Chavarro, J. (2023). Maternal mortality in the United States: Trends and opportunities for prevention. *Annual Review of Medicine, 74*, 199–216. https://doi.org/10.1146/annurev-med-042921-123851

World Health Organization. (2018, August 27). *Reproductive health.* Who.int; World Health Organization: WHO. https://www.who.int/westernpacific/health-topics/reproductive-health

Yarger, J., Schroeder, R., Cabral, M. A., Lamme, J. S., McCulloch, C. E., Trieu, S. L., de Jounge, A., & Harper, C. C. (2022). An educational intervention to raise awareness of contraceptive options among young people. *Journal of Women's Health, 31*(2), 252–260. https://doi.org/10.1089/jwh.2020.8753

Yuan, B., Li, J., & Wang, Z. (2019). The development of global women's rights and improvements in reproductive health intervention access of females with different socio-economic status. *International Journal of Environmental Research and Public Health, 16*(23), 4783. https://doi.org/10.3390/ijerph16234783

# Chapter 10
# Correlates of Maternal and Child Health in Ernakulam, Kerala, India: A Geospatial Approach

**M. A. Arya, R. Jegankumar, S. Syama, K. Arun, and R. S. Libina**

**Abstract** The state of Kerala, despite its high Human Development Index, still experiences disparities in maternal and child health. This research aims to shed light on the social vulnerabilities that contribute to these discrepancies, specifically within the Ernakulam district and underscores the importance of addressing spatial disparities in maternal and child health. By utilizing WorldPop data, this study seeks to identify key indicators of social vulnerability among mothers and children under the demographic, socio-economic, and healthcare facets by employing geospatial techniques like zonal statistics and overlay analysis using ArcGIS software. The findings revealed profound disadvantages concerning social vulnerability towards maternal-child development within the district, particularly within the Kothamangalam taluk, where the vulnerability status is extremely high. By identifying high-risk areas, policymakers can implement targeted interventions to improve the well-being of mothers and children, ultimately promoting social equity and resilience.

**Keywords** Maternal and child health · Social vulnerability' zonal statistics · Overlay analysis

M. A. Arya (✉)
Research Scholar (UGC - SRF), Department of Geography, Bharathidasan University, Tiruchirappalli, India
e-mail: arya.m.a@bdu.ac.in

R. Jegankumar
Professor and Head, Department of Geography, Bharathidasan University, Tiruchirappalli, India
e-mail: jegankumar@bdu.ac.in

S. Syama · K. Arun
MTech Geoinformatics Student, Department of Geography, Bharathidasan University, Tiruchirappalli, India
e-mail: syamacs24@gmail.com

K. Arun
e-mail: arunjr000@gmail.com

R. S. Libina
Research Scholar, Department of Geography, Bharathidasan University, Tiruchirappalli, India
e-mail: libina001@gmail.com



P. Chouhan et al. (eds.), *Women's Health Dynamics in South Asia*, Asian Perspectives on Public Health, https://doi.org/10.1007/978-981-95-2321-4_10

## 10.1 Introduction

Mothers and children, particularly in underdeveloped and developing nations, encounter vulnerabilities caused by a combination of prevailing demographic, social, economic influences that can lead to various vulnerabilities impacting their physical well-being, mental health, and overall social development. Ernakulam District in Kerala, India embodies a socially intricate terrain where different communities have differing levels of vulnerability. Mothers and children are regarded as especially vulnerable groups who confront the intersectional challenges at both individual and community-wide levels due to their biological dependence, developmental needs, and their restricted ability to choose and control their circumstances. It is imperative to comprehend these one-of-a-kind obstacles experienced by mothers and children since they aid in creating efficient measures that aim to promote equity alongside resilience.

In recent years, social vulnerability research pertaining to mothers and children has seen significant growth. Multiple studies have investigated various facets such as socio-economic hardship (Evans & Wachsmuth, 2013), restricted access to health-care and education (Sankoh et al., 2017), exposure to environmental risks (Basu et al., 2019) along with inadequate support networks around them (Benner et al., 2021). Commonly mentioned factors contributing to socio-economic disparities, include poverty, limited educational achievement, and inadequate healthcare access (Sebastian & Jayan, 2018; Radhakrishnan & Nair, 2020). Living conditions play a crucial role in increasing vulnerability, especially for marginalized individuals. Subpar housing, overcrowding and lack of essential services are some factors that contribute to the same (Gokhale & Menon, 2019). Women's access to resources and decision-making authority are unconventionally influenced by patriarchal norms and discriminatory practices, subsequently impacting their own well-being as well as that of their children. This highlights the dynamics of gender (Radhakrishnan, 2016). There exists a pivotal impact of variables such as access to healthcare services, household income, and maternal education on shaping the overall wellness outcomes for mothers and children. The intricate relationship between socio-demographic factors and MCH outcomes has been extensively studied across diverse contexts (Marmot & Wilkinson, 2006; Braveman & Gottlieb, 2014). Several health issues such as inadequate diet, absence of hygienic water and sanitation facilities, and insufficient awareness about proper hygiene practices can result in maternal and child health complications (Kurian & John, 2017).

Kerala has a low infant mortality rate of 6%, a high doctor-population ratio, and a network of hospitals and clinics, contributing to favourable maternal health; Kerala's Maternal Mortality Ratio (MMR) is considerably lower than the countrywide benchmark at 19%. However, healthcare accessibility discrepancies exist between urban and rural areas, and socio-demographic factors like economic disparities and cultural barriers may hinder some mothers from seeking healthcare services, potentially impacting regional maternal health outcomes.

With 68.04% of its population residing in urban areas, Ernakulam is among the most highly urbanized districts in Kerala (Census of India, 2011). Despite potentially positive developments such as improved healthcare access for mothers and children, this trend may also yield negative effects like heightened living expenses and social isolation concerns. While boasting a robust economy bolstered by the IT services industry's presence to some extent, income disparity remains prevalent throughout the area (Kerala State Planning Board, n.d.). This inequality can create obstacles that impede certain families' ability to procure quality nutrition and medical care. Moreover, Kerala's low Total Fertility Rate (TFR) of 1.46 marks an impactful socio-demographic development with lasting implications for maternal and child-related support systems (Family Registration System SRS Report 2020). However, Ernakulam holds high female literacy rates at 91.18% (Census of India, 2011), positioning it favourably towards better outcomes relating to health metrics. Meanwhile, evidence data proceeds further centralizing accomplishments made towards reducing infant mortality within Kerala in recent years. Although specific district data pertaining to IMR may not be readily available, measures portend well regarding improving overall infant survival chances in Ernakulam compared to the state average. Ernakulam's maternal mortality rate data may be limited to just the district level, akin to IMR. Nevertheless, Kerala has an MMR of 19, which indicates a favourable trend in achieving positive outcomes for maternal healthcare (National Health Systems Resource Centre, 2021).

Studies indicate that undernutrition still persists in certain pockets of children residing in Kerala (Headey & Babu, 2016). Despite having good infrastructure for healthcare in Ernakulam, areas with uneven urban–rural distributions might face challenges when accessing it. Ernakulam's coastal location makes it susceptible to natural disasters, posing a hazard that increases the vulnerability of women and children (Rao & Nair, 2022). There exist notable differences among socio-demographic groups in their access to and utilization of antenatal care services (Ramachandran et al., 2013; Sebastian & Jayan, 2018). Such research emphasizes the need for multifaceted approaches taking into account social vulnerabilities. Additionally, studies have called for considering district-specific spatial variations and specific populations like single mothers (Jayadevan & Joseph, 2023; Menon & Pillai, 2021). To enhance decision-making power among women in Ernakulam microfinance programs community engagement should be initiated along with skill development courses (Joseph & Mathew, 2019). The establishment of additional healthcare facilities, implementation of child nutrition programs, and the assurance of safe homes are vital actions to undertake (Gopal & Nair, 2020). Nevertheless, this line of exploration has primarily revolved around national or regional contexts instead of specific investigations into the vulnerabilities faced by urban populations in diverse settings like Ernakulam, India.

The present study explores the social vulnerability status of mothers and children in Ernakulam District, focusing on key social, demographic, and health factors. It contributes to existing knowledge and has policy implications for tailored interventions and strategies, thereby building a more resilient and equitable society.

## 10.2 Materials and Methods

This study utilizes secondary data for the year obtained from WorldPop, an open-source, high-resolution demographic, social, and environmental dataset platform. Although using the latest census data would be optimal, WorldPop 2015–16 data remains important in the current scenario for assessing socio-demographic and health factors in Ernakulam district. This is because it provides valuable insights in the absence of the recent census enumeration, enabling researchers to identify trends and potential problem areas related to maternal and child welfare. Although the exact sample size for the Ernakulam district is not explicitly stated within the dataset, the estimates are based on robust methodologies that ensure accuracy at fine spatial scales. The WorldPop project states that the estimations along with their associated uncertainties, measured as standard deviations (SD), are calculated following the methodology detailed in Utazi et al. (2021, 2022, 2023). The WorldPop project uses a combination of machine learning and statistical interpolation methods to produce population distributions, which are then validated against known population counts. Data on key indicators with a spatial resolution of 1 km, namely, 'demographic', 'health', and 'socio-economic' facets were taken for the study, including sub-indicators like 'Proportion of children aged 12–23 months born to large ($\geq$ 9 members) households', 'Children born to mothers who did not attend antenatal care (ANC)', 'Children born to mothers who did not receive/recall post-natal care within 2 months after birth', 'Mothers with no health insurance', 'Children—not delivered by a skilled birth attendant', 'Children underweight (malnutrition)', 'Children born to poorest/poor households according to DHS /MICS—NICS classifications', 'Born to mothers who had no formal education', and 'Proportion of women aged 15–49 years who did not participate in decision making in their households' were considered along with additional variables like 'women of child bearing age (15–49 years old)', 'No. of live births', and 'No. of pregnancies' (Fig. 10.1). Although 1 km resolution gridded data may not capture the intricate characteristics of each location in Ernakulam District, it still significantly represents socio-demographic and health factors on a larger scale.

As the value of each indicator increases, favourable conditions for the quality of life of mothers & children decrease, leading to an overall increase in degree of vulnerability. Zonal statistics and overlay analysis using ArcGIS 10.5 have been used for analysing the data where the variables were categorized accordingly into five groups, namely: Extremely/Very-High/Good, High/Good, Medium, Low/Poor, and Extremely/Very-Low/Poor. This was based on quantile classification which ensures an equal representation, providing a statistically robust analysis of the spatial pattern of variable distribution. This aided in figuring out the interplay or association they have in the context of social vulnerability among the mothers and children in Ernakulam District. Utilizing ArcGIS, zonal statistics and overlay analysis offers potent means for comprehending the spatial correlations amid maternal and child health outcomes along with development indicators. These techniques allow researchers to locate vulnerable regions by superimposing relevant datasets,

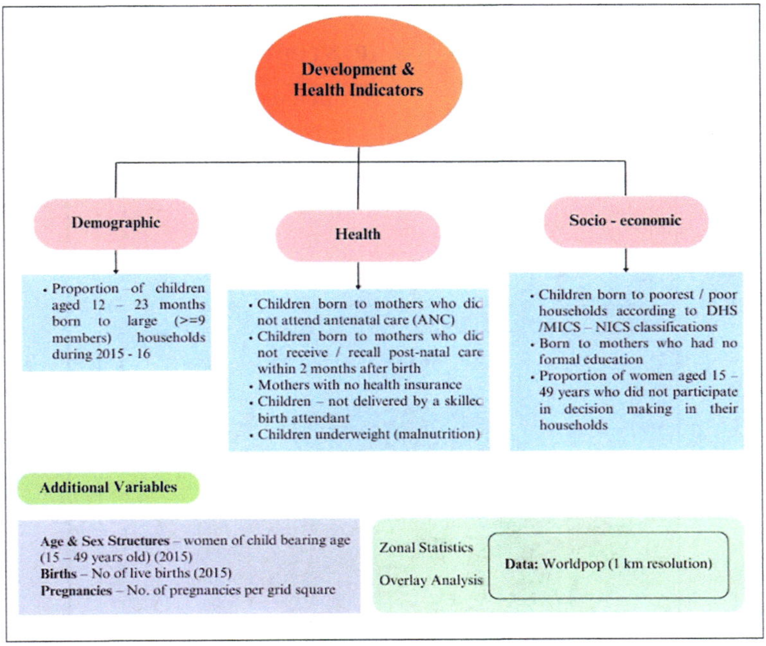


**Fig. 10.1** Conceptual framework of the study

highlighting disparities as well as suggesting targeted interventions. Policymakers can leverage these analyses to effectively allocate resources leading towards better maternal and child healthcare results while providing valuable insights into it.

### *10.2.1 About the Study Area*

The district of Ernakulam encompasses approximately 7.9% of the state's total land area, situated within latitudes 9° 47′ N to 10° 18′ N and longitudes 76° 9′ E to77° 6′ E, with borders shared by Thrissur, Idukki, Kottayam, and Alappuzha districts (SPB, n.d.). According to 2011 census, the total population of the district is 3,282,388, out of which 16,62,831 are females (Government of Kerala, 2011). The population of children aged 0–6 years in the Ernakulam District is a total of 304,242, which accounts for approximately 9% of the entire population. Of this number, there are roughly 155,182 male and 1,49,060 female children (Census India, 2011). Comprising of 7 taluks (Fig. 10.2) and a total of 124 villages, the district is made up of two revenue divisions. Muvattupuzha revenue division covers Kothamangalam, Muvattupuzha, and Kunnathunad taluks with its 53 villages; while Fort Kochi's revenue division

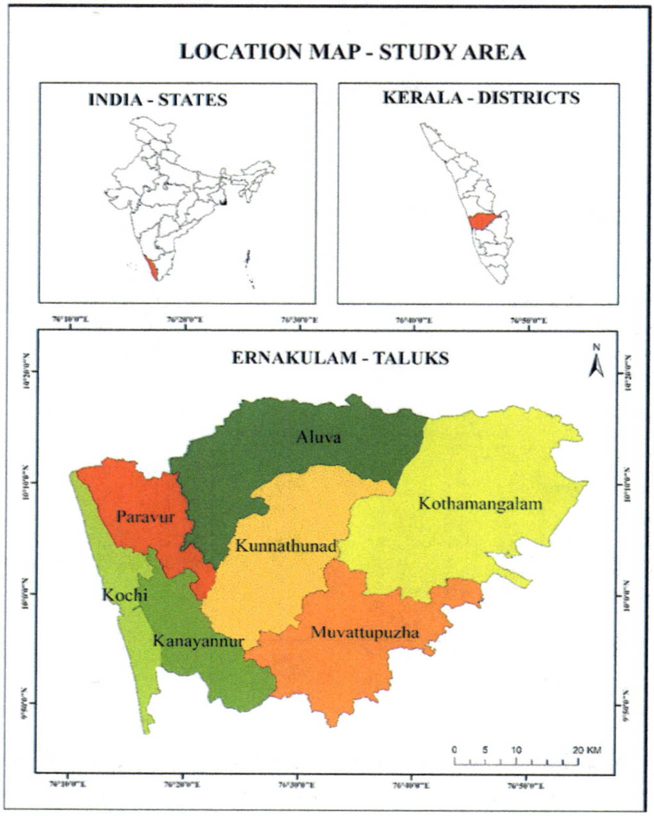


**Fig. 10.2** Location map of the study area

includes Aluva, Paravur, Kochi, and Kanayannur taluks, with their corresponding 71 villages (Government of Kerala, 2011).

## 10.3 Results and Discussions

### *10.3.1 Development Indicators—Demographic: Taluk Level Perspective*

By scrutinizing demographic development indicators under demographic, health, and socio-economic facets, significant metrics can offer a glimpse into the population dynamics and reproductive health of specific regions. These crucial indicators throw light on the trends in childbearing, maternal, and child health, and the overall well-being of the population further leads to meaningful insights for both policymakers and researchers alike.

#### 10.3.1.1 Women of Childbearing Age (15–49 Years Old)

India has a substantial female population in their reproductive age group. Roughly 253.2 million women aged between 15 and 49 makeup around one-fifth (22.2%) of India's total populace (Population Reference Bureau, 2020) and are crucial to maintaining the country's overall population growth rate. Despite this fact, Kerala stands out by defying conventional trends through declining fertility levels, as indicated by the SRS Report from 2020, which highlighted an alarmingly low total fertility rate of just 1.46% (Sample Registration System Report, 2020), implying fewer births than deaths over time and falling below the replacement level.

The demographic analysis of women aged 15–49 provides valuable insights into reproductive capabilities and overall health, aiding in understanding population demographics, fertility levels, and maternal healthcare needs, and suggesting strategies to improve women's health and well-being.

The proportion of women of childbearing age (15 to 49 years) in Ernakulam District (Fig. 10.3) is dominated with a 'very low' status across all the seven taluks except Kochi, Kanayannur, and Paravur taluks; where certain areas within Kochi and Kanayannur taluks falls under the category of 'very high'.The interplay of urbanization, economic opportunities, and migration tendencies can be cited as the possible reasons behind this phenomenon. Regions that are heavily urbanized, like Kochi taluk, tend to draw younger populations, such as women in their reproductive years. Alternatively, areas with less favourable economic opportunities may witness an exodus of young adults—particularly females—which leads to lower representation within this age group.

#### 10.3.1.2 Number of Live Births

Live births are a key indicator of demographics, revealing population growth and fertility rates. They influence healthcare plans and social welfare programs, aiming to improve childbirth outcomes and strengthen families. India grapples with a significant number of live births, holding the top spot for most annual births worldwide at an estimated 25 million each year, accounting for almost one-fifth of global births, according to United Nations estimates (UNICEF India, nd). However, Kerala portrays a unique contrast as it has displayed evidence of declining birth rates. According to the Annual Vital Statistics Report released in 2021 by the Department of Economics and Statistics based in Kerala, its Total Fertility Rate (TFR) stands at only 1.46, which is below replacement-level statistics (Department of Economics and Statistics, Kerala, 2021).

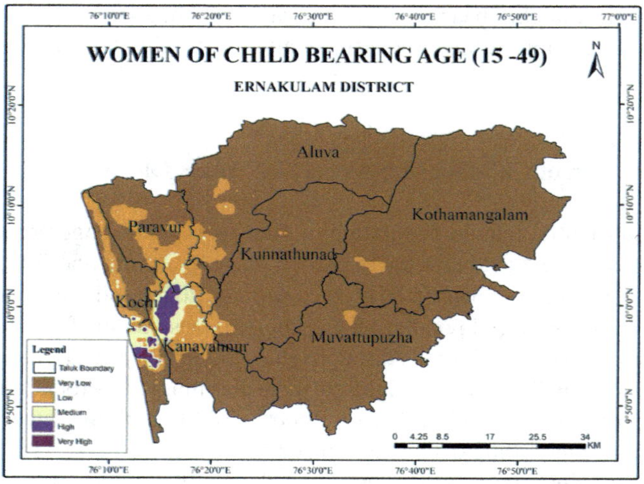


**Fig. 10.3** Women of childbearing age (15–49 years)

The live birth rates in Ernakulam district (Fig. 10.4) display a spatial contrast, with the majority of taluks falling under the "very low" category. This trend is consistent with Kerala's decreasing TFR (Department of Economics and Statistics, Kerala, 2021). Possible contributing factors to this phenomenon include socio-economic conditions and urban development. Notwithstanding, some pockets within Kochi, Kanayannur, and Kunnathunad taluks exhibit very high birth rates that can be attributed to various reasons, such as the concentration of young couples due to career prospects, particularly within urban areas where there have been significant inward migration patterns observed. There exists the possibility of the influence of improved education among women alongside economic empowerment opportunities that could lead them towards delaying childbirth decisions or having fewer children overall (Cleland & Sathar, 2008).

#### 10.3.1.3 Number of Pregnancies per Grid Square

When monitoring the number of pregnancies within each grid square (1 km spatial resolution), one can gain spatial knowledge about where these occurrences are more prevalent in various regions. This information is helpful as it allows for the identification and examination of areas with higher pregnancy concentrations or probable disparities related to reproductive health access. This indicator helps in healthcare planning, systems for resource allocation, and targeted interventions that aim at promoting healthy childbirth results while addressing maternal care needs locally. Every year, India grapples with a significant number of pregnancies, at around 48.5 million (Guttmacher Institute, 2015–2019). Nevertheless, Kerala resists this pattern and distinguishes itself from other Indian states due to its exceptional circumstances:

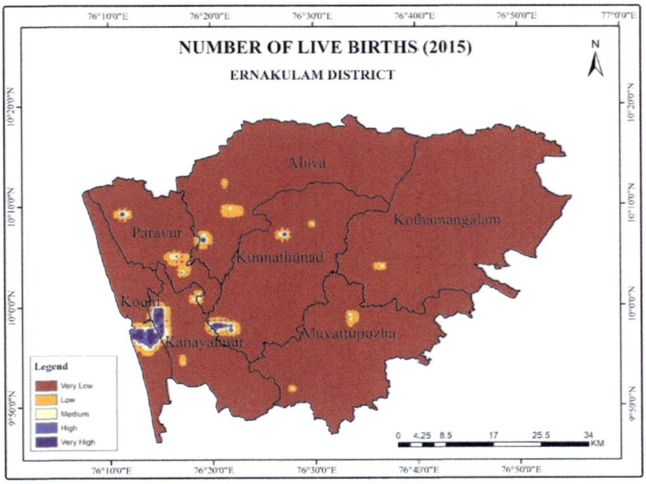


**Fig. 10.4** Number of live births

the total fertility rate in Kerala is lower than the national average according to the National Family Health Survey-5 (NFHS-5) (International Institute for Population Sciences [IIPS] and Ministry of Health and Family Welfare [MoHFW], 2019). Thus, indicating that comparatively fewer instances of pregnancy arise within this state.

The distribution of number of pregnancies per grid square in Ernakulam District (Fig. 10.5) is generally classified as 'very low'. However, there are exceptional areas within Kochi, Kanayannur, and Kunnathunad Taluks that fall under the category of 'very high' status. This zonal statistic appears to resemble the case of the variable 'number of live births. The observed trend of generally 'very low' pregnancies across Ernakulam's taluks may be linked to socio-economic conditions and urban development, which is in line with Kerala's decreasing fertility rate. However, certain pockets within Kochi, Kanayannur, and Kunnathunad taluks show a contrasting pattern of 'very high' birth rates possibly due to the concentration of young couples attracted by career prospects mainly found in areas experiencing substantial migration. Additionally considering improved female education and economic empowerment as potential factors contributing to later childbirth or smaller families overall (Cleland & Sathar, 2008) is crucial.

#### 10.3.1.4 Proportion of Children Aged 12–23 Months Born to Large (≥ 9 Members) Households

There is a decline in the average household size in India, which varies between different states (Chandrasekhar & Sharma, 2014). Assessing the percentage of children aged 12 to 23 months residing in households with nine or more individuals is an integral metric for evaluating living conditions and challenges faced by families

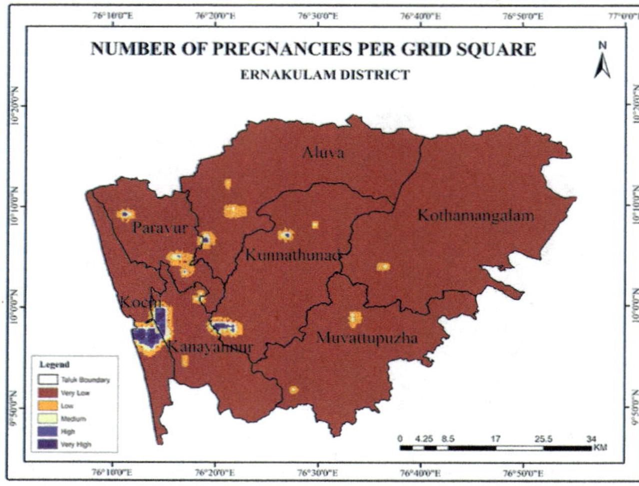


**Fig. 10.5** Number of pregnant women per grid square

within a community. This evaluation can highlight issues like overcrowding, resource scarcity, and socio-economic disparities commonly found in larger family setups that may pose threats to child welfare and development prospects.

The classification of 'very high' pertains to the major regions in Kothamangalam, Kanyannur, and Muvattupuzha taluks while Kochi and Paravur taluks predominantly have a 'very low' categorization (Fig. 10.6). In contrast to Kochi and Paravur; Kothamangalam, Kanayannur (excluding the urban pockets), and Muvattupuzha have a more rural character. In households that centre around agriculture as their livelihood, larger families are often seen as an asset since children can contribute to labour. Certain rural communities may place greater importance on having bigger families due to cultural preferences. Meanwhile, in urban areas where living expenses tend to be higher, the limited space available for residing quarters might influence couples' decisions regarding family size; those prioritizing career advancement might opt for fewer offspring or postpone childbearing altogether instead. Furthermore, city dwellers typically enjoy better access compared to less-populated regions when it comes to planning services and guiding family sizes, which could lead to smaller-sized household formations.

### *10.3.2 Health Indicators Pattern Across the Taluks of Ernakulam District*

By analysing crucial health metrics on a taluk level, we gain valuable insight into the well-being and social vulnerabilities of communities. This evaluation allows us to

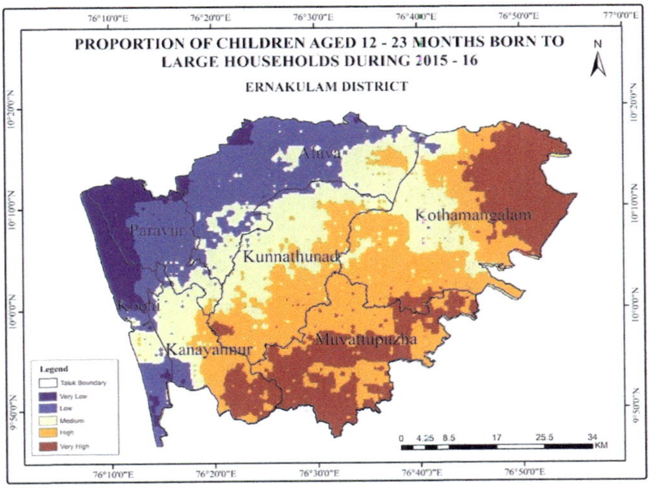


**Fig. 10.6** Proportion of children aged 12–23 months born to large households

identify areas that need improvement and inform policies aimed at reducing healthcare inequality for mothers and children who face specific challenges in these areas. This study concentrates specifically on five health indicators associated with mothers and children: infants born to mothers who did not attend antenatal care (ANC), infants whose mothers did not receive or recall post-natal care within two months after birth, mothers with no health insurance, newborns delivered by unskilled professionals, and underweight children due to malnutrition. The results reveal significant hurdles faced by moms & kids in these regions related particularly to access to healthcare facilities as well as quality concerns.

#### 10.3.2.1 Children Born to Mothers Who Did Not Attend Antenatal Care (ANC)

Maternal and child health outcomes may suffer adversely when antenatal care is absent for mothers. A dearth of ANC services could pave the way to unnoticed medical conditions, escalate pregnancy and childbirth complications risk, as well as insufficient readiness towards a healthy delivery. India continues to face a significant challenge with regard to the number of children born without antenatal care (ANC), despite nationwide efforts aimed at improving ANC utilization. According to estimates from the National Family Health Survey-5 [NFHS-5], approximately 22% of women giving birth in India received no ANC (IIPS & MoHFW, 2019). However, Kerala offers more hopeful statistics; NFHS-5 data shows that an increased proportion of women living in Kerala access essential ANC services compared to national averages, as reported by IIPS and MoHFW in 2019. This higher rate translates into

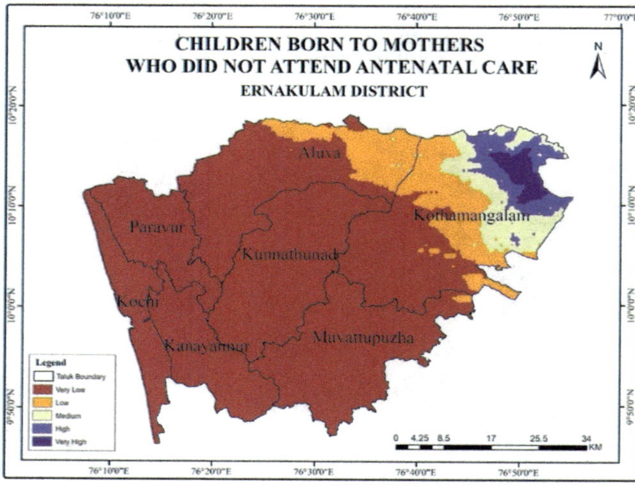


**Fig. 10.7** Children born without ANC visits

fewer instances where mothers skip out on critical prenatal medical intervention when delivering babies than elsewhere across India's broader population centres.

A major portion of Kothamangalam taluk has been categorized as 'very high', while the remaining taluks, excluding Kothamangalam and a part of Aluva taluk, have concentrated on achieving a 'very low' status (Fig. 10.7). In Kothamangalam, lower socio-economic status can hinder the ability to obtain healthcare services such as ANC. Certain areas in Kothamangalam categorized under 'very high' may have limited access to medical facilities or a higher prevalence of poverty due to the majority population being tribal. Additionally, a lack of awareness regarding the significance of ANC might cause mothers living in rural regions to not prioritize these services. Cultural beliefs or social norms could also discourage women from attending ANC appointments. Moreover, transportation difficulties arising from hilly terrain and forest cover, along with distance challenges related to healthcare facilities, pose hindrances for mothers from less privileged backgrounds.

#### 10.3.2.2 Children Born to Mothers Who Did Not Receive/Recall Post-Natal Care Within 2 Months After Birth

Ensuring adequate postpartum care is essential to overseeing the well-being of both mother and newborn, detecting any potential complications arising after delivery, and offering vital guidance during early motherhood. Failing to receive proper medical attention could result in missed chances for timely intervention or support with detrimental consequences on the health outcomes of both individuals. Low utilization of post-natal care (PNC) is a challenge faced by India. Only 44% of mothers in the country receive any form of PNC within two days after giving birth, according to data from the National Family Health Survey-5 (NFHS-5) (IIPS & MoHFW, 2019). Consequently, a significant number of mothers and infants miss out on vital post-natal checkups during this crucial period. However, Kerala bucks this trend with higher usage rates than India's average; NFHS-5 data indicates that more mothers access PNC services there compared to elsewhere across the nation, indicating fewer children and mothers are missing essential healthcare checks within the critical 2-month window.

The category of 'very high' predominates in Kothamangalam taluk, Muvattupuzha, and Kanayannur taluks with regard to children born to mothers who did not receive or recall post-natal care. Lower socio-economic status, like with ANC utilization, may hinder access to PNC services. Within the Kothamangalam and Muvattupuzha regions, the 'very high' category poses added barriers. However, Kanayannur's predominantly urban areas are divided between the 'high' and 'very high' categories, which require a closer evaluation on the ground. Limited awareness about crucial checkups in rural areas might lead to a lower prioritization of PNC, while cultural or social beliefs also play a role. Moreover, transportation difficulties coupled with distance from healthcare facilities pose major challenges for mothers coming from less privileged backgrounds, particularly in these taluks. Recalling PNC within 2 months might be challenging for some mothers. The data might not necessarily reflect a complete absence of PNC, but rather difficulty in remembering the exact timing. On the other hand, areas within Paravur and Aluva taluk exhibit a status classified as 'very low'. Government programs promoting PNC services and improving healthcare infrastructure might be more successful in these areas, making it easier for mothers to access PNC checkups (Fig. 10.8).

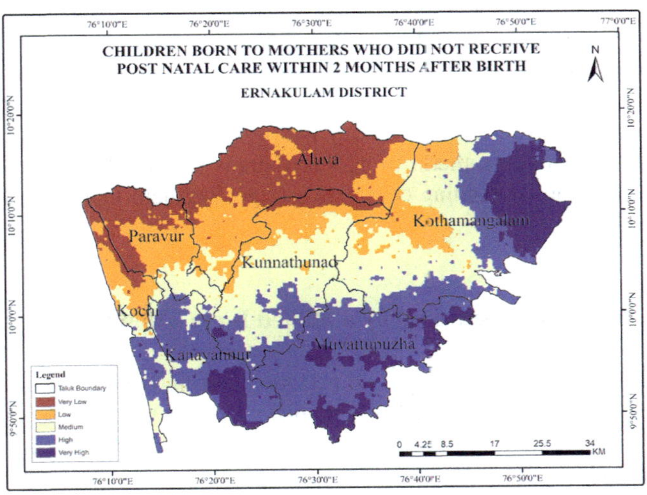


**Fig. 10.8** Children born to mothers who did not receive PNC visits

#### 10.3.2.3 Mothers with no Health Insurance

Access to quality healthcare services for mothers and children heavily relies on health insurance. The absence of proper medical coverage can result in financial constraints, which hinder timely medical attention thereby causing unmet healthcare needs, delayed treatment, and increased susceptibility to various health risks. Current national surveys, such as the NFHS, mainly concentrate on health insurance ownership at the household level rather than individual coverage for mothers. Nevertheless, some states have introduced health insurance programs that focus specifically on pregnant women and mothers. Kerala's Karunya Arogya Suraksha Padhathi (KASU) is one of them, which caters to pregnant women and mothers by offering them medical coverage (SHA, Kerala Government n.d.). Such a program implies that, in comparison to other regions across India, there could possibly be a lower proportion of mothers without health insurance.

A significant number of mothers residing in Kothamangalam and Aluva taluks are without health insurance, resulting in their placement within the 'very high' category. Access to health insurance is impeded by lower socio-economic status, particularly in areas such as Kothamangalam with a significant tribal population and parts of Aluva where poverty prevails. For families struggling financially, the cost of premiums can be prohibitive. Lack of access to employer-sponsored programs could also affect those working informally. Furthermore, mothers may fail to enrol due to limited awareness about available insurance options, especially in rural regions. It's important not just to focus on maternal coverage but overall household insurance coverage too; family health plans are potentially crucial here. Conversely, Kochi, Paravur, Kanayannur, Aluva, and Kunnathunad taluks showcase low instances under the 'very low' classification in this context (Fig. 10.9).

The higher degree of urbanization in Kochi, Paravur, and certain regions of Aluva and Kunnathunad could result in a greater number of salaried workers who benefit from employer-sponsored healthcare policies that also cover their families. State-led programs may demonstrate more efficacy within specific taluks, leading to a lower proportion of uninsured mothers. In addition, areas classified as urban or pockets with elevated economic standing comprise a larger segment that can afford private health insurance.

#### 10.3.2.4 Children not Delivered by a Skilled Birth Attendant

A trained birth attendant is an absolute necessity during delivery as it ensures the safety of labour and lowers the risk of complications for both mothers and babies. Untrained personnel carrying out births run a higher risk of suffering injuries or illnesses that could compromise their overall health. India struggles with a significant proportion of deliveries lacking the presence of skilled birth attendants (SBAs). Data from the National Family Health Survey-5 (NFHS-5) indicates that 28% of births in India take place without an SBA. However, Kerala presents a more promising scenario, with only approximately 5% estimate for unattended childbirths by SBAs

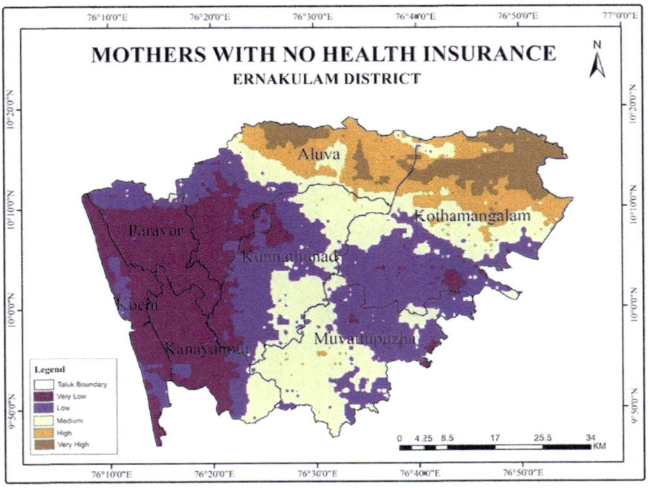


**Fig. 10.9** Mothers with no health insurance

according to NFHS-5 data (IIPS & MoHFW, 2019). This suggests that there is a much higher prevalence of skilled attendance during births in Kerala as compared to the national average.

With the exception of Aluva and Kothamangalam, all taluks are classified as "very low", with Kothamangalam taluk falling into the "very high" category in relation to this development index (Fig. 10.10). Taluks with a good network of hospitals, maternity centres, and well-equipped primary healthcare facilities likely have a higher concentration of SBAs like doctors, nurses, or midwives. This can increase access to expert support during deliveries. Government initiatives that encourage institutional births and incentivize SBAs may be more effective in some taluks due to their higher concentration of skilled delivery resources. Taluks with better socio-economic status tend to prioritize professional medical assistance for childbirth; they are also likelier to have private facilities available for this purpose. The availability of competent personnel at Kothamangalam, if indeed present, might be hampered by inadequate means or the remoteness due to highland topography and forest cover. Certain indigenous birthing practices may discourage tribal people, especially in Kothamangalam taluk from using healthcare amenities adding to the already existing unavailability of services.

#### 10.3.2.5 Children Underweight (Malnutrition)

Proper nutrition is crucial for children's health and prevents underweight conditions. Insufficient nourishment can lead to stunted growth, weak immunity, and increased

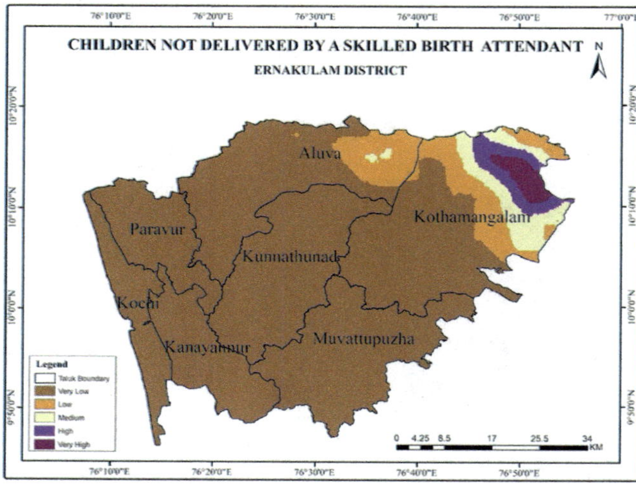


**Fig. 10.10** Children not delivered by skilled birth attendant

illness susceptibility. Eliminating malnourishment is essential for optimal development and quality of life. Despite national efforts, India still faces a significant number of underweight children.

The latest National Family Health Survey-5 (NFHS-5) data reveals that 32.1% of Indian kids aged five and below fall in this category, highlighting the severity of public health concerns. Nevertheless, there is hope as Kerala has demonstrated substantial improvements by boasting considerably lower estimates than the national average of around 19.3%, according to NFHS-5 (IIPS & MoHFW, 2019). This discrepancy suggests successful progress in addressing childhood malnourishment within Kerala's borders.

The distribution of children who are malnourished (Fig. 10.11) falls under 'very low' category within Kochi and Kanayannur taluks. Having a higher socio-economic status in these taluks could lead to greater availability of nourishing food, enhanced sanitation habits, and better medical care, collectively resulting in reduced rates of malnutrition. Moreover, due to increased urbanization levels within Kochi and certain areas of Kanayannur, they may have improved access to government programs aimed at enhancing child nutrition through means such as fortifying foods with nutrients or promoting healthy eating initiatives among the public.

Regions within Kothamangalam and Aluva taluks fall under 'very high' category. A primary cause of malnutrition in these taluks may stem from disadvantaged socio-economic settings. Impoverishment can create barriers to obtaining clean water, proper nutrition, and access to sanitation facilities, ultimately raising the likelihood of malnutrition. Heightened food insecurity in rural areas due to limited supplies of healthy and affordable food is also an important issue that must be addressed. Additionally, ignorance concerning appropriate child nutrition practices, hygiene

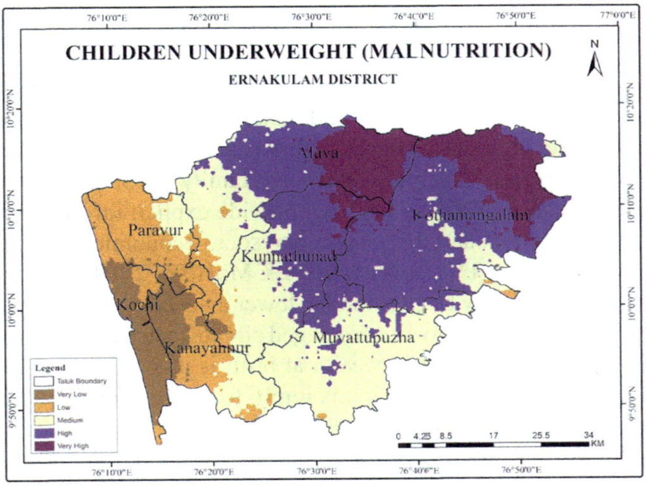


**Fig. 10.11** Underweight children

standards, and dietary diversity could further exacerbate cases of undernourished individuals among certain populations.

### *10.3.3 Socio- Economic Development Indicators: Taluk Level Analysis*

Assessing progress and challenges faced by communities within the socio-economic development realm requires a deep understanding of key indicators at the taluk level. This research aims to analyse significant metrics that provide insight into the socio-economic landscape, including Children born to the poorest/poor households according to Demographic and Health Surveys (DHS) & Multiple Indicator Cluster Surveys (MICS) classifications, born to mothers who had no formal education, the proportion of women aged 15–49 years who did not participate in decision-making in their households. Conducting a comprehensive examination of socio-economic development indicators at the taluk level, considers points to highlight impediments, imbalances, and prospects for progression in advancing all-encompassing and persevering advance over the locale. The resulting results and discussions will dive advance into these markers' repercussions, conveying profitable points of view for policy-making as well as mediation techniques adapted towards cultivating comprehensive socio-economic development and empowerment.

#### 10.3.3.1 Children Born to Poorest/Poor Households

An essential element in the progress of socio-economic development involves scrutinizing children who are born into households categorized as poorest or poor based on DHS/MICS-NICS standards. This metric offers valuable insights into the difficulties encountered by disadvantaged families and how a family's economic situation affects their child's welfare. The NFHS-5 does not provide explicit information on household wealth at birth, but it can offer insight into socio-economic status through data on asset ownership such as TVs and cars (IIPS & MoHFW, 2019). This suggests that many Indian households may be classified in lower asset categories, with a considerable number of children born into disadvantaged circumstances. In Kerala, direct data about the distribution of household wealth at birth is unavailable, although higher literacy rates and social welfare programs imply fewer newborns from the poorest quintiles compared to national levels (UNDP, 2005).

The distribution of children who are born to the poorest or poor households (Fig. 10.12) is 'very low' in all taluks except the portions of Kothamangalam and Aluva taluks whereas it is 'very high' in Kothamangalam taluk. Taluks that exhibit a higher level of socio-economic development may experience lower poverty rates due to factors such as improved infrastructure, better job prospects, and higher average incomes.

In certain taluks within Ernakulam district, social welfare programs aimed at alleviating poverty or providing subsidized food supplies could be more effective in reducing the number of children who are born into low-income households. Conversely, areas like Kothamangalam and parts of Aluva might encounter difficulties accessing high-paying employment opportunities, instead contending with an upsurge in informal work opportunities offering meagre wages. This can

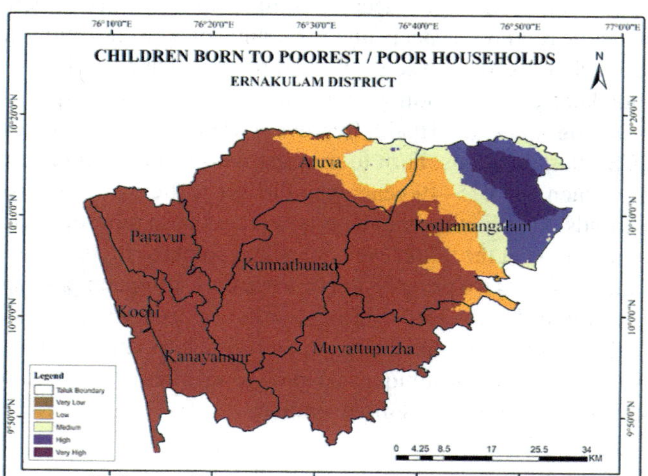


Fig. 10.12 Children born to poorest/poor households

impede economic progress while keeping families entrenched in financial insecurity. Although undergoing urbanization changes, regions throughout Aluva still retain aspects associated with rural communities; conversely, Kothamangalam bears strong similarities to a rural setting and associated activities for income-generation purposes, resulting in low-income-generating households. Crucially limited access to education, along with medical facilities, and a lack of financial options available specifically across these regions serve only to make things even harder, restricting people's abilities to become prosperous beyond the current circumstances they face.

#### 10.3.3.2 Children Born to Mothers with No Formal Education

A significant factor currently being closely examined is the proportion of infants born to mothers without formal education. This measure sheds light on how maternal health and education intersect, revealing critical information regarding the challenges faced by uneducated mothers in attaining healthcare for their offspring and ensuring both parties' welfare. Current data suggests that mothers with limited education face significant challenges across the country. Only around 36% of adult females in India have completed secondary education (UNESCO Institute for Statistics, n.d.), meaning a high probability exists of children being born to uneducated women. While specific national statistics on mothers' childbirth education aren't available for comparison purposes, Kerala's female literacy rate surpasses the average, standing at 78.9% in the 2011 census. This implies potential differences between Kerala and other Indian states where fewer children are probably born to uneducated moms due to higher rates of educational attainment among their populations (Directorate of Census Operations, Kerala, 2011).

Except for the portions of Kothamangalam and Aluva taluks, the distribution of children who are born to mothers with no formal education is 'very low' in all other taluks whereas it is 'very high' in Kothamangalam taluk. Taluks that exhibit higher levels of female literacy rates generally have lower instances of mothers devoid of formal education. This could be attributed to either successful governmental initiatives promoting girls' learning or greater cultural importance laid on educating females. More urbanized taluks may provide better access to educational resources, potentially contributing to enhanced female academic achievements. Compared with other areas, Kothamangalam and certain parts of Aluva report a less impressive rate in terms of women's literacy. Such bleak statistics can likely be attributed to socioeconomic factors like poverty constraining opportunities for girl child education or deep-rooted sociocultural norms placing domestic responsibilities over schooling among young girls (Fig. 10.13).

#### 10.3.3.3 Women's Participation in Household Decision-Making

Examining the percentage of women aged 15–49 who are not involved in household decision-making, reveals the imbalances in female agency and independence within

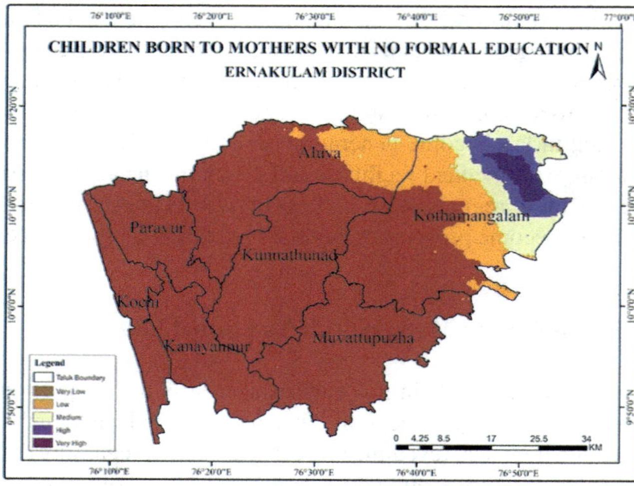


**Fig. 10.13** Children born to mothers with no formal education

a taluk. The study reveals that 88.7% of married women participate in at least three important household decisions, such as healthcare, major purchases, or visiting relatives; however, there is room for improvement. Kerala shows a more encouraging trend, with 94.1% of married women showing greater empowerment compared to the national average.

The general trend in the distribution of the proportion of women aged 15–49 who did not participate in decision-making in their households within the Ernakulam District (Fig. 10.14) is heterogeneous. Areas within Aluva taluk fall under the 'very high' category, whereas regions within Kochi, Kanayannur, and Kothamangalam taluks fall under the 'very low' category. Taluks that are more developed, such as Kochi, may see a higher level of female education and economic participation. This could lead to greater autonomy for women and enable them to have a stronger voice in decision-making processes. In contrast with other taluks where gender roles might be enforced traditionally, progressive social environments associated with urbanization in certain areas like Kochi promote the empowerment of women through exposure to media and social movements. Pockets within Aluva still grapple with ramifications from lower socio-economic statuses, which drastically restrict opportunities available towards educational or monetary independence, further limiting their authority over household-based power dynamics due to the predominantly strong patriarchal tradition. Despite the rural and tribal nature of Kothamangalam taluk with a significant forest cover, which could imply low female involvement in decision-making activities, certain communities or areas within the region may contradict this trend. Within these pockets in Kothamangalam's countryside or among specific tribes are cultural traditions that advocate for more balanced gender roles where women have

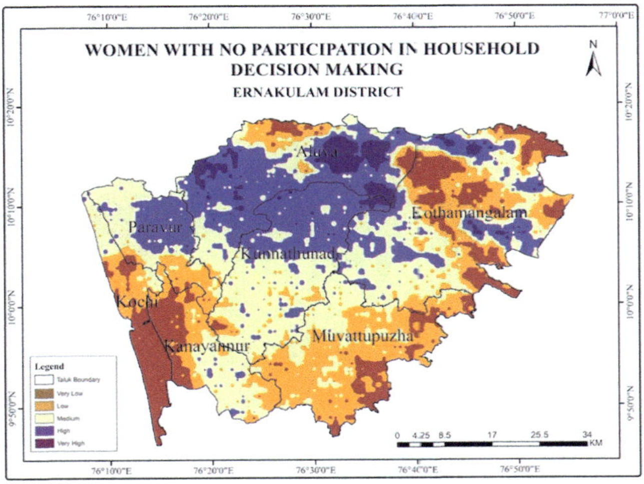


**Fig. 10.14** Women with no participation in household decision-making

increased power to make decisions at home. This is because societal values recognize contributions by females to agriculture, resource management, or community decision-making.

### *10.3.4 Association of Socio-Demographic and Health Determinants Among Mothers and Children in Ernakulam District*

The development of Ernakulam District is significantly influenced by the socio-demographic and health factors affecting mothers and children. The demographic indicators include the population characteristics of women of childbearing age (15–49 years old), the number of live births, and the number of pregnancies. The health indicators encompass the well-being of mothers and children, with a focus on factors such as antenatal and post-natal care, skilled birth attendance, underweight children, and health insurance coverage. Additionally examining socio-economic indicators illuminates how financial stability affects overall wellness for families on different ends of this spectrum—with a particular emphasis on children born to the poorest or poor households, mothers with no formal education and women's participation in household decision-making. By examining these determinants and their interplay, this study seeks to provide a comprehensive understanding of the socio-economic landscape in Ernakulam District, informing policy-making and intervention strategies aimed at promoting inclusive and sustainable development.

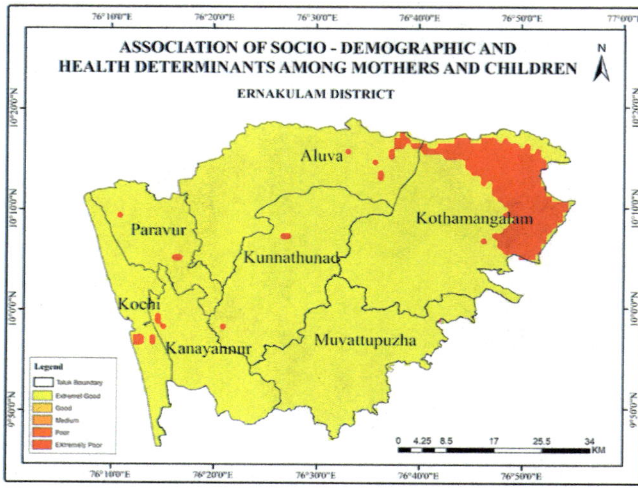


**Fig. 10.15** Association of socio-demographic and health determinants among mothers and children

In the context of identifying the social vulnerability among mothers and children in Ernakulam district based on development indicators (Fig. 10.15), Kothamangalam taluk falls under the 'extremely poor' status, even though patches under the same category are identified within the other taluks. Muvattupuzha taluk in particular falls under the 'extremely good' status along with other taluks in general.

The social vulnerability of mothers and children in Ernakulam district varies across taluks due to various factors. A dense population of childbearing-age women can overburden healthcare resources, affecting access to antenatal care and resulting in higher birth rates among disadvantaged groups. Inadequate nutrition or quality medical attention may also be a concern. Poverty cycles can prevent resource accessibility, contributing to poor health outcomes. In areas with balanced populations, permit allocation optimization can improve midwifery support and preventative treatment, reducing malnutrition rates and promoting upward mobility towards more prosperous living conditions. This leads to maternal and overall quality of life improvements in qualifying neighbourhoods.

Investments in expanding access to essential services like antenatal and post-natal care, skilled birth attendants, and healthcare coverage for underprivileged households can strengthen healthcare infrastructure. Addressing socio-economic discrepancies by improving women's education levels and promoting active participation in household decision-making processes is crucial. Supporting impoverished families with childcare needs is another key aspect. Regular surveillance and assessment of health and socio-economic metrics are essential for monitoring progress and identifying opportunities for improvement.

Various initiatives and schemes at both the central and state levels have been implemented to promote maternal and child care. The Indira Gandhi Matritva Sahodary Yojana (IGMSY) provides financial assistance for improved nutrition to pregnant or lactating women (Ministry of Women and Child Development, Government of India, n.d.), while the Janani Suraksha Yojana (JSY) offers cash incentives to promote institutional deliveries (Ministry of Health and Family Welfare, Government of India, n.d.). Similarly, the Poshan Abhiyan aims to reduce malnutrition among children and mothers across India (Ministry of Women and Child Development, Government of India, n.d.). In Kerala specifically, there are multiple programs such as the Kerala Maternity Benefit Scheme (KMBS), which gives financial aid for proper prenatal care; Sneha Jaalaka, which provides institutional support during difficult pregnancies; the Balashree Karyakram, which offers scholarships promoting holistic development in children (Government of Kerala, Department of Women and Child Development, n.d.); and the Aardram Mission, which aims at strengthening primary healthcare systems and thus improving access to maternal-childcare services overall (Government of Kerala, Department of Health and Family Welfare, n.d.). The implementation challenges of these initiatives can cause discrepancies in their effectiveness across different regions, resulting in difficulty for intended beneficiaries such as mothers and children residing within susceptible communities to receive aid.

Due to insufficient awareness among beneficiaries, the effectiveness of programs and policies in Ernakulam district may be limited causing discrepancies. Flaws in funding and human resources could impede program sustainability. Specialized healthcare professionals and equipment are scarce while geographical inaccessibility further hinders the effective implementation of these initiatives. Although Balashree Karyakam aims at holistic child development, complementary interventions addressing malnutrition, early childhood education, as well as healthcare might improve its impact. Moreover, inadequate grassroots level execution raises concerns about overall program delivery competency, which can exacerbate disparities in maternal-child health indicators across the region due to inadequate monitoring mechanisms during their implementation processes within Ernakulam district specifically.

A collaborative approach involving government agencies, NGOs, and community-based groups is essential to address complex issues in Ernakulam District. A comprehensive perspective at the grassroots level can provide a holistic understanding of the situation.

## 10.4 Conclusion

Factors such as economic status, educational access, and healthcare resources are found to play a complex role in health and well-being outcomes. Taluks with good status in the context of social vulnerability among mothers and children may have better social indicators as in case of the 6 taluks within Ernakulam except Kothamangalam, while those with poor status may have areas with ongoing development initiatives. Persistent disparities in maternal and child health identified, emphasizes the need for targeted interventions that address key vulnerabilities like poverty, limited education opportunities, and restricted healthcare access. The implications extend far beyond district borders leading towards a broader discourse about maternal/child care accessibility, fostering equal opportunity distribution throughout society alongside proactive policy implementation promoting equal and fair resilience development among all.

**Acknowledgements** The authors express their gratitude to the WorldPop Project (2015-16) for providing a valuable population dataset for their study, and to the Department of Geography at Bharathidasan University, Tiruchirappalli, Tamil Nadu, India for their constant support.

## References

Basu, S., Sharma, B., Mukhopadhyay, R., & Dutta, M. (2019). Social vulnerability to environmental hazards in coastal West Bengal, India. *International Journal of Disaster Risk Reduction, 37*, Article 101237.

Benner, L. A., Lee, K., Sass, L. C., & Trentacoste, C. L. (2021). Social vulnerability and maternal social support: Associations with maternal mental health and child behavior problems. *Children's Health Care, 50*(3), 339–354.

Braveman, P., & Gottlieb, L. (2014). The social determinants of health: Evidence for policy and practice. *Public Health Reports, 129*(1), 123–134.

Census of India. (2011). https://www.censusindia.gov.in/

Census India. (2011). Ernakulam District, Kerala. https://www.censusindia.co.in/district/ernakulam-district-kerala-595#:~:text=Also%20the%20Sex%20Ratio%20of,the%20age%200%2D6%20years

Chandrasekhar, C. P., & Sharma, A. (2014). Changing household size in India. *Population Research and Policy Review, 33*(1), 1–22. https://www.ncbi.nlm.nih.gov/pmc/articles/PMC1971249/

Cleland, J., & Sathar, Z. (2008). The effect of rising female education on fertility in developing countries. *Population and Development Review, 34*(4), 597–628. https://www.ncbi.nlm.nih.gov/pmc/articles/PMC8924343/

Department of Economics and Statistics, Kerala. (2021). Annual vital statistics report 2021. https://www.ecostat.kerala.gov.in/publication-detail/annual-vital-statistics-report-2021

Directorate of Census Operations, Kerala. (2011). Census of India 2011, Kerala—Series 23—Part II—Tables of Population—Literacy Rate. https://www.ecostat.kerala.gov.in/data-subset/292

Evans, G. W., & Wachsmuth, D. (2013). Measuring the economic, social, and environmental determinants of health: A conceptual and empirical framework. *Social Science & Medicine, 89*, 8–17.

Gokhale, S., & Menon, R. (2019). Housing conditions and social vulnerability in Ernakulam district, Kerala: A study of selected slums. *Journal of Social Welfare and Management, 10*(4), 231–242.

Gopal, K., & Nair, S. (2020). Improving access to maternal healthcare services in rural Ernakulam: A community-based approach. *International Journal of Community Health and Nursing, 9*(2), 123–132.

Government of Kerala, Department of Health and Family Welfare. (n.d.). Aardram Mission. https://arogyakeralam.gov.in/2020/04/01/aardram/

Government of Kerala, Department of Women and Child Development. (n.d.). https://wcd.kerala.gov.in/

Government of Kerala. (2011). District Census Handbook: Ernakulam (Part-A & B). New Delhi: Office of the Registrar General & Census Commissioner, India.

Headey, D., & Babu, S. (2016). *State-level trends in child undernutrition in India: Evidence from household surveys, 1993–2014*. International Food Policy Research Institute. https://www.ncbi.nlm.nih.gov/pmc/articles/PMC7116138/

International Institute for Population Sciences (IIPS) & Ministry of Health and Family Welfare (MoHFW). (2019). National Family Health Survey-5 (NFHS-5).

Jayadevan, C., & Joseph, K. (2023). Spatial variations in social vulnerability of children in Ernakulam district: A GIS-based analysis. *Journal of the Indian Society of Remote Sensing, 51*(2), 315–324.

Joseph, S., & Mathew, T. (2019). Empowering single mothers through microfinance: A case study from Ernakulam district, Kerala. *Journal of Gender Studies, 28*(4), 421–433.

Kerala State Planning Board. (n.d.). https://spb.kerala.gov.in/

Kurian, J., & John, L. (2017). Malnutrition and health status of children under five in Ernakulam district, Kerala: A community-based study. *Indian Journal of Public Health, 61*(3), 203–208.

Marmot, M., & Wilkinson, R. G. (2006). *Social determinants of health*. Oxford University Press.

Menon, A., & Pillai, R. (2021). Challenges faced by single mothers in Ernakulam district, Kerala: A qualitative study. *Journal of Family Welfare, 67*(3), 312–320.

Ministry of Health and Family Welfare. (n.d.). Janani Suraksha Yojana (JSY). https://nhm.gov.in/index1.php?lang=1&level=3&lid=309&sublinkid=841

Ministry of Women and Child Development. (n.d.). Indira Gandhi Matritva Sahodary Yojana (IGMSY). https://chhindwara.nic.in/en/scheme/indira-gandhi-maternity-support-scheme-i-g-m-s-y/

Ministry of Women and Child Development. (n.d.). Poshan Abhiyan (National Nutrition Mission). https://wcd.nic.in/schemes/poshan-abhiyaan

National Health Profile. (2018). [Available distribution and utilization of health services in Kerala]. State Planning Board, Government of Kerala. https://spb.kerala.gov.in/sites/default/files/inline-files/AvailDistribUtilisationHSKerala_0.pdf

National Health Systems Resource Centre. (2021). https://nhsrcindia.org/

Population Reference Bureau. (2020). 2020 World Population Data Sheet. https://www.prb.org/2020-world-population-data-sheet/

Radhakrishnan, P., & Nair, S. M. (2020). Socioeconomic inequalities in healthcare access and utilization in urban Kerala: A cross-sectional study. *Journal of Public Health, 28*(8), 1421–1428.

Radhakrishnan, S. (2016). *Gender, caste, and health in India: A reader*. Routledge.

Rao, K. N., & Nair, S. M. (2022). The impact of natural disasters on maternal and child health in coastal Kerala, India: A case study of Ernakulam district. *International Journal of Disaster Risk Reduction, 81*, Article 104032.

Ramachandran, P., George, K., Zachariah, R., Jayalekshmi, K. V., & Kumar, P. G. (2013). Socioeconomic inequality in access to and utilization of maternal health care services in Kerala, India: A cross-sectional study. *International Journal of Equity in Health, 12*(1), 30.

Sample Registration System SRS Report. (2020). https://www.ecostat.kerala.gov.in/

Sankoh, S., Banerjee, A., Okonofua, F. C., Akorli, V., Otoo, S., & Mbuthia-Ngonze, L. K. (2017). Social vulnerability and access to maternal healthcare in sub-Saharan Africa: A systematic review. *International Journal for Equity in Health, 16*(1), 37.

Sebastian, T., & Jayan, P. K. (2018). Socioeconomic and caste inequalities in maternal and child health indicators in Kerala, India: A cross-sectional study. *International Journal for Equity in Health, 17*(1), 161.

SHA, Kerala Government. (n.d.). Karunya Arogya Suraksha Padhathi. https://sha.kerala.gov.in/

SPB. (n.d.). District Profile—SPB Home. Ernakulam district, one of the administrative divisions in Kerala, India. http://www.old.spb.kerala.gov.in/index.php/district-profile-ernakulam.html#:~:text=Ernakulam%20district%2C%20one%20of%20the,77o%206'%20east%20longitudes.

UNESCO Institute for Statistics. (n.d.). UIS Data Browser. https://uis.unesco.org/

United Nations Development Programme. (2005). Report on Kerala's Development Experience 2005.

UNICEF India. (n.d.). Key data. https://www.unicef.org/india/key-data

Utazi, C. E., Aheto, J. M. K., Chan, H. M. T., Tatem, A. J., & Sahu, S. K. (2022). Conditional probability and ratio-based approaches for mapping the coverage of multi-dose vaccines. *Statistics in Medicine, 41*(29), 5662–5678.

Utazi, C. E., Chan, H. M. T., Olowe, I., Wigley, A., Tejedor-Garavito, N., Cunningham, A., Bondarenko, M., Lorin, J., Boyda, D., Hogan, D., & Tatem, A. J. (2023). A zero-dose vulnerability index for equity assessment and spatial prioritization in low-and middle-income countries. *Spatial Statistics*, 100772.

Utazi, C. E., Nilsen, K., Pannell, O., Dotse-Gborgbortsi, W., & Tatem, A. J. (2021). District-level estimation of vaccination coverage: Discrete vs continuous spatial models. *Statistics in Medicine, 40*(9), 2197–2211.

# Chapter 11
# Examining Inequalities in Caesarean Section Deliveries in Maharashtra, India: Socio-Economic Determinants and Regional Disparities

**Rushikesh Premdas Khadse** and **Dhananjay W. Bansod**

**Abstract** Global caesarean section (C-section) delivery is unevenly distributed and results in more than 15% of all abdominal deliveries. The present study aims to investigate the socio-demographic and economic determinants of C-section deliveries in Maharashtra. The fifth round of the National Family Health Survey 2019–21 was used to estimate the determinants of C-section. Oaxaca decomposition was used to find inequality in the C-section among public and private health facilities. The proportion of C-section deliveries in Maharashtra during 2019–21 was observed to be 25.4%, with 18.3% of the deliveries occurring at public health facilities, while 38.9% of the deliveries took place in private health care settings. Nandurbar (7.9%) had the lowest prevalence of C-section deliveries while Kolhapur (38.1%) in the western region had the maximum prevalence of deliveries through C-section procedure. About 7% of the total inequality was explained by women's economic status followed by the mother's birth order (5.2%) and the mother's educational attainment (5%). The study found an overall increase in the prevalence of C-section delivery among all the different geographical regions of Maharashtra. A huge gap between C-sections among different districts of the state, along with women's economic status, mother's birth order, and mother's education were also observed which might be the major contributing factors to the increasing gap in C-section delivery among health facilities.

**Keywords** C-section · Inequality · Region · Maharashtra · India

---

R. P. Khadse (✉)
Department of Public Health and Mortlity Studies, International Institute for Population Sciences, Mumbai, India
e-mail: rushikeshkhadse@gmail.com

D. W. Bansod
Department of Public Health and Mortality Studies, International Institute for Population Sciences, Mumbai, India



P. Chouhan et al. (eds.), *Women's Health Dynamics in South Asia*, Asian Perspectives on Public Health, https://doi.org/10.1007/978-981-95-2321-4_11

## 11.1 Introduction

The United Nations General Assembly in 2015 adopted the Sustainable Development Goals (SDGs), with a key focus on reducing the maternal mortality ratio to less than 70 per 100,000 live births by 2024 (UN, 2023). Despite global and national interventions aiming at reducing maternal mortality related to pregnancy and childbirth, the rates remain high. Southern Asia achieved the greatest overall reduction in maternal mortality ratio (MMR), a decline in maternal mortality ratio to 67% (from 408 down to 134) in 2020 (World Health Organization, 2024).

India has a very wide variation in Caesarean Section (C-section) rates across the country. The focuses on the state-wise variation in C-section deliveries, Telangana having 60% of C-section deliveries followed by Andhra Pradesh at 42% and Tamil Nadu at 36% shows the topmost state, while another side Bihar at 7%, Madhya Pradesh at 10% and Jharkhand 11% reported at the bottom end (Roy et al., 2021). National Family Health Survey (NFHS) 2019–21 reported 21% of C-section delivery performed at the national level, focusing on state-level Maharashtra experience of around 25% of C-section deliveries (International Institute for Population Sciences [IIPS] & ICF, 2021) (National Family Health Survey, 2019–21).

There are several medical factors playing an important role in increasing C-section deliveries, women having access to more than 4 antenatal care visits, tall stature, and overweight or obese are foremost determinants of C-section (Pandey et al., 2023). As well as breech presentation of the unborn child, the age of the mother at the time of birth, size of the unborn at birth are the key elements of C-section (Islam et al., 2022; Nakinobe et al., 2023). Nowadays prevalence of emergency C-section deliveries has increased, hence the demand for C-section delivery is more prominent and reduces to chances of maternal and child mortality through improving the quality of obstetric care (Kumari & Thomas, 2013). Even through, C-section numbers are negatively associated with such lack of information on the part of consumers, unskilled training of providers, conveniences of obstetricians, competitive spirit between private and public sector, etc. (Mor, 2020; Shabnam, 2009). Women having a first child through C-section delivery are more likely to have subsequent delivery through a C-section (Islam et al., 2022).

Socio-economic factors also influence to increasing the C-section deliveries, women belonging to higher socio-economic strata, women giving preference to C-section delivery, etc. Observing the upward trend in C-section deliveries, it was found that the rate of C-sections is higher in private healthcare facilities compared to public ones (Das & Sahoo, 2019). Additionally, non-medical factors influence women's decisions regarding their mode of delivery (Bansod et al., 2018; Nakinobe et al., 2023). According to Bansod et al. (2018), key determinants of C-section delivery include a mother's education, age, religion, wealth quintile, and place of delivery (Bansod et al., 2018). Maharashtra in Western India is a socio-economically developed state, reporting 25% of C-section deliveries which is substantially higher than the WHO threshold, along with there being huge differences for C-section delivery in districts and different geographical regions. Kolhapur has 38% of C-section delivery which is the highest in the state, and lowest in the Nandurbar district 7.9%. This study is therefore to investigate the socio-demographic and economic determinants of C-section delivery and differential within the state, and also to estimate inequalities in the health care facility for C-section delivery in the state.

## 11.2 Materials and Methods

The study uses data from the fifth round of the National Family Health Survey (NFHS) conducted during 2019–21. The NFHS provides information on fertility, infant and child mortality, family planning, maternal and child health, reproductive health, nutrition, anaemia, etc. obtained from representative household samples at the federal, state, and district across India. The International Institute for Population Sciences (IIPS), Mumbai has been assigned as the nodal agency to conduct different rounds of the national health family survey in India. The complete analysis was carried out on the 9520-sample size recent birth delivery for Maharashtra.

C-section among married women aged 15–49 years was taken as the dependent variable. Information on C-section delivery was obtained by asking the respondents the following two questions asked to currently married females: "Was the child delivered by C-section?" or "Did they cut your belly open to take the baby out?". Responses were recorded as "Yes" or "No." Women and household characteristics such as wealth index, birth order, mother education, body mass index, place of delivery, financial assistance to delivery, caste, age of mother, ultrasound test, antenatal visit, religion, and geographical regions of the state were included as predictor variable.

Univariate and bivariate methods are used to find the prevalence of C-section delivery and its association with the independent variable. The chi-square test of association was used to determine the relationship between the observed and expected frequencies in one or more categories, denoted by x and described as:

$$\chi^2 = \sum (xi - mi)^2/mi, xi \quad (\text{for} i = 1, 2 \ldots, K)$$

The Blinder-Oaxaca decomposition technique helps to explain the between-group differentials in outcome variables using a set of predictors. Initially, this technique was applied to decompose labor market outcomes between various groups, such as sex and race. The same method can be used to study group differences for any other variable (O'Donnell et al., 2021).

$$\Delta\overline{Y} = \underbrace{(\overline{x}_A - \overline{x}_B)'\hat{\beta}_B}_{} + \underbrace{\hat{\beta}'_B(\hat{\beta}_A - \hat{\beta}_B)}_{}$$

Explained Component Unexplained Component (Residual).

$\Delta\overline{Y}$ is the difference in mean outcomes between groups A and B.

$\bar{x}_A$ and $\bar{x}_B$ are the mean value of the observable characteristics for groups A and B.
$\hat{\beta}_A$ and $\hat{\beta}_B$ are the estimated coefficient vectors for the two groups (usually obtained through regression analysis).

The analysis was carried out using STATA version 16 as well as ArcGIS 10.8 was used to prepare a district-level map of Maharashtra while Microsoft Excel was used to prepare graphs.

## 11.3 Results

Table 11.1 provides the frequency distribution of C-section delivery with different background characteristics in Maharashtra, 2019–21. Women belonging to the richest household reported 38.8% highest rate of C-sections, and household wealth positively associated with C-section delivery. Children's birth order experience 31.1% of C-section delivery compared to second (25.7%) and third (15.1%). As per the mother education increases, C-section deliveries also increase, with women without education having 10.2% of C-section deliveries, and other side women with higher education reported 39.9% C-sections. Likewise, C-section delivery was found higher in private hospitals (38.9%) than public hospitals (18.3%). Other backward classes have 29.1% C-section delivery and the lowest among the scheduled tribe (14.1%). Women aged 35 and more delivered at 33.6% C-section delivery. C-section deliveries are higher among women belonging to other religions (47.8%) followed by Buddhist (26.5%) and Hindu (26%). The western region reported the highest C-section delivery (32%), followed by Konkan (28.2%), Vidarbha (25%), North-Maharashtra (20.6%), and lowest in Marathwada (16.2%).

Figure 11.1 presents the share of C-section delivery among public and private health facilities in different geographical regions of Maharashtra during 2019–21. Maharashtra is divided into five distinct regions namely Konkan, Western, Marathwada, North, and Vidarbha. The proportion of C-section deliveries in Maharashtra during 2019–21 is observed to be 25.4%, with 18.3% of the deliveries occurring at public health facilities, while 38.9% of the deliveries take place in private health care settings. Within the state, the highest proportion of C-section deliveries is witnessed to occur in the western region (41.9%) while the Marathwada region is observed to have a low prevalence at 25.1%. C-section deliveries were observed in all the areas of Maharashtra, with maximum increases occurring in the Konkan region (28.2%), Vidarbha (25%), the western part (32%), and lowest in the Marathwada region (16.2%). The western area has the highest C-section deliveries in public sections, whereas the weakest is in the North with 13.2%, and Marathwada with 13.3%.

The percentage of C-section delivery in different districts of Maharashtra during 2015–16 is shown in Fig. 11.2a. C-section deliveries were observed to be lowest in six districts namely Beed, Gadchiroli, Hingoli, Jalana, Nandurbar, and Yavatmal,

**Table 11.1** Percentage and frequency distribution of C-section delivery by different background characteristics in Maharashtra, India 2019–21

| Background Characteristics | No<br>% (n) | Yes<br>% (n) | *P* value |
|---|---|---|---|
| *Wealth Index* | | | |
| Poorest | 92.7(1070) | 7.3 (74) | 46.4*** |
| Poorer | 83.2(1633) | 16.8 (288) | |
| Middle | 76.7(1916) | 23.3 (530) | |
| Richer | 72.9(1790) | 27.1 (700) | |
| Richest | 61.2(952) | 38.8 (567) | |
| *Birth order* | | | |
| 1 | 68.9 (2917) | 31.1 (1128) | 225.4*** |
| 2 | 74.4 (2717) | 25.7 (820) | |
| 3 | 85 (1096) | 15.1 (163) | |
| 4 > | 91.8 (631) | 8.2 (48) | |
| *Mother education* | | | |
| No Education | 89.8 (692) | 10.2 (52) | 395.9*** |
| Primary | 85.5 (743) | 14.6 (102) | |
| Secondary | 75.9 (5038) | 24.1 (1426) | |
| Higher | 60.1 (888) | 39.9 (579) | |
| *Body Mass Index* | | | |
| < 16.0 | 84.9 (367) | 15.1 (69) | 191.5*** |
| 16.0–18.4 | 78.6 (1503) | 21.4 (302) | |
| 18.5–24.9 | 77.6 (4372) | 22.4 (1198) | |
| 25.0–29.9 | 63.6 (693) | 36.4 (385) | |
| ≥30 | 62.4 (426) | 37.6 (205) | |
| *Place of delivery* | | | |
| Public | 81.7 (4850) | 18.3 (980) | 668.5*** |
| Private | 61.1 (1965) | 38.9 (1179) | |
| Missing | 100 (546) | 0 (0) | |
| *Financial assistance for delivery* | | | |
| No | 70.3 (4264) | 29.7 (1578) | 186.3*** |
| Yes | 77.3 (935) | 22.7 (245) | |
| Missing | 85 (2162) | 15 (336) | |
| *Caste* | | | |
| Scheduled caste | 75.4 (1221) | 24.6 (322) | 175.2*** |
| Scheduled tribe | 85.9 (1464) | 14.1 (184) | |
| Other backward class | 70.9 (2025) | 29.1 (766) | |
| Other | 73 (2651) | 27.1 (887) | |

(continued)

**Table 11.1** (continued)

| Background Characteristics | No<br>% (n) | Yes<br>% (n) | *P* value |
|---|---|---|---|
| *Age of mother (years)* | | | |
| ≤19 | 78.3 (273) | 21.7 (68) | 39.08*** |
| 20–24 | 78.8 (2457) | 21.2 (596) | |
| 25–34 | 73.2 (4241) | 26.8 (1330) | |
| ≥35 | 66.4 (390) | 33.6 (165) | |
| *Ultrasound test* | | | |
| No | 89.6 (594) | 10.4 (47) | 92.3*** |
| Yes | 73.8 (6767) | 26.2 (2112) | |
| *Antenatal visit* | | | |
| 0–3 | 78.3 (1544) | 21.7 (363) | 106.3*** |
| ≥4 | 70.7 (3884) | 29.3 (1406) | |
| Don't know/ Missing | 80.9 (1933) | 19.1 (390) | |
| *Religion* | | | |
| Hindu | 74 (5774) | 26 (1745) | 23.79*** |
| Muslim | 80.5 (1080) | 19.5 (251) | |
| Buddhist | 73.5 (441) | 26.5 (125) | |
| Other | 52.2 (66) | 47.8 (38) | |
| *Regions of Maharashtra* | | | |
| Konkan | 71.8 (849) | 28.2 (322) | 169.9*** |
| Western | 68 (1071) | 32 (490) | |
| Marathwada | 83.8 (2199) | 16.2 (421) | |
| North-Maharashtra | 79.4 (1086) | 20.6 (236) | |
| Vidarbha | 75 (2156) | 25 (690) | |
| **Maharashtra** | **74.6 (7361)** | **25.4 (2159)** | |

*Note* Significant Value 95% C. I. *** $P < 0.001$, ** $P < 0.01$, * $P < 0.05$

medium in five districts of Ahmadnagar, Amravati, Dhule, Chandrapur, Mumbai Suburban, Raigarh, Ratnagiri, Sindhudurg, and Thane, and highest among in Akola, Kolhapur, Nagpur, Pune, Sangali, and Satara. Nandurbar at 10.6% had the lowest prevalence while Nagpur 40.8% has the highest occurrence of C-section delivery in Maharashtra. Along with Nandurbar, districts such as Jalana (10.8%), Gadchiroli (11.9%), Beed (13%), and Yavatmal (14%) have C-section prevalence below the WHO cut-off of 15%. The highest prevalence of C-section delivery is found in economically well-off districts such as Nagpur, Amravati, Kolhapur, Pune, Sangli, and Satara and more than 10 districts had a prevalence of C-section deliveries above 25% in 2015–16. Figure 11.2b presents the prevalence of C-section delivery in Maharashtra during 2019–21. Similar to 2015–16, Nandurbar (7.9%) had the lowest prevalence of C-section deliveries while Kolhapur (38.1%) in the western region

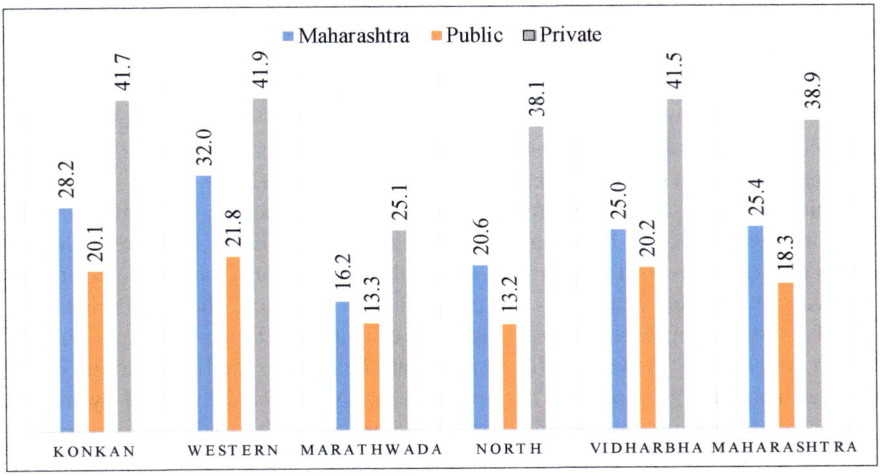


**Fig. 11.1** Percentage of C-section delivery in public and private hospitals by geographical regions in Maharashtra, 2019–21

had the maximum prevalence of deliveries through C-section procedure. Only 3 districts namely Nandurbar, Nanded, and Parbhani have C-section deliveries below 15% while 17 districts have a prevalence of caesarean deliveries above 25%. The change in C-section deliveries between 2015 and 2021 among mothers in Maharashtra is depicted in Fig. 11.2c. Amravati saw the highest percent increase (25.6%) in C-section deliveries among mothers between 15 and 49 years of age followed by Ahmednagar, Gondiya, Mumbai Suburban, Ratnagiri, and Sindhudurg. However, 11 districts witnessed a decline in deliveries through C-section procedures with Nagpur showing the maximum negative growth.

Table 11.2 provides information on the prevalence of C-section deliveries performed in private hospitals in various districts of Maharashtra. In Maharashtra, 38.9% of the C-section deliveries are performed in NFHS-5, whereas 32.8% of C-section deliveries are in NFHS-4, which is a 6.1 percent point over time. The C-section deliveries rapidly increase in the private health facility from NFHS-4 to NFHS-5. District like Amravati (25.6%), Gadchiroli (53.9%), Kolhapur (20.2%),

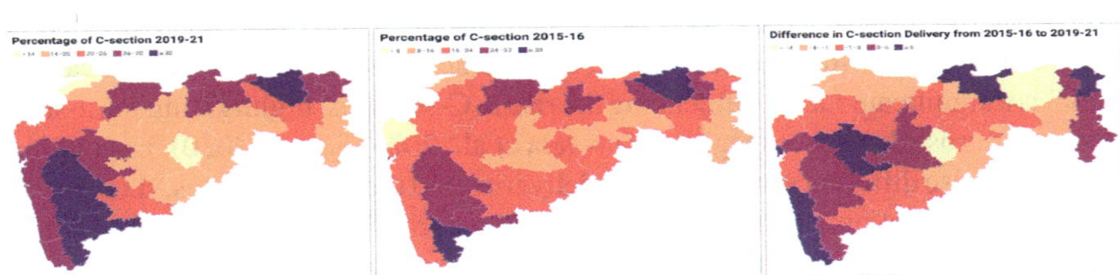


**Fig. 11.2** Change in prevalence of C-section deliveries in different districts of Maharashtra, India from 2015–16 to 2019–21

and Satara (28.2%) has the highest increase, whereas districts Ahmadnagar (9.2%), Nagpur (19.5%), and Wardha (9.6%) negative growth rate of C-section deliveries from NFHS-4 to NFHS-5. If we look at the district level, there is enormous variation among C-sections Amravati (58.9%), Bhandara (53.5%), Gadchiroli (87.2%), Kolhapur (55.8%), Palghar (54.4%), and Satara (53%) has the more than 50% caesarean deliveries at a private health facility in NFHS-5 (2019–21).

Table 11.3 shows the contribution of the endowment effect in explaining the gap in the average C-section between public and private healthcare facilities in Maharashtra during 2019–2021. The negative contribution indicates that the determinants narrowed the gap between public and private health facilities. The economic condition of women is observed to play the most crucial determinant in explaining C-section differentials between public and private healthcare facilities. About 7% of the total inequality is explained by women's economic status followed by mother birth order at 5.2% and mother educational attainment at 5%. 28.2% of the variation between C-section deliveries at public and private healthcare facilities is explained by socio-demographic and economic characteristics of women. In contrast, the negative contribution by the regions of Maharashtra (−1.3%) tends to narrow the difference in the C-section between public and private health facilities.

## 11.4 Discussion

Global C-section deliveries have increased, with one in five live births delivered through C-section (Brown, 2018). Our research identified an increasing trend in C-section deliveries over the last two survey periods. Similarly, Das found that as the state improved institutional birth rates, this indirectly contributed to the rise in C-section deliveries (Das & Sahoo, 2019; Sengupta et al., 2021).

Women from wealthier households had a higher likelihood of undergoing C-sections. Similarly, women with greater decision-making power and better antenatal care attendance were more likely to choose delivery at private health facilities (Gavvala et al., 2024; Quezada-Pinedo et al., 2022; Yaya et al., 2018). These findings align with our results, showing that a higher proportion of C-section deliveries occur in private hospitals compared to public ones. There is a varying prevalence of C-sections across different geographical regions of the state, with the highest rates in the western region and the lowest in the Marathwada region. A study conducted in Andhra Pradesh also found that the choice of medical institution, whether private or public, is a significant factor influencing the rise in C-sections, highlighting intra-state variations across districts or regions (Gavvala et al., 2024; Sarkar, 2020). Examining the district-wise differences in C-section deliveries and their growth rates, six districts reported the lowest prevalence of C-sections. Nandurbar had the lowest prevalence, falling below WHO recommendations, while Kolhapur reported the highest. Carter's research reveals that the choice of delivery method varies based on the availability of adequate facilities to perform C-sections (Carter & Walker, 2022). During the last two survey rounds, the growth of C-section deliveries increased, with Amravati showing

**Table 11.2** Percentage of C-section deliveries in private health facilities by districts in Maharashtra, India 2016–21

| Districts | NFHS-5 | NFHS-4 | Difference |
|---|---|---|---|
| Ahmadnagar | 33.5 | 42.7 | −9.2 |
| Akola | 42.0 | 38.3 | 3.6 |
| Amravati | 58 9 | 33.3 | 25.6 |
| Aurangabad | 19.5 | 22.7 | −3.2 |
| Bhandara | 53.5 | 61.3 | −7.8 |
| Beed | 20.7 | 21.2 | −0.4 |
| Buldana | 27.5 | 32.4 | −4.9 |
| Chandrapur | 41.7 | 48.3 | −6.6 |
| Dhule | 40.4 | 30.3 | 10.2 |
| Gadchiroli | 87.2 | 33.3 | 53.9 |
| Gondiya | 70.7 | 62.1 | 8.6 |
| Hingoli | 29.3 | 20.4 | 8.9 |
| Jalgaon | 39.4 | 40.2 | −0.8 |
| Jalna | 29.6 | 21.3 | 8.4 |
| Kolhapur | 55.8 | 35.6 | 20.2 |
| Latur | 36.5 | 21.7 | 14.8 |
| Mumbai | 39.1 | 33.9 | 5.2 |
| Mumbai Suburban | 41.9 | 43.5 | −1.6 |
| Nagpur | 41.4 | 60.9 | −19.5 |
| Nanded | 28.4 | 28.4 | −0.1 |
| Nandurbar | 28.5 | 26.1 | 2.4 |
| Nashik | 37.6 | 25.8 | 11.8 |
| Osmanabad | 31.9 | 29.2 | 2.7 |
| Palghar | 54.4 | * | * |
| Parbhani | 17.2 | 22.5 | −5.3 |
| Pune | 40.6 | 25.3 | 15.4 |
| Raigarh | 38.5 | 35.2 | 3.3 |
| Ratnagiri | 35.7 | 41.6 | −5.9 |
| Sangli | 43.2 | 46.1 | −2.9 |
| Satara | 53.0 | 24.8 | 28.2 |
| Sindhudurg | 44.3 | 27.9 | 16.4 |
| Solapur | 34.9 | 29.7 | 5.2 |
| Thane | 41.3 | 43.5 | −2.2 |
| Wardha | 38.3 | 47.9 | −9.6 |
| Washim | 29.7 | 29.3 | 0.4 |
| Yavatmal | 32.1 | 26.3 | 5.8 |
| **Maharashtra** | **38.9** | **32.8** | **6.1** |

**Table 11.3** Oaxaca Decomposition showing the contribution of different predictor variables to C-section differences between public and private health facilities in Maharashtra, India 2019–2021

| Contributing factors | Coef | Level of Significant | 95% CI | Contribution (%) |
|---|---|---|---|---|
| *Caesarean delivery* | | | | |
| Differential | | | | |
| Prediction_ Goverment Hospital | 0.181 | *** | (0.170,0.193) | |
| Prediction_Private Hospital | 0.400 | *** | (0.381,0.420) | |
| Difference (Public Hospital-Private Hospital) | 0.219 | *** | (0.196,0.242) | |
| *Explained* | | | | |
| Wealth Index | 0.015 | *** | (0.005, 0.026) | 7.0 |
| Birth Order | 0.011 | *** | (0.007, 0.015) | 5.2 |
| Mother Education | 0.011 | *** | (0.005, 0.018) | 5.0 |
| Body Mass Index | 0.009 | *** | (0.006, 0.013) | 4.3 |
| Place of Residence | 0.007 | *** | (0.002, 0.011) | 3.1 |
| Financial Assistance for Delivery | 0.004 | ** | (0.000, 0.008) | 1.8 |
| Caste | 0.003 | * | (−0.001, 0.007) | 1.3 |
| Age of Mother | 0.002 | *** | (0.001, 0.004) | 1.0 |
| Ultrasound Test | 0.001 | * | (−0.001, 0.003) | 0.5 |
| Antenatal visit | 0.001 | * | (−0.001, 0.002) | 0.4 |
| Religion | 0.000 | * | (0.000, 0.000) | 0.0 |
| Regions of Maharashtra | −0.003 | * | (−0.007, 0.001) | −1.3 |
| **Total** | **0.062** | *** | (0.050, 0.073) | **28.2** |
| **Unexplained** | | | | |
| **Total** | **0.157** | | | **72.1** |

*Note* Significant Value 95% C. I. *** $P < 0.001$, ** $P < 0.01$, * $P < 0.05$

the highest growth rate, while eleven districts reported a decline. The prevalence of C-sections is influenced by both maternal demand and the decisions of physicians and other healthcare providers. Social narratives and the medical necessity for surgical procedures also contribute to the variation in C-section rates (Hallgrimsdottir et al., 2017).

The study reveals that women from the wealthiest households, those experiencing their first pregnancy, women with higher education levels, and those with a body mass index above normal are more likely to undergo C-section deliveries. A recent study also indicated that non-medical factors play a significant role in influencing women's decisions to opt for C-sections (Acharya & Paudel, 2021; Chauhan & Radkar, 2023; Nakinobe et al., 2023). Previous research has similarly shown that overweight women are more likely to have C-section deliveries (Pandey et al., 2023). Moreover, women experiencing their first pregnancy are also at higher risk of undergoing a C-section (Idris & Menghisteab, 2022). Social groups have a significant influence on C-section rates, with women from other backward classes experiencing more C-sections compared to other groups. Similarly, religion affects C-section deliveries, with women from certain religious backgrounds reporting higher rates than those from Buddhist, Hindu, and other communities. Age is also a significant factor, as older women are more likely to undergo C-sections compared to those in younger reproductive age groups. Rajabi's study found that maternal age, age at marriage, and socio-economic factors such as family income and education are associated with C-section deliveries (Rajabi et al., 2015). The higher rate of C-section deliveries in private hospitals highlights significant disparities between public and private healthcare settings. The increasing number of C-sections in private hospitals is concerning, with more than half of these deliveries occurring in private healthcare facilities (Sarkar, 2020). Economic status, birth order of children, and maternal education are key factors contributing to the disparity between healthcare facilities. The rising C-section rates in private health facilities are closely associated with family income, maternal education, the number of children, and previous C-section risks (Carlotto et al., 2020; Rajabi et al., 2015). Given that C-sections typically pose more medical risks than benefits, they should be performed only when medically necessary, following a comprehensive evaluation of the potential risks and benefits (Mahapatra, 2015; Niino, 2011).

## 11.5 Conclusion

The proportion of C-section deliveries has been increasing over time, with a significant concentration occurring in private healthcare settings. There are notable disparities in C-section rates across different districts and geographical regions within the state. Factors such as women's economic status, education, body mass index, caste, religion, and access to healthcare facilities contribute to these differences. In private hospitals, C-section rates are primarily influenced by women's economic status, education, and the number of children, which in turn exacerbate existing inequalities.

## 11.6 Ethical Approval

The present study used secondary data, which is available in the public domain. The dataset has no identifiable information about the survey participants. Therefore, no ethical approval is required for conducting this study.

**Acknowledgements** Thankful to Indian Association for Population Studies gave the opportunity to present the same chapter at a regional level conference, 2022.

**Conflict of Interest** Conflicts of interest, the authors declare that they have no conflict of interest.

## References

Acharya, K., & Paudel, Y. R. (2021). Trend and sociodemographic correlates of cesarean section utilization in Nepal: Evidence from Demographic and Health Surveys 2006–2016. *BioMed Research International, 2021.* https://doi.org/10.1155/2021/8888267

Bansod, D., Paswan, B., & Lhungdim, H. (2018). Increasing trends of caesarean deliveries in India: Does private sector contributes it? *SSRN Electronic Journal*, 1–19. https://doi.org/10.2139/ssrn.3112190

Brown, C. (2018). C-section rate rises globally as "costly intervention" replaces "natural process." *CMAJ: Canadian Medical Association Journal = Journal de l'Association Medicale Canadienne, 190*(50), E1489–E1490. https://doi.org/10.1503/cmaj.109-5686

Carlotto, K., Marmitt, L. P., & Cesar, J. A. (2020). On-demand cesarean section: Assessing trends and socioeconomic disparities. *Revista de Saude Publica, 54*, 1–9. https://doi.org/10.11606/S1518-8787.2019053001466

Carter, E. D., & Walker, P. N. (2022). Estimating C-section coverage: Assessing method performance and characterizing variations in coverage. *Journal of Global Health, 12*, 1–8. https://doi.org/10.7189/JOGH.21.08002

Chauhan, B. G., & Radkar, A. (2023). Trends and inequalities in caesarean section delivery in India. *Journal of Public Health, 0123456789.* https://doi.org/10.1007/s10389-023-01888-3

Das, S., & Sahoo, H. (2019). Caesarean section delivery in India: Public and private dichotomy. *Demography India, 48*(1), 36–48.

Gavvala, N., Thomas M, B., & Jennifer H, G. (2024). Disparities in elective and emergency caesarean section rates among public and private hospitals in the districts of Andhra Pradesh, India. *Cureus, 16*(2), 1–13. https://doi.org/10.7759/cureus.54320

Hallgrimsdottir, H., Shumka, L., Althaus, C., & Benoit, C. (2017). Fear, risk, and the responsible choice: Risk narratives and lowering the rate of caesarean sections in high-income countries. *AIMS Public Health, 4*(6), 615–632. https://doi.org/10.3934/publichealth.2017.6.615

Idris, I. M., & Menghisteab, S. (2022). Cesarean section delivery rates, determinants, and indications: A retrospective study in Dekemhare Hospital. *Global Reproductive Health, 7*(1), e56–e56. https://doi.org/10.1097/grh.0000000000000056

International Institute for Population Sciences (IIPS) and ICF. (2021). *National Family Health Survey (NFHS-5), 2019–21: India.* Mumbai: IIPS. http://rchiips.org/nfhs/factsheet_NFHS-5.shtml

Islam, M. A., Shanto, H. H., Jabbar, A., & Howlader, M. H. (2022). Caesarean section in Indonesia: Analysis of trends and socio-demographic correlates in three demographic and health surveys (2007–2017). In *Dr. Sulaiman Al Habib Medical Journal* (Vol. 4, Issue 3, pp. 136–144). https://doi.org/10.1007/s44229-022-00011-0

Kumari, P. S., & Thomas, V. (2013). A cross-sectional study of rates and determinants of Cs in Hyderabad. *IJMPS, 03*(05), 14–19.

Mahapatra, P. (2015). *Rising cesarean sections: Causes & concerns. Towards a Public Health Agenda for Quality & Safety of Maternity Services. A White Paper.* 0–1.

Mor, N. (2020, May). *Addressing high caesarean section rates in parts of India.* https://www.researchgate.net/publication/339998810

Nakinobe, F. G., Lwanga, C., Ojiambo Wandera, S., Kalule-Sabiti, I., & Mangombe, K. (2023). Caesarean delivery in Uganda: Do non-clinical factors explain the trend? *Journal of Biosocial Science, 55*(5), 980–993. https://doi.org/10.1017/S0021932022000359

Niino, Y. (2011). The increasing caesarean rate globally and what we can do about it. *BioScience Trends, 5*(4), 139–150. https://doi.org/10.5582/bst.2011.v5.4.139

O'Donnell, O., van Doorslaer, E., Wagstaff, A., & Lindelow, M. (2021). Analyzing health equity using household survey data. *The World Bank*. https://doi.org/10.1016/B978-0-323-48410-7.00012-5

Pandey, A. K., Raushan, M. R., Gautam, D., & Neogi, S. B. (2023). Alarming trends of cesarean section-time to rethink: Evidence from a large-scale cross-sectional sample survey in India. *Journal of Medical Internet Research, 25*. https://doi.org/10.2196/41892

Quezada-Pinedo, H. G., Cajachagua-Torres, K. N., Guzman-Vilca, W. C., Tarazona-Meza, C., Carrillo-Larco, R. M., & Huicho, L. (2022). Flat trend of high caesarean section rates in Peru: A pooled analysis of 3,376,062 births from the national birth registry, 2012 to 2020: Caesarean section rates in Peru. *The Lancet Regional Health - Americas, 12*, Article 100293. https://doi.org/10.1016/j.lana.2022.100293

Rajabi, A., Maharlouei, N., Rezaianzadeh, A., Rajaeefard, A., & Gholami, A. (2015). Risk factors for C-section delivery and population attributable risk for C-section risk factors in Southwest of Iran: A prospective cohort study. *Medical Journal of the Islamic Republic of Iran, 29*(1), 1150–1158.

Roy, A., Paul, P., Chouhan, P., Rahaman, M., & Kapasia, N. (2021). Geographical variability and factors associated with caesarean section delivery in India: A comparative assessment of Bihar and Tamil Nadu. *BMC Public Health, 21*(1), 1–15. https://doi.org/10.1186/s12889-021-11750-4

Sarkar, S. (2020). Prevalence and determinants of the use of caesarean section (CS) in the dichotomy of 'public' and 'private' health facilities in West Bengal, India. *Clinical Epidemiology and Global Health, 8*(4), 1377–1383. https://doi.org/10.1016/j.cegh.2020.05.017

Sengupta, A., Sabastin Sagayam, M., & Reja, T. (2021). Increasing trend of C-section deliveries in India: A comparative analysis between southern states and rest of India. *Sexual and Reproductive Healthcare, 28*(September 2020), 100608. https://doi.org/10.1016/j.srhc.2021.100608

Shabnam, S. (2009). Caesarean Section Delivery in India: Causes and Concerns. *Session 221: Assessments of Facility-Based Delivery Services*, 1–20. http://iussp.org/sites/default/files/event_call_for_papers/Caesarean%20section%20delivery%20in%20India_0.pdf

UN. (2023). The Sustainable Development Goals Report. In *United Nation Suistanable Development Goals*.

World Health Organization. (2024). *Maternal mortality*. World Health Organization.

Yaya, S., Uthman, O. A., Amouzou, A., & Bishwajit, G. (2018). Disparities in caesarean section prevalence and determinants across sub-Saharan Africa countries. *Global Health Research and Policy, 3*(1), 1–9. https://doi.org/10.1186/s41256-018-0074-y

# Chapter 12
# Study of Postpartum Amenorrhea Period and Its Determinants: A Hazard Analysis Approach

**Ravi Kant Maurya, Anuj Singh, and Aman Kr Tiwari**

**Abstract** Postpartum amenorrhea (PPA), the temporary cessation of menstruation following childbirth, is a critical parameter that reflects physiological recovery post-delivery and provides insights into fertility, maternal, and child health. The return of a woman's menstrual cycle after childbirth is particularly significant in developing countries with high population growth rates. This chapter used all rounds of the National Family Health Survey (NFHS) to identify covariates affecting postpartum amenorrhea in India. Preliminary basic statistics provide a descriptive understanding of these covariates. The primary analytical method employed is the hazard ratio, a statistical tool used in survival analysis to compare the risk of an event (the return of menstruation) occurring in different groups or conditions over time. The analysis reveals several covariates significantly influencing the duration of postpartum amenorrhea. Maternal age, breastfeeding practices, socioeconomic status, and regional differences emerged as key factors. For instance, extended breastfeeding was associated with longer periods of amenorrhea, while higher socioeconomic status correlated with a quicker return of menstrual cycles. Regional disparities highlighted the impact of cultural and healthcare access factors. Understanding the factors influencing postpartum amenorrhea is vital for developing targeted interventions to improve maternal and child health in India. This study highlights the importance of breastfeeding and socioeconomic factors in determining the duration of PPA. Policymakers should consider these findings to support women's health and family planning initiatives, particularly in regions with limited healthcare access.

**Keywords** Postpartum amenorrhea · Hazard analysis · NFHS · India

R. K. Maurya
Department of Statistics, Mahatma Gandhi Kashi Vidyapith, Varanasi, India
e-mail: ravikantmaurya07@gmail.com

A. Singh (✉)
Department of Mathematics (Sciences), Indian Institute of Information Technology Ranchi, Ranchi, India
e-mail: anujsingh11185@gmail.com

A. K. Tiwari
Krantisinh Nana Patil College of Veterinary Science, MAFSU, Shirwal, Maharashtra, India

 
P. Chouhan et al. (eds.), *Women's Health Dynamics in South Asia*, Asian Perspectives on Public Health, https://doi.org/10.1007/978-981-95-2321-4_12

## 12.1 Introduction

The study of postpartum amenorrhea, a critical facet of reproductive health, serves as a barometer for understanding the complex interplay of biological, sociocultural, and healthcare factors within a population (Bongaarts & Potter, 1983; Gray et al., 1990). Postpartum amenorrhea (PPA), the temporary cessation of menstruation following childbirth, is a crucial parameter that reflects not only the physiological recovery of women post-delivery but also provides insights into broader aspects of fertility, maternal and child health (Labbok & Krasovec, 1990). The return of a woman's menstrual cycle after giving birth is a notable consideration in developing countries marked by high rates of population growth. In these regions, rapid population growth is a major obstacle to comprehensive national development. As India undergoes demographic shifts, socioeconomic changes, and advances in healthcare infrastructure, examining the trajectory of postpartum amenorrhea becomes essential for interventions that cater to the evolving needs of women in the reproductive age group (Nath & Goshawmi, 1996).

As we know, PPA is a natural physiological phenomenon influenced by a multitude of factors such as breastfeeding practices, maternal age, parity, and access to healthcare. In particular, maternal education is inversely related to the duration of Postpartum Amenorrhea (PPA) (Huffman et al., 1987; Singh et al., 1994). Concurrently, previous study showed a positive correlation between the duration of breastfeeding and the duration of postpartum amenorrhea (Santow, 2012). However, it's important to note that this correlation doesn't necessarily imply that extended breastfeeding directly causes a delay in the return of menstruation (Corsini, 1979). Other factors, including overall health and nutrition, likely play a role in this relationship. The early introduction of supplementary foods is likely to reduce the frequency of breastfeeding (Huffman et al., 1980), which, in turn, affects the length of PPA. The age of the mother can indeed influence the duration of PPA. Several studies, including those conducted by (Huffman et al., 1987; Jones, 1990) have demonstrated that amenorrhea tends to be of longer duration in older women compared to their younger counterparts. It's widely recognized that breastfeeding has the effect of inhibiting a mother's natural ovulatory cycle, making it a critical means of preventing pregnancy, especially in low-income nations (Knodel, 1977). The location where a woman resides can impact the duration of her PPA through its influence on the production of prolactin. Frequent and intense breastfeeding leads to higher levels of prolactin that suppresses ovulation (Lunn et al., 1984). Prolactin also affects the ability of a fertilized egg to attach to the uterine wall, suggesting that extended breastfeeding might be associated with a longer period of PPA. Two crucial factors that determine the length of this infertile period are the duration of exclusive breastfeeding (un-supplemented lactation) and the overall duration of breastfeeding (McCann et al., 1981). It's worth noting that it has long been established that the time it takes for ovulation to return and for proper luteal function to resume is significantly longer in women who practice exclusive breastfeeding compared to those who practice partial or no breastfeeding (Howei & McNeilly, 1982; Perez et al., 1971). Furthermore, research by Habicht et al. in 1985 demonstrated that a month of exclusive breastfeeding, on average, extends the period of ovulation by more than a month.

Women's nutrition and overall health status have also a significant impact on the duration of PPA. Poor nutrition can affect a woman's reproductive health and lead to a delay in the resumption of her menstrual cycles, as indicated by research conducted by (Singh et al., 2021). A mother's occupation is also expected to have an impact on the duration of PPA. Women working in modern sectors of the economy are more likely to introduce supplementary foods to their infants' diets earlier, resulting in less frequent and shorter breastfeeding sessions compared to women primarily engaged in household work (Labbok & Krasovec, 1990). Additionally, the socioeconomic status of women plays a role in the duration of PPA. Women in higher socioeconomic status groups tend to have access to more nutritious foods, which can affect their milk production (Dewey & Brown, 2003). In contrast, poorly nourished mothers may produce less milk, leading their hungry infants to breastfeed more frequently and intensively. Consequently, mothers from lower socioeconomic status groups are expected to experience longer periods of PPA (McNeilly et al., 1982).

Some authors have been used the determinants of PPA, a multi-state hazard approach (Aguirre, 1996). While some studies have used socio-demographic correlates of PPA in an urban society in India (Nath & Goshawmi, 1996). Odimegwu (2001) utilized the hazard model to analyze the determinants of postpartum behavior among Igbo women in south-eastern Nigeria. In the Indian context, where diverse demographic and cultural dynamics shape the landscape of maternal health, an in-depth analysis spanning multiple National Family Health Surveys (NFHS) becomes imperative. Therefore, the present chapter aims to investigate the prevalence, duration, and associated determinants of PPA offering a comprehensive perspective on how this phenomenon has evolved over the past few decades. Firstly, we have calculated the mean of PPA with background characteristics to see if there is any variation among them or not. Further, the next objective is to focus on the determinants influencing PPA by using the hazard ratio model.

## 12.2 Materials and Methods

The NFHS is a comprehensive and nationally representative survey conducted in India to gather data on various aspects of public health, including maternal and child health. One of the essential aspects covered by the NFHS is postpartum amenorrhea, which is the absence of menstruation in the months following childbirth. The NFHS records the duration of postpartum amenorrhea for women who experience it (IIPS & ICF, 2021). This information helps in understanding how long postpartum amenorrhea typically lasts and when women are likely to resume their menstrual cycles. Additionally, demographic and socioeconomic variables have been included to facilitate a nuanced analysis of the determinants influencing postpartum amenorrhea. By using all rounds of the NFHS, authors have identified the covariate which affects postpartum amenorrhea. After identifying the covariates, inferential statistics have been shown in the recent round of the National Family Health Survey, i.e., NFHS-5.

### 12.2.1 Dependent Variable

Postpartum amenorrhea of women (15–49 years) is our explained variable.

### 12.2.2 Independent Variables

Caste is a traditional social stratification system in India that divides people into hierarchical groups based on their birth. It is crucial to include caste as an independent variable in the study of postpartum amenorrhea (PPA) in India because it significantly influences socioeconomic status, access to healthcare, nutrition, and breastfeeding practices, all of which are critical determinants of PPA (Mishra et al., 2021; Nath & Goshawmi, 1996; Singh et al. 1994). Understanding the role of caste can provide insights into disparities in maternal and child health outcomes and help tailor interventions to reduce these inequalities (Table 12.1).

### 12.2.3 Statistical Analyses

Univariate and bivariate Statistics have been used to get a descriptive idea about the covariates of PPA. A hazard ratio is a statistical method used in survival analysis to compare the risk of an event or outcome occurring in different groups or conditions over time. It is a fundamental concept in epidemiology, clinical research, and various other fields to assess the effect of a particular intervention, exposure, or variable on the time-to-event outcomes, such as the time until a disease occurs, the time until an event happens, or the time until death. The most common method for estimating hazard ratios is the Cox-proportional hazards model. This model doesn't make any assumptions about the shape of the baseline hazard function, which is a crucial advantage. It allows for the inclusion of multiple covariates in the analysis.

The mathematical form of the hazard ratio (HR) typically arises is expressed using mathematical notation.

$$h_1(t) = h_0(t) * \exp(\beta_1 * X)$$

where,

- $h_1(t)$ is the hazard function for the treatment group.
- $h_0(t)$ is the baseline hazard function for the reference group.

**Table 12.1** Description of independent variables, coding scheme, and references used in the analysis

| Independent variables | Definition | Sub-category | Coding | Reference |
|---|---|---|---|---|
| Age-group | Age of the women (years) | 15–24<br>25–29<br>≥30 years | Recode v012 (15/24 = 1 "15–24 year") (25/29 = 2 "25–29 year") (30/49 = 3 " > 30 year"), gen(ag) | Aguirre, 1996; Mishra et al., 2021 |
| Caste | Caste of the women | SC/ST<br>OBC<br>Others | Recode s116 (1/2 = 1 "SC/ST") (3 = 2 "OBC") (4 = 3 "Others") (else = .), gen (caste) | Nath & Goshawmi, 1996; Mishra et al., 2021 |
| Residence | Place of residence of the women | Rural<br>Urban | v025 | Nath & Goshawmi, 1996; Mishra et al., 2021 |
| Mother education | Education of the women | No education<br>Primary<br>Secondary<br>Higher | v106 | Nath & Goshawmi, 1996; Mishra et al., 2021 |
| Breastfeeding | Duration of breastfeeding of women after given birth | 0–6 months<br>> 6 months | Recode m4_2 (0/6 = 1 "0–6 month") (7/60 = 2 " > 6 month") (94/98 = .),gen(bf) | Nath & Goshawmi, 1996; Singh et al.1994 |
| Body Mass Index | Women's BMI based on height and weight | Underweight<br>Normal<br>Overweight/ Obese | Gen bmi = v445/100 if v445! = 9998<br>Gen BMI =<br>Replace BMI = 1 if bmi < = 18.499 & bmi! =<br>Replace BMI = 2 if bmi ≥ 18.50 & bmi < = 24.999<br>Replace BMI = 3 if bmi ≥ 25.00 & bmi! =<br>Replace BMI = . if bmi = = 9998<br>Label define T 1 "Underweight" 2 "Normal" 3 "Overweight/ Obese"<br>Label values BMI T<br>ta BMI | Nath & Goshawmi, 1996; Aguirre, 1996 |
| Wealth index | Composite measure of household assets and amenities | Poorest<br>Poorer<br>Middle<br>Richer<br>Richest | V190 | Nath & Goshawmi, 1996; Mishra et al., 2021 |

- $\beta_1$ is the coefficient associated with the treatment group in the Cox model.
- $X$ represents the vector of covariates (e.g., age, caste, etc.).

The exponential term, $\exp(\beta_1 * X)$ quantifies how the hazard in the treatment group differs from the reference group based on the values of the covariates.

## 12.3 Results

Table 12.2 presents the mean of postpartum amenorrhea (mPPA) for the last but one birth with the socio-demographic covariates of the study population from the first round to the fifth round of the National Family Health Survey (NFHS) in India. In the case of the age group of the women, results show that mPPA has increased as the age of women increases across all rounds of NFHS. Furthermore, results show that higher mPPA was found among the 35–39 years of aged women with 7.5 and 5.33 months from the first and fourth round of NFHS, respectively, and among 40–44 years of aged women with 7.41 and 5.62 months of mPPA from the third and fifth round of NFHS, respectively. Caste of the women shows that scheduled tribe (ST) women had the higher mPPA across all rounds of NFHS and general women had lower mPPA across the rounds of NFHS. Afterwards, results for religion show that Hindu women had higher mPPA (5.01, 6.2, 4.86 and 4.96 months) across all rounds of NFHS except the first round (5.67 months) of NFHS as compared to Muslim women. Rural areas women had higher mPPA across all rounds of NFHS than urban areas women. Moreover, in the case of maternal education, results show that as the education of the mother increased the level of mPPA decreased over the period of time, i.e., a mother with no education had a higher level of mPPA and a higher educated mother had a lower level of mPPA over the period of time. Women with more than six months of breastfeeding showed a higher level mPPA as compared to the women with less than 6 months of breastfeeding across all rounds of NFHS, i.e., higher the duration of breastfeeding, higher the level of mPPA, and lower the duration of breastfeeding caused the lower the level of mPPA. Additionally, results of body mass index show that underweight women had higher levels of mPPA and overweight women had lower levels of mPPA across all rounds of NFHS. In the case of the wealth status of the women, the poorest women had the highest level of mPPA and the richest women had the lowest level of mPPA across all rounds of NFHS.

Table 12.3 analyzed the duration and determinants of postpartum amenorrhea (PPA) among women in India using NFHS-5 data. The results showed that women aged 15–24 years had a mean PPA of 4.67 months, with 75.81% experiencing PPA for 0–6 months. In contrast, women aged 25–29 had a mean PPA of 4.99 months, and those aged 30 years and above had a mean PPA of 5.30 months. Caste-wise, Scheduled Castes/Scheduled Tribes (SC/ST) women had the longest mean PPA of 5.42 months, while women from other castes had a mean PPA of 4.46 months. Rural women had a mean PPA of 5.09 months, whereas urban women had a mean PPA of 4.48 months. Educational attainment influenced PPA duration, with women having

**Table 12.2** Mean postpartum amenorrhea with the socio-demographic covariates of the population for India from NFHS-1 (1992–93) to NFHS-5 (2019–2021)

| Covariates | PPA | | | | |
|---|---|---|---|---|---|
| | NFHS-1 | NFHS-2 | NFHS-3 | NFHS-4 | NFHS-5 |
| | Mean | Mean | Mean | Mean | Mean |
| *Age-group* | | | | | |
| 15–19 | 5.7 | 4.7 | 5.4 | 4.7 | 4.7 |
| 20–24 | 5.9 | 4.7 | 5.6 | 4.7 | 4.8 |
| 25–29 | 6.0 | 5.1 | 6.2 | 4.9 | 5.0 |
| 30–34 | 6.8 | 5.6 | 6.7 | 5.1 | 5.2 |
| 35–39 | 7.5 | 5.0 | 7.3 | 5.3 | 5.5 |
| 40–44 | 7.2 | 5.3 | 7.4 | 5.2 | 5.6 |
| *Caste* | | | | | |
| SC | 6.6 | 5.0 | 6.4 | 4.8 | 4.8 |
| ST | 6.7 | 5.5 | 6.8 | 5.6 | 6.1 |
| OBC | - | 5.1 | 6.3 | 4.7 | 4.7 |
| GEN | 5.9 | 4.5 | 5.2 | 4.4 | 4.5 |
| *Residence* | | | | | |
| Urban | 5.18 | 4.37 | 5.19 | 4.45 | 4.48 |
| Rural | 6.50 | 5.15 | 6.63 | 4.98 | 5.09 |
| *Mother education* | | | | | |
| No education | 6.71 | 5.26 | 6.86 | 5.03 | 5.14 |
| Primary | 5.99 | 5.00 | 6.27 | 5.05 | 5.18 |
| Secondary | 4.77 | 4.51 | 5.39 | 4.76 | 4.95 |
| Higher | 3.23 | 4.09 | 4.12 | 4.18 | 4.49 |
| *Duration of breastfeeding* | | | | | |
| < 6 months | 3.5 | 3.21 | 3.76 | - | 4.21 |
| > 6 months | 6.8 | 5.55 | 6.74 | - | 5.24 |
| *Body mass index* | | | | | |
| Underweight | - | 4.99 | 6.79 | 5.24 | 5.43 |
| Normal | - | 4.98 | 6.01 | 4.84 | 4.98 |
| Overweight/ Obese | - | 3.58 | 4.35 | 4.15 | 4.46 |
| *Wealth index* | | | | | |
| Poorest | - | - | 7.77 | 5.34 | 5.64 |
| Poorer | - | - | 6.83 | 5.06 | 5.05 |
| Middle | - | - | 6.24 | 4.75 | 4.79 |
| Richer | - | - | 5.21 | 4.35 | 4.48 |
| Richest | - | - | 4.22 | 3.93 | 3.89 |

no education showing a mean PPA of 5.18 months, and those with higher education having a mean PPA of 4.49 months. Breastfeeding for more than 6 months was associated with a longer mean PPA of 5.24 months, compared to 4.21 months for those breastfeeding for 0–6 months. Body mass index (BMI) also played a role, with underweight women having a mean PPA of 5.43 months, while overweight/obese women had a mean PPA of 4.46 months. The wealth index showed that the poorest women had the longest mean PPA of 5.64 months, whereas the richest had the shortest mean PPA of 3.89 months. Overall, the total sample had a mean PPA of 4.99 months, with 74.16% of women experiencing PPA for 0–6 months.

Table 12.4 shows the association between postpartum amenorrhea and women's selected covariates using Cox-proportional hazard analysis. Women aged 25–29 years and those aged 30 years or older have a significantly lower hazard of experiencing postpartum amenorrhea compared to the reference group of 15–24 years. In both adjusted and unadjusted models, the hazard ratio for women aged 25–29 years is 0.28, and for women aged 30 years or older, it is between 0.02 and 0.03, indicating a significantly reduced likelihood of experiencing postpartum amenorrhea as maternal age increases. Compared to women from SC/ST backgrounds, women from Other Backward Classes (OBC) have a higher hazard ratio of experiencing postpartum amenorrhea in the unadjusted model (1.75). However, in the adjusted models, the hazard ratio for OBC women drops to 1.03, indicating a minimal increase in likelihood after adjusting for other factors. Women from other castes have consistently higher hazard ratios (1.97) across all models, suggesting a greater likelihood of experiencing postpartum amenorrhea compared to SC/ST women. Women residing in rural areas have a higher hazard of postpartum amenorrhea compared to those living in urban areas. The unadjusted hazard ratio for rural women is 1.37, which decreases to approximately 1.05 in the adjusted models. Women with no education, and those with primary education initially show a higher hazard ratio (1.21) in the unadjusted model, which becomes lower than 1 (0.89) in the adjusted models. Women with higher education have the highest hazard ratio (2.23) in the unadjusted model, which reduces to around 1.84–1.88 in the adjusted models, indicating that higher education is associated with a greater likelihood of postpartum amenorrhea. Women who breastfeed for more than six months have a reduced hazard of postpartum amenorrhea, with a hazard ratio of 0.74 across all models. Compared to women with normal BMI, underweight women have a reduced hazard of postpartum amenorrhea (0.47) in the unadjusted model. In the adjusted model II, this hazard ratio is 0.74, indicating a protective effect. Overweight/obese women have a higher hazard ratio in the unadjusted model (1.46), which slightly decreases to around 1.056 in the adjusted model II. Higher wealth is consistently associated with an increased hazard of postpartum amenorrhea. Compared to the poorest category, the hazard ratios increase progressively from 1.53 (poorer) to 1.87 (richest) in the unadjusted model, with similar increases in the adjusted models.

In the adjusted model, all the predictor variables contribute to maximizing the log-likelihood of the model and it is observed that in Model-II, pseudo-likelihood is reduced after considering the body mass index (BMI) as a predictor. It indicates

**Table 12.3** Descriptive Statistics of postpartum amenorrhea with background characteristics for India using NFHS-5 data

| PPA | 0–6 months | > 6 months | Mean PPA |
|---|---|---|---|
| | *n*<br>(percentage) | *n*<br>(percentage) | |
| **Covariates** | | | |
| *Age-group* | | | |
| 15–24 | 11,786<br>(75.81) | 3,760<br>(24.19) | 4.67 |
| 25–29 | 15,356<br>(74.13) | 5,359<br>(25.87) | 4.99 |
| ≥30 years | 7,840<br>(71.86) | 3,070<br>(28.14) | 5.30 |
| *Caste* | | | |
| SC/ST | 14,042<br>(70.03) | 6,010<br>(29.97) | 5.42 |
| OBC | 14,340<br>(76.33) | 4,447<br>(23.67) | 4.72 |
| Others | 5,094<br>(79.76) | 1,293<br>(20.24) | 4.46 |
| *Residence* | | | |
| Rural | 28,645<br>(73.12) | 10,529<br>(26.88) | 5.09 |
| Urban | 6,337<br>(79.24) | 1,660<br>(20.76) | 4.48 |
| *Mother education* | | | |
| No education | 9,001<br>(73.32) | 3,275<br>(26.68) | 5.18 |
| Primary | 4,974<br>(72.11) | 1,924<br>(27.89) | 5.14 |
| Secondary | 17,262<br>(74.20) | 6,003<br>(25.80) | 4.95 |
| Higher | 3,745<br>(79.14) | 987<br>(20.86) | 4.49 |
| *Breastfeeding* | | | |
| 0–6 months | 432<br>(80.15) | 107<br>(19.85) | 4.21 |
| > 6 months | 1,260<br>(71.84) | 494<br>(28.16) | 5.24 |
| *Body Mass Index* | | | |
| Underweight | 6,789<br>(70.11) | 2,894<br>(29.89) | 5.43 |

(continued)

Table 12.3 (continued)

| PPA | 0–6 months | > 6 months | Mean PPA |
|---|---|---|---|
| | n (percentage) | n (percentage) | |
| Normal | 22,094 (74.35) | 7,623 (25.65) | 4.98 |
| Overweight/Obese | 5,158 (78.56) | 1,408 (21.44) | 4.46 |
| *Wealth Index* | | | |
| Poorest | 10,225 (68.27) | 4,753 (31.73) | 5.64 |
| Poorer | 8,567 (73.64) | 3,066 (26.36) | 5.05 |
| Middle | 6,816 (75.68) | 2,190 (24.32) | 4.79 |
| Richer | 5,553 (78.95) | 1,481 (21.05) | 4.48 |
| Richest | 3,821 (84.54) | 699 (15.46) | 3.89 |
| **Total** | **34,982 (74.16)** | **12,189 (25.84)** | **4.99** |

that Model-II provides a better explanation for PPA with the proposed predictor, i.e., BMI show a significant impact on the PPA.

## 12.4 Discussion

This study provides a comprehensive analysis of the PPA period in India, utilizing data from all rounds of the National Family Health Survey (NFHS). By examining various socio-demographic factors, we have identified key determinants influencing the duration of PPA. One of the most striking findings is the influence of maternal age on PPA duration. Our results indicate that older women tend to have longer periods of PPA. This observation aligns with previous studies suggesting that older maternal age is associated with delayed resumption of menstrual cycles postpartum. Biological factors may partly explain this, as older women might experience slower hormonal recovery after childbirth. Additionally, older women may have different breastfeeding practices compared to younger mothers, contributing to longer PPA durations (Begum & Donta, 2017; Singh et al., 2014).

The study reveals a complex relationship between socioeconomic status, maternal education, and PPA duration. Higher socioeconomic status and maternal education are linked to shorter PPA durations. This may be attributed to better access to health-care, improved nutrition, and greater health awareness among women of higher

**Table 12.4** Unadjusted and Adjusted hazard ratio for postpartum amenorrhea with selected background characteristics for India using NFHS-5 data

| Variables | Unadjusted Model | | Adjusted Model-I | | Adjusted Model-II | |
|---|---|---|---|---|---|---|
| | Haz. Ratio | Confidence-interval | Haz. Ratio | Confidence-interval | Haz. Ratio | Confidence-interval |
| **PPA (0–6 months)** | **ref** | | | | | |
| *Mothers-age* | | | | | | |
| 15–24 year | ref | | | | | |
| 25–29 year | 0.28* | 0.28–0.29 | 0.28* | 0.27–0.29 | 0.28* | 0.28–0.29 |
| ≥30 year | 0.03* | 0.02–0.02 | 0.03* | 0.02–0.03 | 0.02* | 0.02–0.03 |
| *Caste* | | | | | | |
| SC/ST | ref | | | | | |
| OBC | 1.75* | 1.73–1.78 | 1.03* | 1.01–1.05 | 1.03* | 1.01–1.06 |
| Others | 1.97* | 1.95–2.00 | 1.964* | 1.93–1.99 | 1.97* | 1.93–2.00 |
| *Place of residence* | | | | | | |
| Urban | ref | | | | | |
| Rural | 1.37* | 1.34–1.41 | 1.06* | 1.03–1.09 | 1.05* | 1.01–1.08 |
| *Mother education* | | | | | | |
| No education | ref | | | | | |
| primary | 1.21* | 1.17–1.25 | 0.89* | 0.86–0.92 | 0.89* | 0.86–0.93 |
| secondary | 1.65* | 1.61–1.69 | 0.96* | 0.93–0.99 | 0.98 | 0.95–1.00 |
| higher | 2.23* | 2.15–2.32 | 1.84* | 1.76–1.92 | 1.88* | 1.80–1.97 |
| *Breastfeeding* | | | | | | |
| 0–6 months | ref | | | | | |
| > 6 months | 0.74* | 0.67–0.83 | 0.74* | 0.66–0.83 | 0.74* | 0.66–0.83 |
| *Body Mass Index* | | | | | | |

(continued)

**Table 12.4** (continued)

| Variables | Unadjusted Model | | Adjusted Model-I | | Adjusted Model-II | |
|---|---|---|---|---|---|---|
| | Haz. Ratio | Confidence-interval | Haz. Ratio | Confidence-interval | Haz. Ratio | Confidence-interval |
| Normal | ref | | | | | |
| Underweight | 0.47* | 0.45–0.48 | - | - | 0.74* | 0.71–0.76 |
| Overweight/Obese | 1.46* | 1.45–1.53 | - | - | 1.056* | 1.03–1.09 |
| *Wealth Index* | | | | | | |
| poorest | ref | | | | | |
| poorer | 1.53* | 1.50–1.54 | 1.77* | 1.74–1.81 | 1.74* | 1.70–1.78 |
| middle | 1.63* | 1.61–1.65 | 1.77* | 1.74–1.80 | 1.81* | 1.78–1.84 |
| richer | 1.69* | 1.67–1.71 | 1.79* | 1.77–1.82 | 1.82* | 1.79–1.85 |
| richest | 1.81* | 1.78–1.83 | 1.86* | 1.84–1.89 | 1.87* | 1.85–1.91 |
| **Log likelihood** | | | **-50,056.24** | | **-48,432.086** | |

socioeconomic status and education levels. These women may also have different breastfeeding practices, potentially opting for shorter breastfeeding periods due to work commitments or access to alternative feeding options. The disparity in PPA duration across socioeconomic groups highlights the need for equitable healthcare access and targeted support for lower socioeconomic groups. Interventions should focus on improving healthcare services, nutrition, and breastfeeding support for disadvantaged populations to reduce health disparities and enhance maternal and child health outcomes (Kravdal, 2004; Sahoo et al., 2015).

Women from rural areas and those belonging to Scheduled Tribes (ST) tend to have longer PPA durations compared to their urban and higher caste counterparts. These differences may reflect variations in healthcare access, socioeconomic conditions, cultural practices, and breastfeeding behaviors across regions and caste groups. Rural areas and marginalized communities often face limited healthcare resources, lower educational attainment, and poorer economic conditions, contributing to longer PPA durations (Kishor & Parasuraman, 1998; Subramanian et al., 2006).

Body Mass Index (BMI) also plays a significant role in determining PPA duration, with underweight women experiencing longer PPA periods. This finding aligns with existing research linking nutritional status and reproductive health. Underweight women may have lower energy reserves and altered hormonal profiles, contributing to delayed resumption of menstruation postpartum. Addressing malnutrition and improving overall nutritional status among women, particularly in lower socioeconomic groups, is essential for enhancing reproductive health outcomes. Nutritional interventions should focus on promoting balanced diets, providing nutritional supplements where necessary, and educating women about the importance of maintaining a healthy weight for reproductive health (Billewicz & Thomson, 1973; Frisch, 1984).

### *12.4.1 Limitations of the Study*

The major limitation of the study is that some of the information within the category of wealth index, i.e., poorest, poorer, middle, richer, and richest is not given in NFHS-1 and 2. And body mass index of women in NFHS-1 had not been given. The cross-sectional nature of the NFHS data limits the ability to establish causal relationships. Longitudinal studies are needed to better understand the causal pathways and long-term impacts of the identified determinants on PPA duration. Additionally, the study relies on self-reported data, which may be subject to recall bias and reporting inaccuracies. Future research should explore the potential biases and validate the findings using other data sources.

## 12.5 Conclusion

Postpartum amenorrhea (PPA) in India exhibits notable variations influenced by socioeconomic, cultural, and demographic factors. PPA, the period after childbirth during which a woman does not menstruate, is largely impacted by breastfeeding practices, maternal health, and healthcare access. These influences vary widely across India's diverse regions and communities. Breastfeeding significantly affects PPA duration, as prolonged breastfeeding is associated with extended amenorrhea. Rural areas, where traditional practices prevail, see longer breastfeeding durations compared to urban areas, where early weaning is more common, leading to shorter PPA periods. Socioeconomic status also plays a critical role; women from lower socioeconomic backgrounds often experience longer PPA due to prolonged breastfeeding and limited access to contraceptives and healthcare services. In contrast, women from higher socioeconomic backgrounds have shorter PPA durations due to better access to healthcare and family planning services. Demographic factors such as age and parity also impact PPA. Younger women and first-time mothers may have longer PPA due to prolonged breastfeeding and lack of family planning experience, while older women with multiple children typically have shorter PPA due to better knowledge and experience. Policymakers must consider these determinants to develop targeted, equitable, and culturally sensitive interventions aimed at improving maternal and child health outcomes. By addressing these factors, India can make significant strides in enhancing the well-being of mothers and children, thereby contributing to broader national development goals.

## References

Aguirre, G. P. (1996). *The determinants of postpartum amenorrhea: a multi-state hazard approach*. University of Wisconsin, Madison Center for Demography and Ecology Working Paper, 96-03.

Begum, S., & Donta, B. (2017). Maternal age and pregnancy outcome: A review of the literature. *Maternal and Child Health Journal, 21*(2), 247–256.

Billewicz, W. Z., & Thomson, A. M. (1973). The relationship of birth-weight, parity, and maternal age to perinatal mortality and to the duration of the menstrual cycle. *Annals of Human Biology, 1*(3), 367–376.

Bongaarts, J., & Potter, R. G. (1983). *Fertility, biology, and behavior: An analysis of the proximate determinants*. Academic Press.

Corsini, C. A. (1979). Is the Fertility-reducing Effect of Lactation Really Substantial? In *Natural Fertility. Liege: Ordina Editions* (Chapter 9, pp. 195–215). Published for the International Union Are Breastfeeding Patterns in Pakistan Changing, 311.

Dewey, K. G., & Brown, K. H. (2003). Women in higher socio-economic status groups tend to have access to more nutritious foods, which can affect their milk production. *Journal of Nutrition, 133*(1), 303–308. https://doi.org/10.1093/jn/133.1.303

Frisch, R. E. (1984). Body fat, menarche, fitness and fertility. *Human Reproduction, 1*(1), 45–52.

Gray, R. H., Campbell, O. M. R., Apelo, R., Eslami, S. S., Zacur, H., Ramos, R. M., & Labbok, M. H. (1990). Risk of ovulation during lactation. *The Lancet, 335*(8680), 25–29.

Habicht, J. P., DaVanzo, J., Butz, W. P., & Meyers, L. (1985). The contraceptive role of breastfeeding. *Population Studies, 39*(2), 213–232.

Howie, P. W., & McNeilly, A. S. (1982). Effect of breast-feeding patterns on human birth intervals. *Reproduction, 65*(2), 545–557.

Huffman, S. L., Chowdhury, A. K. M. A., Chakraborty, J., & Simpson, N. K. (1980). Breast-feeding patterns in rural Bangladesh. *The American Journal of Clinical Nutrition, 33*(1), 144–154.

Huffman, S. L., Ford, K., Allen, H. A., Jr., & Streble, P. (1987). Nutrition and fertility in Bangladesh: Breastfeeding and post-partum amenorrhoea. *Population Studies, 41*(3), 447–462.

International Institute for Population Sciences (IIPS) and ICF. (2021). *National Family Health Survey (NFHS-5), 2019–21: India*. Mumbai: IIPS.

Jones, R. E. (1990). The effect of initiation of child supplementation on resumption of post-partum menstruation. *Journal of Biosocial Science, 22*(2), 173–189.

Kishor, S., & Parasuraman, S. (1998). Mother's employment and infant and child mortality in India. *National Family Health Survey Subject Reports, 8*, 1–38.

Knodel, J. (1977). Breast-feeding and population growth. *Science, 198*(4322), 1111–1115.

Kravdal, Ø. (2004). Child mortality in India: The community-level effect of education. *Population Studies, 58*(2), 177–192.

Labbok, M. H. (2016). Postpartum breastfeeding and longer-term maternal health. *Breastfeeding Medicine, 11*(2), 56–59.

Labbok, M. H., & Krasovec, K. (1990). Toward consistency in breastfeeding definitions. *Studies in Family Planning, 21*(4), 226–230.

Lunn, P. G., Austin, S., Prentice, A. M., & Whitehead, R. G. (1984). The effect of improved nutrition on plasma prolactin concentrations and postpartum infertility in lactating Gambian women. *The American Journal of Clinical Nutrition, 39*(2), 227–235.

McCann, M. F., Liskin, L. S., Piotrow, P. T., Rinehart, W., & Fox, G. (1981). Breast-feeding, fertility, and family planning. *Population reports Series J, Family Planning Programs, 24*, J525–J575.

McNeilly, A. S., Glasier, A., Jonassen, J., & Howie, P. W. (1982). Evidence for direct inhibition of ovarian function by prolactin. *Reproduction, 65*(2), 559–569.

Mishra, R., Singh, K. K., & Singh Brijesh, P. (2021). Duration of Post-partum Amenorrhoea: A Model-based Approach. *Indian Journal of Population and Development, 1*(1), 41–50.

Nath, D. C., & Goshawmi, G. (1996). The socio-demographic correlates of post-partum amenorrhoea in an urban society of India. *Genus*, 105–123.

Odimegwu, C. (2001).Determinants of post-partum behavior among IGBO women of south-eastern nigeria: A hazard model analysis.

Perez, A., Vela, P., Potter, R., & Masnick, G. S. (1971). Timing and sequence of resuming ovulation and menstruation after childbirth. *Population Studies, 25*(3), 491–503.

Rollins, N. C., Bhandari, N., Hajeebhoy, N., Horton, S., Lutter, C. K., Martines, J. C., & Victora, C. G. (2016). Why invest, and what it will take to improve breastfeeding practices? *The Lancet, 387*(10017), 491–504.

Sahoo, H., Pradhan, M. R., & Bhuyan, S. K. (2015). Maternal education, female autonomy and fertility in India. *Journal of Biosocial Science, 47*(6), 749–764.

Santow, G. (2012). *A simulation approach to the study of human fertility* (Vol. 5). Springer Science & Business Media.

Singh, K. K., Suchindran, C. M., & Singh, K. (1994). Effect of breast-feeding on post-partum amenorrhea: experience of an Indian population. *Journal of Biosocial Sciences*, Forthcoming issue.

Singh, A., Chalasani, S., Koenig, M. A., & Mahapatra, B. (2014). The consequences of unintended births for maternal and child health in India. *Population Studies, 68*(1), 15–29.

Subramanian, S. V., Nandy, S., Irving, M., Gordon, D., Lambert, H., & Davey Smith, G. (2006). The mortality divide in India: The differential contributions of gender, caste, and standard of living across the life course. *American Journal of Public Health, 96*(5), 818–825.

Victora, C. G., Bahl, R., Barros, A. J., França, G. V., Horton, S., Krasevec, J., & Rollins, N. C. (2016). Breastfeeding in the 21st century: Epidemiology, mechanisms, and lifelong effect. *The Lancet, 387*(10017), 475–490.

# Chapter 13
# Barriers Associated with Maternal Healthcare Among the Migrant Slum Dwellers

**Suchismita Mishra, Bontha V. Babu, and T. Rajendra Prasad**

**Abstract** The present chapter reports the barriers associated with maternal healthcare services among the interstate migrants living in the slums of Bangalore city of Karnataka, India. The study used the mixed-method approach. Quantitative data were collected by interviewing 100 mothers having a <2-year-old child or pregnant during data collection. Qualitative data were collected through in-depth interviews with mothers and healthcare providers, such as doctors, and peripheral health workers, such as ASHA. The study found more vulnerable to accessing maternal healthcare services due to socio-cultural barriers like distance to the government healthcare centre, financial constraints, lack of awareness about the availability of government healthcare services, lower educational literacy, and language barrier to communicating with the healthcare providers. Some institutional barriers are also noticed, including the unavailability of free-of-cost medicines, lack of infrastructure like enough space, provision of drinking water, and toilet facilities and less access to reproductive health information due to their migratory status. Another important drawback was unreachable by the health workers working in their area due to their remote location and unrecognized slum identity. Hence, the study warrants developing a system to strengthen maternal healthcare services in this marginalized slum population by incorporating migrant-sensitive policies and improving government healthcare services to improve the utilization level.

**Keywords** Maternal health · Migrants · Barriers

S. Mishra (✉) · T. R. Prasad
Department of Economics, Bangalore University, Bangalore, Karnataka, India
e-mail: suchismita44@gmail.com

B. V. Babu
Socio-Behavioural, Health Systems and Implementation Research Division, Indian Council of Medical Research, New Delhi, India

 
P. Chouhan et al. (eds.), *Women's Health Dynamics in South Asia*, Asian Perspectives on Public Health, https://doi.org/10.1007/978-981-95-2321-4_13

## 13.1 Introduction

Maternal health comprises family planning, preconception, prenatal, and postnatal care in order to ensure a positive and fulfilling experience in most cases and reduce maternal mortality and morbidity in other cases (WHO). Even though South Asia has made significant progress in maternal healthcare services, there are 38% of neonatal deaths in the world occur in South Asia (Dayal et al., 2021). Migrant populations living in urban slums are more vulnerable towards health due to various reasons like diverse cultural identity, substandard ways of living, poor financial conditions, lack of basic amenities, etc. Even though a higher concentration of healthcare services with many facilities is found in urban areas, the slum population's health is not satisfactory. Inadequate healthcare access is found among socioeconomically disadvantaged women (Furler et al., 2002; McLean et al., 2015; I. G. H Origlia et al., 2019; P. Origlia et al., 2017). Education and wealth status are the most important factors among other socioeconomic factors of maternal healthcare services, as found in the study by Paul and Chouhan (2020) using the National Family Health Survey (NFHS-4) data. Emphasizing migrant health, WHO calls upon its member states to promote migrant-sensitive health policies, equitable access to health promotion, and disease prevention and healthcare programmes for migrants (World Health Assembly, 2008). Hence, migrants are more vulnerable in terms of maternal health in the urban area.

### *13.1.1 Rationale of the Study*

According to the WHO (2023), South Asian countries contribute one-fifth of total global maternal deaths, and India shares 8% of all global maternal deaths. Studies from developing countries, which have experienced greater rates of urbanization, revealed that the use of maternal healthcare services was associated with migration status, and utilization was less among the recent migrants compared to the host society and the native rural population (Babu et al., 2018). Bangalore is one of the fastest-growing cities in India because of its rapid urbanization. According to the 2001 census, out of 44,977,201 people (total population), 879,106 people migrated to Bangalore. A majority of migrants come not only from neighbouring states like Andhra Pradesh, Tamil Nadu, and Kerala but also from other farther states like Uttar Pradesh, Bihar, Gujarat, and Madhya Pradesh in search of better livelihood strategies. Although higher income quartiles represent a higher proportion of migrants in India, there is a very substantial chunk of poorer migrants involved in low-paid and low-earning jobs, principally in the informal sector, and they suffer from various deprivations and handicaps which also have to do with the nature of urban policies and absence of employer support (Srivastava, 2011). Many programmes and schemes are available for maternal health in Karnataka, including Janani Suraksha Yojana, Thayi Bgaya Scheme, and Pradhan Matri Matru Bandana Yojana. A study conducted by Bellad et al. (2017) in Karnataka found that the maternal mortality ratio was 103 (per 100,000 livebirths), neonatal mortality ratio was 25 per 1,000 livebirths, and perinatal mortality ratio was 50 per 1,000 livebirths which shows the real maternal health scenario. In this chapter, the term migrants refer to socioeconomically disadvantaged urban migrants. It is anticipated that the migrants from rural to urban areas change their treatment-seeking behaviour (including maternal healthcare seeking) due to their low awareness, accessibility, and availability of healthcare services. There must be various socio-cultural reasons associated with maternal healthcare seeking along with the financial barriers. Along with this background, the present study is proposed with a broader objective to explore the barriers associated with maternal healthcare services among poorer migrant women living in Bangalore.

Bengaluru, often referred to as the "Silicon Valley of India", is the capital city of Karnataka and a major hub for technology and innovation (Fig. 13.1). As of 2023, Bengaluru has an estimated population of over 13 million, making it one of India's largest and fastest-growing cities. The city attracts a significant number of migrants from various parts of the country due to its booming IT industry and employment opportunities. However, this rapid urbanization has also led to challenges, particularly in housing. A considerable portion of Bengaluru's population lives in slums, with estimates suggesting that over 1.5 million people reside in such areas. These slums are often inhabited by low-income migrants who move to the city in search of better livelihoods. The living conditions in these slums are typically poor, with inadequate access to basic amenities like clean water, sanitation, and healthcare, highlighting the stark contrast between the city's economic growth and its socioeconomic disparities.

## 13.2 Materials and Methods

The present study is community-based and used a mixed-method approach for data collection. Secondary data was collected from the municipal corporation and other development authorities to identify the notified and non-notified slums of Bangalore City (Fig. 13.1). During the pilot study, clusters were identified from newer slums, de-notified slums, and camps. Only the slum locations that have more than 100 households with interstate migrants were considered as a cluster. From them, 5 locations/clusters were identified based on the availability of migrants living for not less than six months and not more than seven years. Quantitative data were collected by interviewing 100 mothers having a <2-year-old child or pregnant during data collection. The qualitative data were collected through in-depth interviews with mothers (17) and the healthcare providers, namely, government (3) and private doctors (4) and Peripheral health workers (7) working in the study area.

Data obtained from quantitative surveys were entered into the computer through MS Excel, and analyses were done using SPSS for Windows v.22.0. Qualitative data analysis software ATLAS/ti for Windows V.4.1 was used to analyse qualitative data. All in-depth interviews were conducted in the respondents' local languages, i.e., Telugu, Tamil, and Hindi, by the researcher. The entire interview/discussion was recorded. At the end of each interview/discussion, the audiocassettes were played

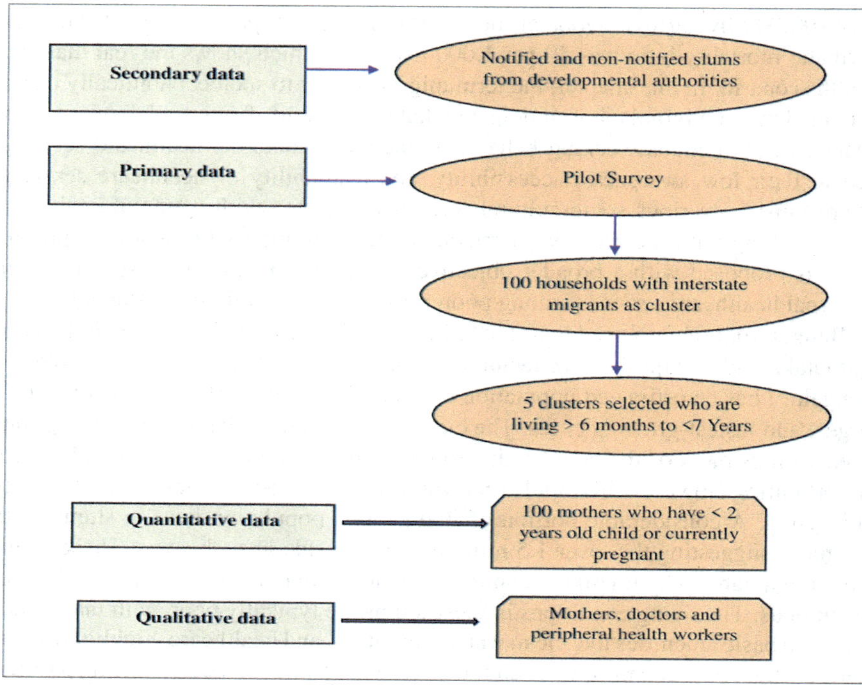


**Fig. 13.1** Schematic presentation of the study

back, and the scripts were translated into English. During the transcription and translation of qualitative data, the guidelines of Mergenthaler and Stinson (1992) and Mclellan et al. (2003), respectively, were followed.

## 13.3 Results

The study slum population belongs to two types of slums: non-notified slums (50%) and migrant camps (50%). It is evident from Table 1 that most respondents (60%) were from the recent migrant category, i.e., six months to three years. More than 50% of the study respondents were illiterate. Some respondents (18%) had completed their primary school education, and a considerable number of respondents studied more than the $6^{th}$ standard. A majority of the respondents belonged to the Hindu community (76%) and from other backward class categories (44%) (Table 13.1). A considerable number of respondents (40%) were more than 25 years of age. Interestingly, more than 60% of the respondents got married below the age of 18 years.

A maximum (54%) of respondents travelled half an hour to 1 hour to avail of the antenatal care services. Out of that, more (57.4%) number of respondents were

**Table 13.1** Distribution of respondents by their socioeconomic status

| Variable | Years of migration | | Total ($n = 100$) |
|---|---|---|---|
| | 0.6–3 years ($n = 60$) | 4–7 years ($n = 40$) | |
| *Education* | | | |
| Illiterate | 33 (55.0%) | 22 (55.0%) | 55 (55.0%) |
| 1–5 years education | 11 (18.3%) | 07 (17.5%) | 18 (18.0%) |
| More than 6 years of education | 16 (26.7%) | 11 (27.5%) | 27 (27.0%) |
| *Caste* | | | |
| Schedules castes | 13 (21.7%) | 10 (25.0%) | 23 (23.0%) |
| Scheduled tribes | 14 (23.3%) | 8 (20.0%) | 22 (22.0%) |
| Other backward classes | 26 (43.3%) | 18 (45.0%) | 44 (44.0%) |
| Others | 7 (11.7%) | 4 (10.0%) | 11 (11.0%) |
| *Religion* | | | |
| Non-Hindu | 19 (31.7%) | 05 (12.5%) | 24 (24.0%) |
| Hindu | 41 (68.3%) | 35 (87.5%) | 76 (76.0%) |
| *Age* | | | |
| Less than 20 years | 17 (28.3%) | 05 (12.5%) | 22 (22.0%) |
| 20–24 years | 26 (43.3%) | 12 (30.0%) | 38 (38.0%) |
| More than 25 years | 17 (28.3%) | 23 (57.5%) | 40 (40.0%) |
| *Age at marriage* | | | |
| 14–17 years | 45 (75.0%) | 22 (55.0%) | 67 (67.0%) |
| 18 years and above | 15 (25.0%) | 18 (45.0%) | 33 (33.0%) |

*Source* Primary Survey

found in the recent groups of migrants, whereas 42.6% of respondents were found in the older group of migrants. Following this, 16% of respondents travelled more than one hour, and the rest, 12%, travelled less than half an hour. As this migrant population is poor in general, they try to get government health services. Even though the accessibility of government health services is less, they still prefer to go despite a long distance of travel, i.e., more than half an hour. Hence, the preference to avail of the services from government health centres due to their low cost is evident from Table 13.2.

Table 13.3 provides the utilization of the transport system when availing of the ANC services. We can observe from the table that the majority of people (43%) used public transport, and out of that, recent migrants (23) used more compared to the settled migrants (20). If we calculate the years of migration of recent migrants, i.e., out of 60, many respondents (38.3%) and out of 40 settled migrants, many respondents (50%) utilized the public transport system while getting ANC service. Some respondents (20%) hired a vehicle, and some others (14%) went by walking.

**Table 13.2** Distribution of respondents by duration of migration and distance travelled to seek antenatal checkups

| Distance travelled | Years of migration | | Total |
|---|---|---|---|
| | 0.6–3 years | 4–7 years | |
| NA | 12 (66.7%) (20.0%) | 6 (33.3%) (15.0%) | 18 (18.0%) |
| Less than 30 min | 8 (66.7%) (13.3%) | 4 (33.3%) (10.0%) | 12 (12.0%) |
| 30 min-1 h | 31 (57.4%) (51.7%) | 23 (42.6%) (57.5%) | 54 (54.0%) |
| More than 1 h | 9 (56.3%) (15.0%) | 7 (43.8%) (17.5%) | 16 (16.0%) |
| **Total** | **60** | **40** | **100** |

*Source* Primary Survey

Very few (5%) went by bicycle. As they are from poor socioeconomic backgrounds, their utilization of public transport is high compared to other transport systems.

Regarding the reason behind not getting ANC services, out of 100 respondents, some (18%) respondents did not avail of the ANC services. Among them, a majority of the respondents (77.78%) said they were right only, so there was no need to spend money on the ANC services. Other reasons cited by the respondents were that nobody was at home to look after the other children in the city, and they were new to the place and did not know where to go to get ANC services.

When the healthcare service provider asked whether the people in this area were satisfied with the services, most of the health workers agreed that the migrant people coming to them were satisfied with their services. At the same time, they revealed that they take time to accept them as after repeatedly visiting them, they cooperate and understand things. They do not feel free to discuss their health issues. Interestingly,

**Table 13.3** Distribution of respondents by duration of migration and transport facilities utilized for ANC services

| Transport facilities utilized | Years of migration | | Total |
|---|---|---|---|
| | 0.6–3 years | 4–7 years | |
| NA | 12 (66.7%) (20.0%) | 6 (33.3%) (15.0%) | 18 (18.00%) |
| Walking | 8 (57.1%) (13.3%) | 6 (42.9%) (15.0%) | 14 (14%) |
| Bicycle | 2 (50.0%) (3.3%) | 3 (50.0%) (5.00%) | 5 (5%) |
| Public Transport | 23 (53.4%) (38.3%) | 20 (46.6%) (50.0%) | 43 (43%) |
| Hired Vehicle | 12 (60.0%) (20.0%) | 8(40.0%) (20.0%) | 20 (20%) |

*Source* Primary Survey

one Junior Health Assistant said, "I do not know whether they are satisfied or not. We are trying our best, but they are not following our instructions. They always miss the card and are not serious about their health. They demand that they do not have permanent housing, so we should help them get voter cards and space to stay. We are helpless in this matter.

> One respondent said, "*We do not know where the govt. hospitals, in our native place, it is free, even here, govt also takes money for vaccination. Once I experienced this, they charged 100 rupees for vaccination. Hence, I do not feel like going to govt.*

Table 13.4 provides the data on the satisfaction level of the respondents by their migration status. A maximum (46%) of respondents replied the service was good and there is no significant difference between the recent and settled migrants with regard to their opinion. Following this, many respondents (32%) said yes, it was okay kind, and in this maximum, 25 (78.1%) respondents were from a recent category, whereas some 7 (21.9%) were from the settled migrants' category. With regard to the very good response category, very few respondents agreed. This shows that the highest satisfaction level and the total dissatisfaction level are found to be low.

Most respondents said they were satisfied as the doctor treated them well (this is generally private clinics only). People are not satisfied with government health centres. The first thing is the distance, the second thing is it is not totally free of cost, and the third thing is the nurse's attitude, which is not so friendly. Even the medicines they prescribe are unavailable to them, so they have to purchase them from outside.

> One respondent said, "*During my delivery, the nurses are behaving so rudely, even for small things. Even though I was in pain, they did not care and scolded me.*"
>
> Another respondent said, "*They do not give good quality medicines, so generally, we do not take and many times they won't be available. Whatever the private doctors tell us is good, and we rely on that. But in our native place, the govt doctors are good, and what medicine they give the illness get rid of that means it works better*".

Regarding the extent to which these people are satisfied with your facilities/staff, most of the health workers said that yes, the people are satisfied with their services;

**Table 13.4** Distribution of respondents by satisfaction level of postnatal care services and duration of migration

| Postnatal care | Years of Migration | | Total |
|---|---|---|---|
| | 0.6 to 3 years | 4 to 7 years | |
| Not taken | 10 (66.7%) | 05 (33.3%) | 15 |
| Very Good | 1 (20.00%) | 4 (80.00%) | 5 |
| Good | 23 (50.00%) | 23 (50.00%) | 46 |
| It is okay | 25 (78.1%) | 7 (21.9%) | 32 |
| Bad | 1 (50.00%) | 1 (50.00%) | 2 |
| **Total** | **60** | **40** | **100** |

*Source* Primary Survey

otherwise, they do not come for the next visit. The Anganwadi workers revealed that as the health centres are along with the school premises, no separate facilities are available for them like rooms, toilets or water; the patients and the health staff have to suffer. The govt health workers said that sometimes medicines or other incentives are not available in the health centres, but still people are satisfied with our services.

One of the ASHA workers said, "*Medicines are not a problem. Yes, toilet and drinking water facilities are not there*".

Table 13.5 provides a clear picture of the sample respondents' views about the language problem they faced while availing of maternal health services in the current city. Surprisingly, many (42%) respondents felt the difficulty of language. Out of that, in the recent migrant category, more respondents faced difficulty (55.7%) than the settled migrants' (22.5%). Because of their poor socioeconomic status, it is sometimes difficult for them to get health care services. A few respondents (8%) felt they were treated differently, and many (92%) said no, they did not feel any difference from the healthcare provider (Table 13.5).

Regarding the problems faced by the health workers while disposing of their duties, very few said that they do not face any problem. All the ASHA workers revealed that the absence of basic facilities in the centre is a major drawback. The health workers felt difficulty in completing their work due to the migratory nature of the pregnant women in the study areas. The private and government doctors said these people won't maintain hygiene after repeatedly making them understand.

One ASHA worker said, "*That thing only no separate room for us. With the Anganwadicentre, they tie these services. So kids are also there they shout a lot. When mothers are coming with kids, there is no place to sit also*".

One health assistant said, "*That's what I told you no, they keep moving and do not listen to us seriously*".

One private doctor said, "*Same problem, only they would not visit regularly and not maintain hygiene after repeatedly telling*".

**Table 13.5** Distribution of respondents by duration of migration and problems faced

| Language problem | Years of migration | | Total |
|---|---|---|---|
| | 0.6 to 3 years | 4 to 7 years | |
| Yes | 33 (78.6%) (55.00%) | 9 (21.4%) (22.5%) | 42 (100%) (42.00%) |
| No | 21 (46.6%) 45.0%) | 31 (53.4%) (77.5%) | 58 (100%) (58.00%) |
| *Poor status* | | | |
| Yes | 4 (50.00%) (06.7%) | 4 (50.00%) (10.00%) | 08 (100%) (08.00%) |
| No | 56(60.90%) (93.3%) | 36 (39.10%) (90.00%) | 92 (100%) (92.00%) |
| **Total** | **60** | **40** | **100** |

*Source* Primary Survey

Regarding support, the healthcare service provider gets from community leaders and local politicians. Out of five slums, only two slums ASHA workers reported that they get some benefits from the local political parties. They also provide pencils, bags, toys, mats, etc., to the Anganwadi centres and food packets. All the govt and private doctors and health staff reported that they do not get anything from the political parties. And they also do not want anything from them.

> One ASHA worker said, "*Yes, they give pencils, bags, mats to the Anganwadicentre, and some days they give good food also*".
>
> One private doctor said, "*Nothing we are getting and won't want to be involved with politicians*".

Regarding the problems the healthcare service providers faced in terms of logistics and supplies, all the health staff revealed that no problem is there related to logistics and supply. All the medicines and the groceries are coming at the right time, even the drugs. Sometimes, it comes late, but they inform people and distribute it to the people.

> One of the health workers said, "*Nothing. Sometimes some drugs are not available. But when it comes, we are informing the people*".
>
> One ASHA worker said, "*No, no problem. Tablets and tonics are coming. All dals, groundnut, wheat, rice, milk powder, anarkai, etc., are coming*".

When it was asked to provide suggestions for the more effective functioning of your health facility, the govt hospital staff revealed that they need more staff, as sometimes it is difficult for them to control the patients. They get restless at the end of the day because of work pressure and lack of rest. Only two nurses, one doctor, and one compounder are there in the respective government hospital. The nurse has to visit the Anganwadi centres twice weekly. These days, with one nurse, it is difficult to ensure the smooth functioning of the health centre. The Anganwadi centres said that they need separate rooms and proper drinking water supply with toilet facilities for smooth functioning and ease of use for the patients. Few private doctors highlighted that their services to the migrants can be improved if the local NGOs help together with a better approach. Some others pointed out that the environment outside the clinic is very bad, so improving it will be good for their health centre.

> One of the nurses in the govt hospital said, "*We need more staff with regular functioning. In weekly, twice we will do our service it will be good. Sometimes it too rushes we won't get a little break also*".
>
> One health worker said. "*That's what if a separate room with drinking water and a toilet facility is provided, it will be good only.*
>
> One private doctor revealed, "*If some voluntary organization or local bodies really want to help these poor, if they approach us, then it will be good, and I am ready to do*".

With regard to the problems faced/involved in delivering the services, particularly to migrants and pregnant and lactating mothers, maximum health staff including the health workers and doctors, both government and private, that these migrants do not take their things seriously and in between, they move to their native place for delivery or to help in agricultural work. Even their unhygienic way of living also irritates the health workers. The health workers try their best by repeatedly visiting to make them understand, but they won't follow them.

> One health worker said, "*Staff are cooperative and trying their hard. Those people are not willing to take our service and not understanding*".
>
> One private doctor said, "*Yes, after telling them so many times also they do not follow the hygienic way of living. They are not doing a regular check-ups also. And they usually go to their native place for delivery*".

## 13.4 Discussion

The study population is basically from the lower education attained groups, which indicates their less knowledge and awareness of the health system as well as their health condition. Early at marriage and early age of pregnancy, the study respondents point out an alarming situation which definitely has an adverse effect on women's health. Furthermore, several studies have pointed out that migration is not always permanent, and seasonal and circular migration is widespread, especially among the socioeconomically deprived groups, such as the Scheduled Castes (SCs), Scheduled Tribes (STs) and Other Backward Castes (OBCs), who are asset-poor and face resource and livelihood deficits (Deshingkar & Akter, 2009). Even the present study highlights that most respondents are from SC, ST, and OBC categories.

There are several patterns regarding accessing and utilizing health care services by the present study migrant population. The various barriers identified among the study population are discussed here: From the study, it is clear that more than 50% of the respondents travelled for half an hour to one hour to get the ANC checkup during their last pregnancy. Some cases (16%) even reported that they travelled more than one hour. This shows that ANC services were not so easily available to them, whether in a native place or in the present urban habitat. Regarding transportation facilities, many respondents utilized public transport and hired a vehicle to avail themselves of the ANC checkup. The percentage of travelling long is more may be because both in their native place and current habitat, the government hospital is quite far from their place of staying and they preference to get ANC from the government healthcare centre only. Long-distance travel has even been a disincentive to seeking care, especially in the case of women who need somebody to accompany them, as they do not know the location properly. People in this study area are illiterate, and it is difficult for them to travel alone to distant places. As a result, the factor of distance strongly adheres to other factors such as availability of transport, the total cost of travel, women's illiteracy, and mobility. Even though the study respondents travelled a lot to get the ANC services, nobody said distance is the reason behind not getting ANC, which indicates that distance to the healthcare centre is not the barrier to avail the ANC checkup, but of course, the utilization level can be increased if the government health centres are nearby. When asked about suggestions for improving maternal healthcare services in their locality, the present respondents have already revealed this issue. Similar findings are reported by Zaver and Said (2013).

The majority of respondents who did not avail themselves of ANC checkups during their last pregnancy revealed that they felt no need for them. As these people are poor, they perceive that if something is wrong, then they should do the ANC checkup. Evidence suggests that demand-side barriers such as the cost of services are important barriers to obtaining services, especially in poor and vulnerable groups. However, few respondents pointed out that they faced difficulty in getting healthcare services due to their poor economic situation. The financial constraint limits their utilization of government health services as the transportation charge is higher and medicines are not available free of cost. Similar findings were obtained by Yuyal et al. (2020).

A few respondents said they were unaware of the location of the government health centre as they are new to the current area of living. Moving to a new urban environment makes them vulnerable, and they can miss out on public healthcare services (Mishra et al., 2017). The socioeconomic inequities in an urban environment may affect access to and use of health services (Kusuma et al., 2010; Makinen et al., 2007) and the selection of an appropriate healthcare provider (Srivastava et al., 2009). Accessibility of health services has been shown to be an important determinant of the utilization of health services in developing countries.

The educational level of these respondents was also not very satisfactory. Illiteracy is another barrier for women to seek treatment from private or government hospitals. The illiteracy leads to poor communication between the healthcare provider and the mother. Communication between physician and patient was especially important in increasing compliance (Winnick et al., 2005). Educated women may have more understanding of the physiology of reproduction and be less disposed to accept the complications and risks of pregnancy as inevitable than illiterate or uneducated women. Education has been described as a medication against fatalism (Béhague et al., 2008; Royston & Armstrong, 1989).

Language was found to be one of the most important barriers to healthcare services for the study population because of their migratory status. Many (42%) respondents said they faced difficulty getting healthcare services as the local language, Kannada of Bangalore, is quite different from their language, especially the people who migrated from Bihar, Rajasthan, Assam, and Uttar Pradesh. The recently migrated people faced more difficulty than the settled migrants, obviously because of the duration of their stay in the new area. Due to language problems, the study population sometimes does not get the proper information about the various benefits they get at the Anganwadi health centre. However, most healthcare service providers revealed that they do not feel any difficulty communicating with these migrant populations. However, few said that as some people speak their typical local language, they sometimes have difficulty understanding. In fact, some studies found that barriers to effective and equitable healthcare can result from linguistic differences between patients and clinicians (Chu, 1998; Jacobs et al., 2006; Murray & Skull, 2005).

All the above points show their ignorance as well as unawareness about the importance of ANC services. Socio-cultural, economic and demographic factors, including the behaviour of families and communities, social status, education, culture, income, health decision-making power, age, and access to health facilities compound poorer access to medical services. The availability of health services played a vital role in reducing maternal mortality (Yahaya, 2004). Several socio-demographic characteristics of the individual affect the underlying tendency to seek care.

The qualitative data found that due to the non-availability of free medicines and poor quality of the medicines in the government health centre in the urban area, many respondents are not utilizing the government health centre. However, in contrast to this, none of the healthcare providers accepted that they were not getting medicines at the proper time. In fact, they pointed out that the basic infrastructure, like enough space, provision of drinking water, toilet facility, etc., needs to be improved along with the increase in the staff members. These are some of the factors which greatly impact seeking healthcare services. Less access to information related to healthcare services is another drawback found in the study area. However, the healthcare service providers said they were making the proper announcements in some of the study areas, while others accepted that they informed the people during their visit. In this regard, Gardner and Blackburn (1996) highlighted that there is an increasing concern about migrant women having less access to reproductive health information and services than non-migrants.

### 13.4.1 Limitations of the Study

The study covered only the southern part of Bangalore city due to time and manpower constraints. Few respondents are difficult to trace due to frequent visits to nearby states like Andhra and Tamil Nadu, so they are not included in the study. However, the study's strength is that both qualitative and quantitative methods were used for data collection, so more comprehensive information was collected from the migrants' and institutional points of view.

## 13.5 Conclusions

The study identified several barriers to the availability and utilization of healthcare services for maternal health. These barriers include the distance to healthcare centres, low levels of literacy, lack of awareness about the location of government health centres, financial constraints due to the high costs of healthcare services in urban areas, the unavailability of free medicines at government health centres, and language or communication barriers. Another significant challenge was the inaccessibility of health workers in certain areas due to the remote location and unrecognized status of slums. Additionally, the absence of migrant-sensitive programmes and policies in the study areas further excludes migrants from the formal healthcare system. Therefore, the study emphasizes the need for the development of targeted policies to address these barriers for migrants, particularly concerning maternal health. Furthermore, government healthcare services should be strengthened to improve utilization levels and ensure equitable access to care.

## 13.6 Ethical consideration

The study was approved by the ethical committee of Bangalore University, Karnataka, India.

## 13.7 Conflicts of Interest

There are no conflicts of interest.

**Acknowledgements** The present study is a part of postdoctoral research conducted out by the first author, which is funded by the Indian Council of Social Science Research, New Delhi.

## References

Babu, B. V., Sharma, Y., Kusuma, Y. S., Sivakami, M., et al. (2018). Internal migrants' experiences with and perceptions of frontline health workers: A nationwide study in 13 Indian cities. *The International Journal of Health Planning and Management*. https://onlinelibrary.wiley.com/doi/10.1002/hpm.2538

Béhague, D. P., Kanhonou, L. G., Filippi, V., Légonou, S., & Ronstmans, C. (2008). Pierre Bourdieu and transformative agency: A study of how patients in Benin negotiate blame and accountability in the context of severe obstetric events. *Social Health Illness, 30*, 489–510.

Bellad, M. B., Goudar, S. S., Mallapur, A. A., Sharma, S., Bone, J. F., Charantimath, U. S., ... & Derman, R. J. (2017). Maternal and newborn health in Karnataka state, India: The Community Level Interventions for Pre-Eclampsia (CLIP) Trial's baseline study results. *PLoS One, 12*(1), e0166623.

Chu, C. (1998). Cross-cultural health issues in contemporary Australia. *Ethnicity & Health, 3*(1–2), 125–134. https://doi.org/10.1080/13557858.1998.9961854

Dayal, P., Jimenez-Soto, E., Matthew, R., & Morgan, A. (2021). *Investing in newborn health in South Asia*. UNICEF.

Deshingkar, P., & Akter, S. (2009). Migration and human development in India. UNDP Human Development Research Paper 2009/13. http://hdr.undp.org/en/reports/global/hdr2009/papers/HDRP_2009_13.pdf

Furler, S., Harris, E., Chondros, P., Powell Davies, G., Harris, M. F., & Young, D. Y. (2002). The inverse care law revisited: Impact of disadvantaged location on accessing longer GP consultation times. *Medical Journal of Australia, 177*(2), 80–83.

Gardner, R., & Blackburn, R. (1996). People who move: New reproductive health focus. *Population Reports, 24*(3).

Hart, J. T. (1971). The inverse care law. *The Lancet, 1*(7696), 405–412.
Jacobs, E., Chen, A. H. M., Karliner, L. S., Agger-Gupta, N., & Mutha, S. (2006). The need for more research on language barriers in health care: A proposed research agenda. *Milbank Quarterly, 84*(1), 111–133.
Kusuma, Y. S., Kumari, R., Pandav, C. S., & Gupta, S. K. (2010). Migration and immunization: Determinants of childhood immunization uptake among socioeconomically disadvantaged migrants in Delhi, India. *Tropical Medicine & International Health, 15*(11), 1326–1332.
Makinen, M., Waters, H., Rauch, M., Almagambetova, N., Bitrán, R., & Gilson, L. (2007). Inequalities in health care use and expenditures: Empirical data from eight developing countries and countries in transition. *Bulletin of the World Health Organization, 78*, 55–65.
Mclellan, E., Mac Queen K.M., Naidig J.L. (2003). Beyond the qualitative interview. Data preparation and transcription, *Field Methods. 2003 Feb*, 15(1), 63–84.
McLean, G., Guthrie, B., Mercer, S. W., & Watt, G. C. (2015). General practice funding underpins the persistence of the inverse care law: Cross-sectional study in Scotland. *British Journal of General Practice, 65*(641), e799–e805.
Mergenthaler, E., & Stinson, C. (1992). Psychotherapy transcription standards. *Psychotherapy Research, 2*(2), 125–142.
Mishra, S., Kusuma, Y. S., & Babu, B. V. (2017). Treatment seeking and out-of-pocket expenditure on childhood illness in a migrant tribal community in Bhubaneswar, Odisha state, India. *Journal of Paediatrics and International Child Health, 37*(3), 181–187.
Murray, S. B., & Skull, S. A. (2005). Hurdles to health: Immigrant and refugee healthcare in Australia. *Australian Health Review, 29*(1), 25–29. https://doi.org/10.1071/AH050025
Origlia, I. G. H., Kurth, E., Asafew, F., Pehlke-Milde, J., & Cicnacco, E. (2019). Communication barriers in maternity care of allophone migrants: Experiences of women, healthcare professionals, and intercultural interpreters. *Journal of Advanced Nursing, 75*(10), 2200–2210.
Origlia, P., Jevitt, C., Zu Sayn-Wittgenstein, F., & Cignacco, E. (2017). Experiences of antenatal care among women who are socioeconomically deprived in high-income industrialized countries: An integrative review. *Journal of Midwifery & Women's Health, 62*(5), 589–598.
Paul, P., & Chouhan, P. (2020). Socio-demographic factors influencing utilization of maternal health care services in India. *Clinical Epidemiology and Global Health, 8*(3), 666–670.
Royston, E., & Armstrong, S. (Eds.). (1989). *Preventing maternal mortality*. World Health Organization.
Srivastava, R. (2011). Labour migration, inequality and development dynamics in India: An Introduction. *Indian Journal of Labour Economics, 54*(3), 373–385.
Srivastava, R. K., Kansal, S., Tiwari, V. K., Piang, L., Chand, R., & Nandan, D. (2009). Assessment of utilization of RCH services and client satisfaction at different levels of health facilities in Varanasi district. *Indian Journal of Public Health, 53*(3), 183–189.
World Health Assembly. (2008). *Health of migrants: Resolution WHA61.17*. World Health Organization. https://apps.who.int/gb/ebwha/pdf_files/A61/A61_R17-en.pdf
World Health Organization (WHO). (2023). Trends in maternal mortality 2000 to 2020: Estimates by WHO, UNICEF, UNFPA, World Bank Group and the United Nations Population Division.
Yahaya, M. K. (2004). Analysis of women's reproductive health situation in Bida Emirate of Niger State, Nigeria. *African Journal of Reproductive Health, 6*(1), 50–64.
Yuyal, R., Semwal, J., & Kandal, S. D. (2020). Piecing the evidences: Barriers to utilization of antenatal care services by currently married women in rural Uttarakhand—A community-based study. *Indian Journal of Community Health, 32*(1), 114–119.
Zaver, I. S., & Said, I. Y. (2013). Knowledge and barriers in utilization of maternal health care services in Kano State, Northern Nigeria. *European Journal of Biology and Medical Science Research, 1*(1), 1–14.

# Part IV
# Mental Health, Social Support, and Well-being

# Chapter 14
# Mental Health of Indigenous Women in South Asia: A Scoping Review

**Manisha Gore and Julia Morgan**

**Abstract** Indigenous Peoples globally may have a higher risk of mental health illnesses than the general population with mental health burden often being greater for Indigenous women. This chapter explored the mental health of Indigenous women in South Asia. A scoping review of the literature, utilising Arksey and O'Malley's framework, was undertaken for literature published between 2004 and 2024. Six databases were searched and 333 articles were identified. Title/abstract and full text were screened using inclusion and exclusion criteria which resulted in 17 articles being included in the final review. Fourteen studies took place in India, 2 in Bangladesh and 1 in Pakistan whilst 15 articles were quantitative and 2 were qualitative. A significant burden of mental health issues was identified for Indigenous women. Articles highlighted the importance of the social determinants of health as risk factors. Accesses to interventions to support mental health were limited and there was a preference, among some, for traditional support such as faith healers and herbal remedies. The stigma around mental health was highlighted as a barrier to accessing support and mental health issues were attributed to a wide range of factors including supernatural, biological, and environmental factors. Psychological resilience was supported through community and cultural activities. Interventions need to be culturally responsive reflecting Indigenous worldviews and traditions. Action on the social determinants of health is needed including a focus on reducing social exclusion and structural disempowerment. More research is needed on the mental health of Indigenous women in South Asia.

**Keywords** Indigenous women · South Asia · Mental health

M. Gore (✉)
Faculty of Medical Health Sciences, Symbiosis Community Outreach Programme Extension, Symbiosis International Deemed University, Lavale, India
e-mail: researchofficerscope1@siu.edu.in

J. Morgan
Department of Human Sciences, Public Health and Wellbeing, University of Greenwich, London, UK
e-mail: j.e.morgan@gre.ac.uk



P. Chouhan et al. (eds.), *Women's Health Dynamics in South Asia*, Asian Perspectives on Public Health, https://doi.org/10.1007/978-981-95-2321-4_14

## 14.1 Introduction

Indigenous Peoples represent 6.2% of the global population with approximately 97% of Indigenous peoples living in low- and middle-income countries (LMICs) (International Labour Organisation, 2019). High levels of poverty, human rights violations including dispossession of lands, forced assimilation and erosion of identity, discrimination, and marginalisation are evident (Office of the High Commissioner for Human Rights, 2007); this may be especially the case for Indigenous women, who may be faced with increased inequities because of the intersection of being both a woman and Indigenous (Human Rights Council, 2022; International Labour Organisation, 2019). Indigenous Peoples are more likely to live in ill health, have lower life expectancies at birth, and have poorer access to health care (Morgan & Breau, 2024; United Nations, 2015). Moreover, evidence suggests that Indigenous Peoples may be more likely to experience poorer mental health (Lee et al., 2022; Owais et al., 2020). The Sustainable Development Goals have put emphasis on 'leaving no-one behind' whilst the United Nations (2014: 3) has made a global commitment to ensure 'that Indigenous individuals have equal access to the highest attainable standard of physical and mental health.' This chapter will contribute to these discussions by exploring and mapping the existing literature on the mental health of Indigenous women in South Asia.

### *14.1.1 Indigenous Peoples in South Asia*

Globally, there is no one accepted definition of Indigenous Peoples, and the Global Declaration on the Rights of Indigenous Peoples (Office of the High Commissioner for Human Rights, 2007) does not define Indigeneity. The Indigenous and Tribal Peoples Convention, 1989 (No. 169) (International Labour Organisation, 1989), however, refers to Indigenous Peoples as: (a) Tribal Peoples with distinct socio-economic, traditions, and cultural backgrounds whose way of life is informed by 'special laws or regulations.' (b) People who are descended from those who originally inhabited the country, region, or islands at the time of colonisation. And (c) Self-identification as Indigenous or Tribal.

Self-identification as Indigenous and acceptance by their Indigenous community, therefore, is a key element of Indigenous identity along with relationships and connections to their lands/territories and natural resources (including pre-colonial, pre-settler, or pre-invasion connections to lands), shared traditions, knowledge and worldviews, experiences of domination, marginalisation, and oppression by non-Indigenous groups, shared political systems, and shared culture including language (United Nations, n.d.). Many Indigenous Peoples may be nomadic or migratory and Indigenous identity is not lost if individuals move away, either through choice or force, from their ancestral lands.

Defining who Indigenous Peoples are, however, can be complicated by the different terms used within and between countries for Indigenous Peoples, the diversity of groups within the term and the association of Indigenous Peoples with those who originally inhabited the land. Whilst the latter is relevant to North America, Latin America, Aotearoa, and Australia, it may have less relevance for Asia and Africa (see Thornberry, 2002 for further discussion). However, as we have seen above the Indigenous and Tribal Peoples Convention, 1989 (No. 169) (International Labour Organisation, 1989) definition of Indigenous Peoples is wider than original inhabitants. This is key in relation to understanding Indigenous Peoples within Asia with Mohindra (2017: 582) highlighting that in Africa and Asia, the focus is now increasingly on the self-identification of Indigenous Peoples and their situation in relation to the majority populations as opposed to a focus on 'aboriginality.'

Moreover, identifying Indigenous Peoples can be difficult as many States may not officially recognise groups as Indigenous or the concept of Indigeneity within their borders (Béteille, 1998; Buenavista et al., 2018; Geiger, 2008). This may be especially the case across Asia with some countries recognising Indigeneity globally by signing up to the Declaration on the Rights of Indigenous Peoples (Office for the High Commissioner of Human Rights, 2007) but at the same time not recognising that the concept applies to particular groups within their own country, claiming instead, using the original inhabitants understanding of Indigenous Peoples, that all citizens are indigenous to the country (Baird, 2016). The concept of Indigeneity therefore may be contested across Asia and terminology such as Scheduled Tribes or Adivasis in India, Jummas or Adivasi in Bangladesh, Janajatis or Adivasi in Nepal, or ethnic minorities may be used locally instead of the term Indigenous Peoples (Buenavista et al., 2018; IWGIA, 2024). However, over recent years, some Asian countries have started to recognise the rights of Indigenous groups nationally (Baird, 2016) and many Indigenous Peoples across Asia are increasingly claiming their rights to their Indigenous identity (Chakma et al., 2022).

More than two-thirds of the world's Indigenous Peoples live in the Asian region (Errico, 2017) with approximately 95 million Indigenous Peoples in South Asia (Lama, 2016). However, a lack of data, disaggregated by ethnicity, within some South Asian countries means that any appropriation of numbers of Indigenous Peoples is probably an underestimation (Thresia et al., 2022). The lack of disaggregated ethnicity data also impacts on analysis of between and within-country differences in relation to inequalities (Thresia et al., 2022) including health inequalities. Bearing the issues in data collection in mind, Table 14.1 gives a brief overview of available information on Indigenous groups in the eight countries of South Asia.

Indigenous Peoples in South Asia have poorer health outcomes than the general population (Thresia et al., 2022) and have poorer access to health services throughout Asia (Lama, 2016; Morgan & Breau, 2024). A report on the health of Scheduled Tribes in India has indicated higher rates of malaria and TB including death by malaria, lower life expectancy and higher rates of infant mortality, higher rates of under-nutrition, increased anaemia prevalence rates, and increased smoking and alcohol use (Ministry of Health and Family Welfare, 2018). Similarly, Thresia et al. (2022) found disparities in health status between Indigenous Peoples and the general

**Table 14.1** Indigenous Peoples of South Asia

| | |
|---|---|
| Afghanistan | Afghanistan is a multi-ethnic and multi-Tribal country. There is a lack of data which focuses specifically on Indigenous groups |
| Bangladesh | Over 54 Indigenous groups speaking approximately 35 languages living in the plain's districts and Chittagong Hill Tracts. These groups could include the Santal, Manipuri, Rakhain, Chakma, and Lushai (Dhir, 2015). Indigenous groups make up 1% of the total population according to the census of 2022 (16,504,781 people) but this number is disputed by Indigenous Peoples. The term Indigenous is not used by the Bangladeshi state (IWGIA, 2024) and Bangladesh did not ratify the United Nations Declaration on the Rights of Indigenous Peoples in 2007; the only South Asian country to not sign the declaration (Human Rights Council, 2020) |
| Bhutan | There are several Indigenous groups in Bhutan such as the Monpas and Urap but there is minimum literature or data available |
| India | Approximately 705 groups (8.6% of the population) are officially listed as Scheduled Tribes with the term Adivasis being used in some areas of India. Approximately, 75 Scheduled Tribes (1,702,545 people) are categorised as Particularly Vulnerable Tribal Groups (PVTGs) (IWGIA, 2024). The term Indigenous is not generally used by the Indian government (Dhir, 2015) who state that all Indians are Indigenous (Koreti, 2023). India is a signatory to the Declaration on the Rights of Indigenous Peoples (Office of the High Commissioner for Human Rights, 2007), but not to the Indigenous and Tribal Peoples Convention, 1989 (No. 169) (International Labour Organisation, 1989) |
| Maldives | Information is lacking on Indigenous Peoples in the Maldives |
| Nepal | The government of Nepal has officially recognised fifty-nine Indigenous Peoples in Nepal with another 19 identified in the census 2021 who are still to be officially recognised. The census identifies that 35.08% of the population of Nepal are Indigenous but other estimates by Indigenous groups put this above 51% (Indigenous Navigator, n.d.; IWGIA, 2024). Nepal is a signatory to the Declaration on the Rights of Indigenous Peoples (Office of the High Commissioner for Human Rights, 2007) and to the Indigenous and Tribal Peoples Convention, 1989 (No. 169) (International Labour Organisation, 1989) |
| Pakistan | The government of Pakistan does not use the term Indigenous but refers to Indigenous groups along with other minoritised groups as ethnic minorities (Wagha, 2012). This makes it difficult to estimate the numbers of Indigenous Peoples within Pakistan as they may be grouped together with ethnic minorities or in the category Tribal which could include both Indigenous and non-Indigenous Peoples. Indigenous Peoples within Pakistan are said to include the Baluch, Kehal, Jogi, Kabootra, Sanyasi, Koochis, Rebari, Bakarwal, and Kalash (Cultural Survival, 2017). See Siddiqui (2023) for an overview of the situation of the Kalasha Peoples |
| Sri Lanka | Indigenous Peoples such as the Vedda or Wanniyalaeto make up approximately 0.5% of the population (Ananda & Nahallage, 2022) and are not legally recognised within Sri Lankan legislation (Dhir, 2015) |

population in Nepal, Pakistan, India, and Bangladesh including increases in non-communicable diseases and significant inequalities in life expectancy across all four countries. However, a lack of data about Indigenous populations across Asia is evident and is often reflective of both the health needs of the communities not being national priorities in many countries (Lama, 2016; Morgan & Sengedorj, 2023) and the lack of recognition given to Indigenous groups (Buenavista et al., 2018). Poorer health status is compounded by a range of socio-economic and political factors which impact on Indigenous Peoples across Asia including discrimination, lack of self-determination, food insecurity, forced assimilation, social disadvantage and poverty, lack of citizenship, illiteracy, low levels of education, higher likelihood of informal employment, increased rates of child labour, and displacement or imposed migration due to forced acquisition of ancestral lands (Buenavista et al., 2018; Thresia et al., 2022). Moreover, the degradation of Indigenous lands in India, through mining and other industries, was found to impact on Indigenous livelihoods (Ministry of Health and Family Welfare, 2018) and concerns have been raised about the impact of climate change on Indigenous Peoples in the region (Ahmed et al., 2022; Chakma et al., 2022).

Having given a brief overview of the terminology, numbers of Indigenous groups in South Asia and some of the general health issues which the communities face in the region, the remainder of this chapter explores the available literature on mental health and Indigenous women in South Asia. Global research has indicated that Indigenous Peoples may face increased mental health burdens including higher rates of substance use (Gracey & King, 2009; Hobden et al., 2023). For example, Kisely et al. (2017) in their meta-analysis of studies from Latin America, Canada, and the United States found that Indigenous Peoples reported high levels of Post Traumatic Stress Disorder (PTSD) and phobias whilst a population-based cohort study in Australia, which focused on psychiatric hospitalisations, found that Aboriginal and Torres Strait Islander Peoples were much more likely to be diagnosed with a range of psychiatric conditions including high rates of substance and alcohol use (Ogilvie et al., 2021). Moreover, in Aotearoa, Māori were more likely than any other ethnic group to report high or very high psychological distress with significantly higher rates of suicide reported (Ministry of Health, 2023). Similar findings have been found in Canada with First Nation and Inuit peoples reporting high levels of distress with rates of suicide up to 30 times higher than the general population (Kielland & Simeone, 2014). However, not all studies have found increased mental health risk for Indigenous Peoples and risk may vary according to ethnicity, the particular mental health illness, and socio-economic factors (Black et al., 2017). In relation to Indigenous women, a global systematic review identified an increased risk of depression, anxiety, and substance use during pregnancy (Owais et al., 2020) whilst studies in Canada (Hu & Hajizadeh, 2023), Australia (Australian Institute for Health and Welfare, n.d.), and United States (Ka'apu & Burnette, 2019) have found a gender health gap with Indigenous women more likely to report poorer health including mental health, compared to Indigenous men. Female gender and Indigenous identity, therefore, intersect and Indigenous women may be especially vulnerable to socio-economic factors, disempowerment, climate change, systemic racism, and structural violence including gender-based violence (Chapola et al., 2024; Human Rights

Council, 2022; International Labour Organisation, 2019; Morgan & Choak, 2023; Rogg & Pezzia, 2024; Tauli-Corpuz, 2015). Given the above findings about higher rates of mental health burden in Indigenous populations and in particular Indigenous women, a scoping review of the available literature on mental health and Indigenous women in South Asia will provide valuable information on the situation in the region.

## 14.2 Materials and Methods

A scoping review methodology was chosen to enable a thorough exploration of the available literature on mental health and Indigenous women in South Asia and to identify gaps within the literature (Munn et al., 2018; Peters et al., 2022). The methodology for the scoping review is outlined below following Arksey and O'Malley (2005) framework for scoping reviews. The preferred reporting items for systematic reviews and meta-analyses extension for the scoping reviews checklist (PRISMA-ScR) were also utilised in tandem with Arksey and O'Malley's framework.

***Stage 1:*** *Identifying the research question*

As recommended by Joanna Briggs Institute (Peters et al., 2015) the research question was developed following the 'participants, concept and context' (PCC) approach. P (types of participants): Indigenous women, C (concept): Mental health, and C (context): South Asia. The research review question was 'What is the available literature on mental health and Indigenous women in South Asia?

***Stage 2:*** *Identifying relevant studies*

We searched the following electronic databases: CINAHL Plus with Full Text, MEDLINE, Academic Search Premier, Psychology and Behavioural Sciences Collection, APA PsycInfo, and APA PsycArticles (through EBSO host) for published empirical studies that focused on the research question. The search was performed in June 2024. Limiters were as follows: articles published since 2004, and articles published in Hindi and English. The keywords using Boolean operators were "mental health" OR "mental illness" OR "mental disorder*" OR wellbeing OR "psychiatric illness" OR "Substance Use" OR Suicide AND women OR female* OR woman AND Indigenous OR "Scheduled Tribe*" OR Tribal OR Adivasi OR Jummas OR Janajatis OR Vedda AND "South Asia*" OR India OR Pakistan OR Nepal OR Bangladesh OR Bhutan OR Afghanistan OR Maldives OR Sri Lanka.

***Stage 3:*** *Study selection*

The initial search identified 333 papers. Retrieved articles were transferred to Endnote and duplicates were removed ($n = 105$ duplicates). Article abstracts and titles ($n = 228$) were screened for eligibility according to inclusion and exclusion criteria. One hundred and ninety-eight articles were excluded according to the inclusion and exclusion criteria. Full texts ($n = 30$) were then screened to identify the final articles according to the inclusion and exclusion criteria. The inclusion criteria were articles published in the last 20 years (since 2004) which were written in English and Hindi and focused on Indigenous women, mental health, and wellbeing including suicide and substance use in South Asia. The exclusion criteria were articles written before 2004 in languages other than English or Hindi that related to non-Indigenous women and focused on physical health in countries other than those in South Asia. This left 17 articles in the final review. The PRISMA diagram in Fig. 14.1 outlines each stage and the reasons for exclusion.

As the aim of this scoping review was to map out the main themes from existing literature, provide an overview of key concepts and identify gaps in the evidence, critical appraisal of the final articles was not undertaken (Peters et al., 2021).

***Stage 4:*** *Charting the data*

Data was manually extracted from the articles and presented in an Excel spreadsheet/matrix. The following information was extracted: research aim, study methodology and analysis, sample size and setting, and findings.

***Stage 5:*** *Collating, summarising, and reporting the results*

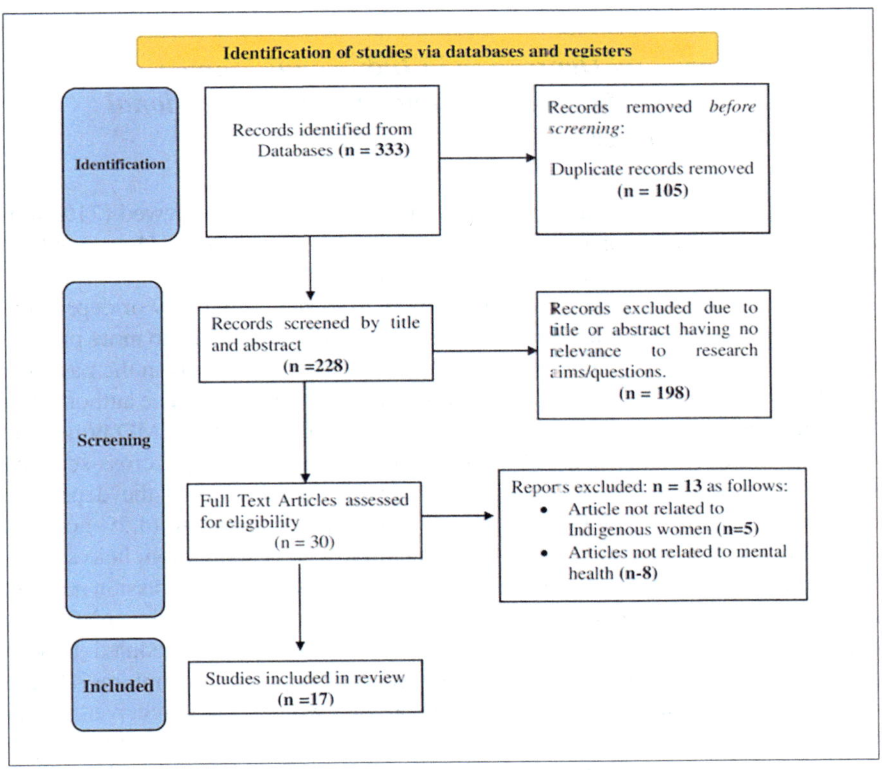


**Fig. 14.1** PRISMA flow diagram detailing method of study selection

The findings were analysed thematically, using Braun and Clarke's (2022) reflexive thematic analysis and themes identified across all articles. Results are reported as follows: description of study characteristics, followed by main findings and thematic analysis. The last section relates to discussion and conclusions.

## 14.3 Results

### *14.3.1 Study Characteristics*

Out of the seventeen studies which focused on Indigenous women, 14 were carried out in India, 2 in Bangladesh and 1 in Pakistan. There were no studies which focused on Indigenous women in the Maldives, Nepal, Afghanistan, and Bhutan. Most of the studies were quantitative ($n = 15$) with 2 studies using qualitative methods. Out of the quantitative studies, most studies utilised a cross-sectional study design. Table 14.2 provides details about 17 studies.

### *14.3.2 Anxiety and Depression in Indigenous Women in South Asia: Social, Economic, and Educational Disadvantage*

At a Tribal hospital in Kerala, India, 721 outpatients were interviewed (71% were female) and measured for weight and haemoglobin concentration. Household and physical health information was collected along with self-reported questionnaires to measure common mental health disorders (CMD) such as anxiety or depression. The analysis revealed that higher SRQ scores for CMD were linked to more physical health symptoms, being female, no education, and more life events in the past year. CMD prevalence was 27% (having an SRQ score greater than 11). The authors highlight the importance of understanding social factors in relation to CMD prevalence in Tribal women (Hackett et al., 2007). Similarly, a population-based cross-sectional survey in North India of 960 people with (50%) females found the depression prevalence was (6%), with (7.9%) of women affected compared to (4.2%) of men. The study used the Patient Health Questionnaire to assess depression, help seeking behaviour and socio-economic status. Significant risk factors for depression included illiteracy, lower caste status (Scheduled Caste/Tribe or Other Backward Castes), temporary housing, and recent loans. Those who identified as Scheduled Tribe or Scheduled Caste have three times of odds of reporting depressive symptoms. Despite a higher rate of healthcare visits among depressed women, none received talking therapy, and only (3.3%) were prescribed antidepressants. The gender difference in depression rates became non-significant after adjusting for education and economic status, highlighting the influence of these factors (Mathias et al., 2015). Another

**Table 14.2** Description of included studies

| Authors | Objective |
|---|---|
| Singh et al. (2013) | To explore previous findings of the high rate of suicides among *Idu Mishmi* and to evaluate psychological traits in India |
| Faruk and Rosenbaum (2023) | To investigate stigma and risk factors in the Chattogram Hill Tracts (CHT) in Bangladesh |
| Richardson et al. (2020) | To estimate the effect of physical and sexual abuse (Intimate Partner Violence) on women's mental distress |
| Hackett et al. (2007) | To examine the association between Common Mental Health Disorders (CMD) and anaemia, malnutrition and physical symptoms |
| Singh and Rao (2018) | To assess impulsive and aggressive behaviours among the Idu Mishmi Tribe |
| Bhattacharjee (2022) | To examine prevalence of depression among Tribal pregnant women |
| Rose-Clarke et al. (2019) | To assess the health, nutrition and wellbeing of adolescent girls |
| Kar et al. (2024) | To measure postnatal depression scores. To compare family care vs. facility care as factors associated with EPDS scores |
| Nadkarni et al. (2022) | To measure psychological distress in Indigenous women and explore associations with individual, household, and socio-political factors |
| Powathil and Parthsarathy (2017) | To study the socio-demographic profile of unwed mothers and assess two psychological parameters, self-esteem and psychological distress and their correlation with demographic factors |
| Mathias et al. (2015) | Assess depression prevalence and associations with healthcare seeking and socio-economic determinants |
| Faruk et al. (2021) | To understand the extent of symptoms of anxiety and depression |
| Pati et al. (2018) | To understand beliefs around alcohol consumption during pregnancy |
| Parihar and Jha (2014) | To examine the role of culture in self-concept of adolescents |
| Choudhry et al. (2018) | To explore cultural protective factors and preferences for interventions |
| Hansda et al. (2021) | To assess supernatural attitudes among Tribal people about mental illness, to explore general practices related to mental health and psychosocial issues |
| Hegde et al. (2022) | To understand knowledge, attitude, cultural beliefs, and practices with regard to mental illness |

cross-sectional survey of 303 women in the Nilgiri Biosphere Reserve, South India which was undertaken with Particularly Vulnerable Tribal Groups, revealed a prevalence of 39.9% for psychological distress. Prevalence for self-reported anxiety was (24.8%), whilst the prevalence for disturbed sleep was (27.1%) and reduced appetite (22.1%). Significant risk factors included social isolation, tobacco use, hypertension (personal and familial), and violent household conflicts. Those experiencing psychological distress were more likely to be older, divorced/separated/unmarried, and landless (Nadkarni et al., 2022).

In a study involving the Marma and Chakma communities in Bangladesh, 240 participants completed standardised anxiety and depression scales. Results showed elevated anxiety and depression scores in both communities, with (59.2%) scoring above the clinical cut-off for anxiety and (58.8%) for depression. Among the Marma, women scored significantly higher on both scales compared to men, whilst in the Chakma community, men scored higher on anxiety with no significant gender difference in depression. These findings emphasise the varying impact of mental health issues across different Indigenous communities and the influence of gender (Faruk et al., 2021). Another study focusing on intimate partner violence was undertaken with 3010 women in rural Tribal communities in Rajasthan, India. Baseline interviews and follow-up interviews 1.5 years later were utilised. Intimate partner violence (IPV) was assessed using questions from the Demographic and Health Survey's Domestic Violence Module, covering physical abuse, psychological abuse, and partner's controlling behaviour. Mental distress was measured with the 12-item General Health Questionnaire. Women reported an average of 2.1 distress symptoms at baseline. Poisson regression models showed that experiencing psychological abuse increased distress symptoms by 0.65 (95% CI 0.32, 0.98), and controlling behaviour increased symptoms by 0.31 (95% CI 0.18, 0.44). Physical abuse was not linked to an increase in distress symptoms (mean difference = −0.15, 95% CI −0.45, 0.15). Psychological abuse and controlling behaviour were found to be more detrimental to mental health than physical abuse. Women reporting physical abuse initially showed higher distress (2.6 vs. 1.6 symptoms), but this association was not significant when accounting for other abuses. The authors suggest that psychological abuse and controlling behaviour are key drivers of mental distress (Richardson et al., 2020).

### *14.3.3 Indigenous Women in South Asia: Mental Health, Alcohol Use, and the Perinatal Period*

A study in Tripura, north-east India, examined the prevalence of depression among pregnant Tribal women, focusing on self-concept, depression, and quality of marital life. The sample included 200 women in their 1st and 3rd trimesters, selected from hospitals and private gynaecological providers. Findings revealed that 70.5% of these women had minimal depression, followed by moderate (13.5%), mild (12.5%), and severe (3.5%) depression. Women in the 1st trimester reported higher depression, lower self-concept, and poorer marital quality of life compared to those in the 3rd trimester (Bhattacharjee, 2022). A fast-track study in the villages of Koraput and Boudh, Odisha, India was undertaken and focused on women with babies aged 1–6 months in Tribal areas. Using the General Health Questionnaire GHQ-12 for familial stress and Edinburgh Postnatal Depression Scale (EPDS) for postnatal depression, the study included 98 women (50 from Boudh, 48 from Koraput). Findings indicated that Koraput had higher postnatal poor mental health, with mean EPDS scores 6 points higher than Boudh. Despite high institutional delivery rates and low out-of-pocket expenses in both villages, Koraput showed lower male participation in family planning. Family stress and socio-demographic characteristics were also significantly associated with rates of postnatal depression. The EPDS and GHQ-12 scores were significantly higher in Koraput compared to Boudh, with a mean EPDS score of $14.56 \pm 3.86$. High EPDS scores ($\geq$15) were found in 54.2% of the women, with 73.9% reported in Koraput. The authors highlight how factors outside the health system itself may need to be addressed including family stressors to support women with postnatal depression (Kar et al., 2024).

Additionally, a study in south India aimed at examining the socio-demographic profile of unwed Tribal mothers assessed their self-esteem and psychological distress. Data collected using the Rosenberg Self-Esteem Scale and the Self-Reporting Questionnaire showed that (60%) of the population reported psychological distress, with a mean self-reporting questionnaire score of 9.2. A significant negative correlation was found between psychological distress and self-esteem ($r = -0.410, p = 0.010$), highlighting the interrelationship between these factors (Powathil & Parthsarathy, 2017). In relation to alcohol use, research in a Tribal-dominated district of Odisha, eastern India explored Tribal women's and community perceptions regarding alcohol consumption during pregnancy. Using the WHO AUDIT tool, in-depth interviews were conducted with 19 women and 18 family members, alongside focused group discussions with community leaders and health workers. The study found that factors such as limited social monitoring, easy access to alcohol, low alcohol literacy, and the normalisation of alcohol in daily customs contributed to unrestricted alcohol intake among pregnant women. The community often perceived homemade alcohol as harmless. The authors highlight how addressing this issue requires culturally sensitive interventions involving community counselling and collaboration among alcohol researchers, mental health specialists, public health workers, and anthropologists (Pati et al., 2018).

### *14.3.4 Suicide and Indigenous Peoples in South Asia*

A study on the Idu Mishmi Tribe from Arunachal Pradesh in north-east India seeks to validate earlier reports of high suicide rates and to evaluate the associated psychological traits. The study involved interviewing 218 individuals from the Idu Mishmi Tribe and administering the Patient Health Questionnaire (PHQ). In the Idu Mishmi population, the suicide attempt rate (14.22%) was significantly higher than in the general urban population, with females at a higher risk. The prevalence of depression (8.26%) was comparable to earlier reports, whilst anxiety syndrome (6.42%), alcohol abuse (36.24%), binge eating (6.42%), and bulimia nervosa (1.38%) were also recorded (Singh et al., 2013). Another study included 177 unrelated Idu Mishmi participants from Arunachal Pradesh state, India which included 39 people who had attempted suicide and 138 non-attempters. Data on demographics and suicide attempts were collected, and participants completed assessments for aggression and impulsivity traits. Among the Idu Mishmi, (22.03%) had attempted suicide, with a significant sex difference: (35.9%) male and (64.1%) female ($p = 0.002^*$). There was a higher frequency of suicide attempts for those aged over 19 years old, those who were in high school education, and those who were married. Moreover, the research found a higher prevalence of students and female housewives in the suicide attempters category; this was statistically significant. In all interviewed female and male participants, the prevalence of suicide attempters was found to be (32.89%) and (13.86%) respectively. Suicide attempters scored higher on aggression than non-attempters (23.93 vs. 18.46, $p \leq 0.05$) and impulsivity (75.53 vs. 71.59, $p \leq 0.05$). When analysed according to gender, the results were statistically significant for females for aggression only. However, impulsiveness showed a stronger difference [F(1, 117) = 7.274] compared to aggression [F(1, 117) = 2.647], indicating its significant role in suicide attempts. Multivariate logistic regression indicated gender (OR = 1.079, $p = 0.05$) and impulsiveness (OR = 3.355, $p = 0.013$) were significant factors in suicide attempts. A sex-wise comparison in the total population showed elevated female impulsivity (Singh & Rao, 2018).

In another study, researchers conducted extensive face-to-face surveys among 3324 adolescent girls aged 10–19 years old from Jharkhand in India. Eighty-two per cent of the girls were from Scheduled Tribes. Their investigation aimed to comprehensively assess various dimensions of health and social conditions affecting them. They found alarming rates of health issues among the participants, including high levels of anaemia, prevalence of thinness, and stunting affecting 45% of the cohort. Educational attainment varied significantly, with 89% attendance among younger girls but only 46% among those aged 15–19, often due to household responsibilities or agricultural work. The study also reported that 40% of the younger participants reported emotional violence, 14% physical violence, and a smaller fraction, 0.7%, reported sexual violence. Mental health concerns were prevalent, with 12% of the girls' experiencing symptoms of depression or anxiety, 3% answering true or somewhat true to indicators of externalising behaviours such as oppositional defiant disorder or conduct disorder, 6% of older girls reporting that they had considered suicide in the last year compared to 4% of younger girls, with most of these girls having attempted suicide at least once (Rose-Clarke et al., 2019).

### *14.3.5 Indigenous Beliefs and Mental Health in South Asia*

A community-based cross-sectional study assessed the supernatural attitudes towards mental illness among Scheduled Tribes in Jharkhand, India. The assessment of supernatural attitudes was carried out using a questionnaire. A total of 60 participants from selected villages in the Ranchi and Pakur districts were included in the study. Around 65% were women; however, the results were not differentiated according to gender. The majority of the 60 participants believed in supernatural powers, attributing common physical and psychological illnesses to bhoot prêt (ghosts), oprikasar (black magic), and devi-devtaprakop (God's curse) and most preferred visiting the faith healers for any type of psychiatric illness (Hansda et al., 2021). Another study in Pakistan's Kalasha Indigenous community was undertaken to understand youths' perceptions towards mental health. The in-depth qualitative study, guided by Bronfenbrenner's ecological system framework, explored mental health among 12 Kalasha adolescents and emerging adults (5 men, 7 women) in the Kalasha valleys, all fluent in Urdu. Three main themes emerged across the 12 participants' interviews. First, psychological resilience was fostered by intra-communal bonding, Kalasha festivals and traditions, purity concepts, and practices promoting happiness. Second, mental health issues were attributed to a mix of biological, psychosocial, supernatural, spiritual, and environmental factors. Lastly, preferred interventions included shamanic treatments, Ta'awiz (amulets), communal sharing, problem-solving, medical treatments, and herbal methods (Choudhry et al., 2018). This study highlighted the Kalasha community's unique integration of cultural, spiritual, and communal influences in understanding and addressing mental health.

Another study compared the knowledge, attitudes, cultural beliefs, and practices regarding mental illness among urban, rural, and Scheduled Tribal populations in Mysuru, India. Using a semi-structured questionnaire, data were collected on their attitudes, beliefs, and understanding of mental illness. Tribal people were more likely than urban and rural people to answer do not know to the question 'what is mental health?' Among the Tribal participants, 25% attributed mental illness to abnormal thinking, 19% to behavioural changes, 5% to abnormal beliefs, 11% to supernatural causes, and 17% identified social withdrawal, isolation, and violence as symptoms. Whilst 20% cited stigma and social implications as reasons for hesitance in seeking treatment for mental illness (Hegde et al., 2022). Another cross-sectional survey in Rangamati, Bangladesh involving Indigenous communities revealed significant differences in mental illness stigma between genders. Using the 28-item Bangla-translated Mental Illnesses Stigma Scale, females reported more stigma ($M = 134.26$) compared to males ($M = 128.12$), with a statistically significant result ($t(347) = -3.580$, $p < 0.05$). This higher stigma among females may stem from their reliance on informal support, which can prevent them from seeking professional mental health care (Faruk & Rosenbaum, 2023). In a separate investigation, researchers explored cultural influences on self-concept among adolescents by comparing 200 Tribal and 200 non-Tribal students in the eleventh grade in Chhattisgarh State, India. Equal numbers of males and females were included in the sample. Using the native self-concept assessment, the study found that cultural background significantly influenced self-perception. Non-Tribal students generally reported higher levels of self-concept compared to their Tribal counterparts (Parihar & Jha, 2014).

## 14.4 Discussion

Our review of the literature on mental health and Indigenous women in South Asia found a significant burden of mental health issues, including depression, anxiety and psychological distress, among women in Indigenous populations in India and Bangladesh (Faruk et al., 2021; Mathias et al., 2015; Nadkarni et al., 2022). In relation to suicide, Indigenous Peoples reported higher levels of suicide attempts than the general population; this was particularly the case for women (Singh & Rao, 2018; Singh et al., 2013). Social determinants of health such as education, literacy levels, temporary housing, economic status, social isolation, lower status and exposure to household conflict were associated with poorer mental health outcomes (Hackett et al., 2007; Kar et al., 2024; Mathias et al., 2015; Nadkarni et al., 2022; Richardson et al., 2020). For alcohol use, risk factors included the normalisation of alcohol in the community, easy access to alcohol and low levels of health literacy around alcohol (Pati et al., 2018). Access to interventions to support mental health was limited (Mathias et al., 2015) with some participants preferring to visit faith healers or shamans and use traditional methods of treatments such as herbal remedies (Choudhry et al., 2018; Hansda et al., 2021). Stigma around mental health was identified as being a potential barrier to take up of interventions (Hegde et al., 2022) with this being especially the case for women (Faruk & Rosenbaum, 2023). Participants attributed mental health issues to a wide range of factors including supernatural and spiritual (Choudhry et al., 2018; Hansda et al., 2021), as well as biological, psychosocial, and environmental factors (Choudhry et al., 2018). Psychological resilience was found to be promoted through community bonding and Indigenous identity including festivals and traditions (Choudhry et al., 2018).

Recommendations to improve the mental health of Indigenous women in South Asia include interventions, such as poverty reduction initiatives, to improve the social determinants of health and initiatives to improve access to psychological therapies and support. The latter must be informed by Indigenous worldviews and practices and be culturally sensitive taking on board the role of traditional healers and Indigenous traditions including the importance of Indigenous cultural activities which promote Indigenous identity and connections to their lands (Choudhry et al., 2018; Ka'apu & Burnette, 2019). South Asian countries have established national mental health programs, policies, strategies, and acts that delineate guidelines aimed at enhancing the mental health of their populations. These frameworks encompass provisions for screening, referral, and treatment. However, there is an evident lack of targeted strategies for Indigenous populations and women within these documents. This gap highlights the potential for expanding and improving the implementation of gender-informed programs to ensure the inclusion and equitable support of Indigenous communities which is culturally relevant and takes on board the situation of women. Moreover, increased training on Indigenous cultural norms including the importance of ancestral knowledge, connections to the land and traditional medicines as well as the factors that impact on Indigenous Peoples' wellbeing should be part of health professionals training. In addition, culturally sensitive and appropriate health literacy education and health promotion that supports community understanding of mental health including interventions and services that are available should be strengthened (Choudhry et al., 2018). This should be undertaken in collaboration with the communities themselves so that health professionals and policy-makers learn from Indigenous Peoples. This is important as it has been highlighted, for example, that Indigenous Peoples' conceptualisations of mental health may differ from those put-forward by the bio-medical model; this may have ramifications for the provision of services to Indigenous populations (Mpofu et al., 2023). Moreover, the use of community health workers, such as Accredited Social Health Activists (ASHAs) in India, could be utilised to build relationships and improve the dissemination of mental health information. Indigenous advocates from the communities could also be trained to support women in accessing services (O'Keefe et al., 2019). At a wider level, governments need to focus on reducing the social exclusion, structural disempowerment, stigmatisation, and marginalisation of Indigenous Peoples including acting on issues which impact the communities including climate change, structural violence, and dispossessions of lands (Office of the High Commissioner for Human Rights, 2007). The latter point is key not only in relation to social justice and human rights but also to promoting psychological resilience.

Limitations of this scoping review include the potential to miss articles, as papers did not always make it clear whether the population was from an Indigenous community. This was especially the case in relation to the term 'Tribal' in Pakistan and Afghanistan. To overcome this issue, extensive research was undertaken on the groups concerned. The exclusion of literature written in languages other than English and Hindi meant that the review may not have covered the full breadth of literature. In terms of future research, there was a lack of research in all countries in South Asia apart from India. More research is needed on Indigenous women in Nepal, Bangladesh, Bhutan, Maldives, Pakistan, and Afghanistan. This scarcity of research on Bhutan, Maldives, Pakistan, and Afghanistan is reflective of a lack of data on Indigenous Peoples in these countries. There was also minimal in-depth qualitative research with almost all studies being quantitative. Understanding the perspectives of Indigenous women is key to supporting holistic wellbeing including promoting resilience and identifying factors which impact on mental health, we would, therefore, advocate for more high-quality qualitative studies. Furthermore, there was a greater level of cross-sectional studies undertaken and thus a need for more in-depth longitudinal and epidemiological studies which differentiate between genders, Indigenous groups, socio-economic status, and compare outcomes to non-Indigenous groups. Research which takes a participatory focus including Indigenous women as collaborators in studies, as opposed to being the subjects of research, would be welcome.

## 14.5 Conclusion

In this chapter, we explored the literature on the mental health of Indigenous women in South Asia. To our knowledge, this is the first review of the literature which has focused on this topic in the region. Our findings highlight a significant mental health burden among Indigenous women in South Asia. However, there is a lack of research on Indigenous women in Nepal, Bhutan, Maldives, Pakistan, and Afghanistan with most studies in the review being undertaken in India and some in Bangladesh. More research on understanding the mental health burden, access to services and risk factors across South Asia for Indigenous women as well as Indigenous constructions of mental health and support mechanisms is needed. This is key to supporting the Sustainable Development Goals and its emphasis on 'leaving no-one behind' and ensuring that Indigenous women have 'equal access to the highest attainable standard of ….mental health' (United Nations, 2014: 3).

## References


Ahmed, M. N. Q., Chowdhury, M. T. A., Ahmed, K. J., & Haq, S. M. A. (2022). Indigenous peoples' views on climate change and their experiences, coping and adaptation strategies in South Asia: A review. In M. F. Mbah, W. Leal Filho, & S. Ajaps (Eds.), *Indigenous methodologies, research and practices for sustainable development* (pp. 285–301). World Sustainability Series. Springer. https://doi.org/10.1007/978-3-031-12326-9_17

Ananda, T., & Nahallage, C. (2022). Present sociocultural status of the Sri Lankan Indigenous people (the Veddas) and future challenges. In U. Chatterjee, A. Kashyap, M. Everard, G. Krishna Panda, D. Mahata (Eds.), *Indigenous people and nature* (pp. 381–398). Elsevier.

Arksey, H., & O'Malley, L. (2005). Scoping studies: Towards a methodological framework. *International Journal of Social Research Methodology, 8*(1), 19–32. https://doi.org/10.1080/1364557032000119616

Australian Institute of Health and Welfare. (n.d.). *Mental health.* https://www.indigenousmhspc.gov.au/topics/mental-health#aboutthistopic. Accessed 22 July 2024.

Australian Institute of Health and Welfare. (2022). *Determinants of health for Indigenous Australians.* AIHW, Australian Government. https://www.aihw.gov.au/reports/australias-health/social-determinants-and-indigenous-health. Accessed 16 July 2024.

Baird, I. G. (2016). Indigeneity in Asia: An emerging but contested concept. *Asian Ethnicity, 17*(4), 501–505. https://doi.org/10.1080/14631369.2016.1193804

Béteille, A. (1998). The idea of Indigenous people. *Current Anthropology, 39*, 187–191.https://doi.org/10.1086/204717

Bhattacharjee, A. (2022). Mental dispositions of tribal pregnant women of Tripura. *Journal of Psychosocial Research, 17*(2). https://doi.org/10.32381/JPR.2022.17.02.22

Black, E., Kisely, S., Alichniewicz, K., & Toombs, M. (2017). Mood and anxiety disorders in Australia and New Zealand's indigenous populations: A systematic review and meta-analysis. *Psychiatry Research, 255*, 128–138. https://doi.org/10.1016/j.psychres.2017.05.015

Braun, V., & Clarke, V. (2022). *Thematic analysis: A practical guide.* Sage.

Buenavista, D. P., Wynne-Jones, S., & McDonald, M. (2018). Asian indigeneity, indigenous knowledge systems, and challenges of the 2030 agenda. *East Asian Community Rev, 1*, 221–240. https://doi.org/10.1057/s42215-018-00010-0

Chakma, A. K., Bijoy, C. R., & Rai, T. B. (2022). *Nationally determined contributions in Asia: Are governments recognizing the rights, roles and contributions of Indigenous Peoples?* Asia Indigenous Peoples Pact (AIPP).

Chapola, J., Datta, R., & Waucaush-Warn, J. (2024). Climate change and its impact on the mental health well-being of Indigenous women in Western cities, Canada. *Journal of Community & Applied Social Psychology, 34*(3), Article e2807. https://doi.org/10.1002/casp.2807

Choudhry, F. R., Khan, T. M., Park, M. S. A., & Golden, K. J. (2018). Mental health conceptualization and resilience factors in the Kalasha youth: An indigenous ethnic and religious minority community in Pakistan. *Frontiers in Public Health, 6*, 187. https://doi.org/10.3389/fpubh.2018.00187

Cianconi, P., Lesmana, C. B. J., Ventriglio, A., & Janiri, L. (2019). Mental health issues among indigenous communities and the role of traditional medicine. *International Journal of Social Psychiatry., 65*(4), 289–299. https://doi.org/10.1177/0020764019840060

Cultural Survival. (2017). *Observations on the State of Indigenous Human Rights in Pakistan Prepared for: The 28th Session of the United Nations Human Rights Council Universal Periodic Review*. https://www.culturalsurvival.org/sites/default/files/PakistanUPR2017.pdf. Accessed 11 July 2024.

Dhir, R. K. (2015). *Indigenous peoples in the world of work in Asia and the Pacific: A status report*. ILO.

Errico, S. (2017). *The rights of Indigenous peoples in Asia. Human rights-based overview of national legal and policy frameworks against the backdrop of country strategies for development and poverty reduction*. ILO.

Faruk, M. O., Nijhum, R. P., Khatun, M. N., & Powell, G. E. (2021). Anxiety and depression in two indigenous communities in Bangladesh. *Global Mental Health, 8*, Article e34. https://doi.org/10.1017/gmh.2021.33.eCollection

Faruk, M. O., & Rosenbaum, S. (2023). Mental illness stigma among indigenous communities in Bangladesh: A cross-sectional study. *BMC Psychology, 11*(1), 216. https://doi.org/10.1186/s40359-023-01257-5

Geiger, D. (2008). Some thoughts on "indigeneity" in the context of migration and conflicts at contemporary Asian Frontiers. In C. Erni (Ed.), *The concept of Indigenous Peoples in Asia*. IWGIA.

Gracey, M., & King, M. (2009). Indigenous health part 1: Determinants and disease patterns. *The Lancet, 374*(9683), 65–75. https://doi.org/10.1016/S0140-6736(09)60914-4

Hackett, R. J., Sagdeo, D., & Creed, F. H. (2007). The physical and social associations of common mental disorder in a tribal population in South India. *Social Psychiatry and Psychiatric Epidemiology, 42*, 712–715. https://doi.org/10.1007/s00127-007-0223-y

Hansda, N. M., Singh, U., Kapse, P. P., & Kiran, M. (2021). Supernatural attitude and mental health practices among the tribal with special reference to Jharkhand. *Indian Journal of Psychiatric Social Work*, 90–95. https://doi.org/10.29120/IJPSW.2021.v12.i2.275

Hegde, S., Chandrashekarappa, S. M., Akbar, S., & Murthy, M. N. (2022). Community perceptions with regard to mental illness in urban, rural, and tribal areas in Mysuru. *Archives of Mental Health, 23*(1), 47–55. https://doi.org/10.4103/amh.amh_107_21

Hobden, B., Freund, M., Rumbel, J., Heard, T., Davis, R., Ying Ooi, J., Newman, J., Rose, B., Sanson-Fisher, R., & Bryant, J. (2023). Mental health and substance use co-occurrence among indigenous peoples: A scoping review. *International Journal of Mental Health and Addiction*. https://doi.org/10.1007/s11469-023-01114-x

Hu, M., & Hajizadeh, M. (2023). Mind the gap: What factors determine the worse health status of indigenous women relative to men living off-reserve in Canada? *Journal of Racial and Ethnic Health Disparities, 10*(3), 1138–1164. https://doi.org/10.1007/s40615-022-01301-x

Human Rights Council. (2020). *Regional consultation on the rights of Indigenous peoples in Asia Report of the Special Rapporteur on the rights of Indigenous peoples*. https://documents.un.org/doc/undoc/gen/g20/193/69/pdf/g2019369.pdf?token=jb7ssbBC1QLNG9Hx2L&fe=true. Accessed 15 July 2024.

Human Rights Council. (2022). *Violence against Indigenous women and girls. Report of the Special Rapporteur on violence against women, its causes and consequences*. https://documents.un.org/doc/undoc/gen/g22/323/90/pdf/g2232390.pdf?token=crGamUKPyAVYqAyHlM&fe=true. Accessed 14 July 2024.

Indigenous Navigator. (n.d.). https://Indigenousnavigator.org/data-explorer/2. Accessed 12 July 2024.

International Labour Organisation. (1989). *Indigenous and Tribal Peoples Convention, 1989 (No. 169)*. https://www.ohchr.org/en/instruments-mechanisms/instruments/indigenous-and-tribal-peoples-convention-1989-no-169. Accessed 19 July 2024.

International Labour Organisation. (2019). *Implementing the ILO Indigenous and Tribal Peoples Convention No. 169: Towards an inclusive, sustainable, and just future*. International Labour Organisation,

IWGIA. (2024). *The Indigenous World, 2024*. IWGIA.

Ka'apu, K., & Burnette, C. E. (2019). A culturally informed systematic review of mental health disparities among adult indigenous men and women of the USA: What is known? *British Journal of Social Work, 49*(4), 880–898. https://doi.org/10.1093/bjsw/bcz009

Kar, S., Samantaray, P. C., Patnaik, L., Mishra, A., & Lakshmi, P. (2024). Family and facility care variables attributing to postnatal depression among women in two tribal-dominated districts of Odisha: Log model analysis to suggest intervention. *Journal of Family Medicine and Primary Care, 13*(3), 958–963. https://doi.org/10.4103/jfmpc.jfmpc_1367_23

Kielland, N., & Simeone, T. (2014). Current issues in mental health in Canada: The mental health of First Nations and Inuit Communities. *Curr Issues Ment Heal Canada., 6*, 1–8.

Kisely, S., Alichniewicz, K. K., Black, E. B., Siskind, D., Spurling, G., & Toombs, M. (2017). The prevalence of depression and anxiety disorders in Indigenous people of the Americas: A systematic review and meta-analysis. *Journal of Psychiatric Research, 84*, 137–152. https://doi.org/10.1016/j.jpsychires.2016.09.032

Koreti, S. (2023). Adivasi's of India as indigenous people in postcolonial world. In B. Sengar & A. M. E. Adjoumani (Eds.), *Indigenous societies in the post-colonial world*. Springer.

Lama, M. (2016). Access to health services by indigenous peoples in Asia. In United Nations (Eds.), *State of the world's indigenous peoples: Indigenous peoples access to health services*. United Nations.

Lee, R. S., Brown, H. K., Salih, S., & Benoit, A. C. (2022). Systematic review of Indigenous involvement and content in mental health interventions and their effectiveness for Indigenous populations. *Australian and New Zealand Journal of Psychiatry, 56*(10), 1230–1251. https://doi.org/10.1177/00048674221089837

Mathias, K., Goicolea, I., Kermode, M., Singh, L., Shidhaye, R., & San Sebastian, M. (2015). Cross-sectional study of depression and help-seeking in Uttarakhand, North India. *BMJ Open, 1;5*(11), e008992.

Ministry of Health and Family Welfare. (2018). *Tribal Health in India*. Ministry of health and family Welfare and the ministry of tribal affairs.

Ministry of Health. (2023). *Health and independence report 2022*. Ministry of Health.

Mohindra, K. S. (2017). Research and the health of indigenous populations in low- and middle-income countries. *Health Promotion International, 32*(3), 581–586. https://doi.org/10.1093/heapro/dav106

Morgan, J., & Breau, G. (2024). Access to maternal health services for Indigenous women in low- and middle-income countries: An updated integrative review of the literature from 2018 to 2023. *Rural and Remote Health, 24*, 8520. https://doi.org/10.22605/RRH8520

Morgan, J., & Choak, C. (2023). Global public health and violence. In V. La Placa and J. Morgan (Eds.), *Social science perspectives on global public health* (pp. 109–118). Routledge.

Morgan, J., & Sengedorj, T, (2023). Nomadic peoples and access to healthcare. In V. La Placa & J. Morgan (Eds.), *Social science perspectives on global public health* (pp. 149–157). Routledge.

Mpofu, E., Doyle, A. K. E., Machina, E., Sefotho, M., & Brune, K. (2023). Mental health and indigenous people. In P. Liamputtong (Ed.), *Handbook of social sciences and global public health* (pp. 1690–1704). Springer.

Munn, Z., Peters, M. D. J., Stern, C., Tufanaru, C., McArthur, A., & Aromataris, E. (2018). Systematic review or scoping review? Guidance for authors when choosing between a systematic or scoping review approach. *BMC Medical Research Methodology, 18*(1), 143. https://doi.org/10.1186/s12874-018-0611-x

Nadkarni, A., Vasudevan, P., & Krishnakumar, J. (2022). Symptoms of psychological distress reported by women from indigenous communities in South India: Implications for methodology and future studies. *Archives of Women's Mental Health, 25*(3), 667–670. https://doi.org/10.1007/s00737-022-01215-x

Office of the High Commissioner for Human Rights. (2007). *UN Declaration on the Rights of Indigenous Peoples*. https://www.ohchr.org/en/indigenous-peoples/un-declaration-rights-indigenous-peoples. Accessed 19 July 2024.

Ogilvie, J. M., Tzoumakis, S., Allard, T., Thompson, C., Kisely, S., & Stewart, A. (2021). Prevalence of psychiatric disorders for indigenous Australians: A population-based birth cohort study. *Epidemiology and Psychiatric Sciences, 10*(30), Article e21. https://doi.org/10.1017/S204579602100010X

O'Keefe, V. M., Cwik, M. F., Haroz, E. E., & Barlow, A. (2019). Increasing culturally responsive care and mental health equity with indigenous community mental health workers. *Psychological Services, 18*(1), 84–92. https://doi.org/10.1037/ser0000358

O'Neill, L., Fraser, T., Kitchenham, A., & McDonald, V. (2018). Hidden burdens: A review of intergenerational, historical and complex trauma, implications for indigenous families. *Journal of Child & Adolescent Trauma, 11*(2), 173–186. https://doi.org/10.1007/s40653-016-0117-9

Owais, S., Faltyn, M., Johnson, A. V. D., Gabel, C., Downey, B., Kates, N., & Van Lieshout, R. J. (2020). The perinatal mental health of indigenous women: A systematic review and meta-analysis. *The Canadian Journal of Psychiatry, 65*(3), 149–163. https://doi.org/10.1177/0706743719877029

Parihar, N., & Jha, M. (2014). Study of self-concept of tribal and non-tribal adolescents. *Indian Journal of Health & Wellbeing, 5*(7).

Pati, S., Chauhan, A. S., Mahapatra, P., Hansdah, D., Sahoo, K. C., & Pati, S. (2018). Weaved into the cultural fabric: A qualitative exploration of alcohol consumption during pregnancy among tribal women in Odisha, India. *Substance Abuse Treatment, Prevention, and Policy, 13*, 1–9. https://doi.org/10.1186/s13011-018-0146-5

Peters, M. D. J., Godfrey, C., McInerney, P., Khalil, H., Larsen, P., Marnie, C., Pollock, D., Tricco, A. C., & Munn, Z. (2022). Best practice guidance and reporting items for the development of scoping review protocols. *JBI Evidence Synthesis, 20*(4), 953. https://doi.org/10.11124/JBIES-21-00242

Peters, M. D. J., Marnie, C., Tricco, A. C., Pollock, D., Munn, Z., Alexander, L., McInerney, P., Godfrey, C. M., & Khalil, H. (2021). Updated methodological guidance for the conduct of scoping reviews. *JBI Evidence Implementation, 19*(1), 3. https://doi.org/10.11124/JBIES-20-00167

Peters, M., Godfrey, C., McInerney, P., Soares, C., Khalil, H., & Parker, D. (2015).*The Joanna Briggs Institute Reviewers' Manual 2015: Methodology for JBI Scoping Reviews*. The Joanna Briggs Institute. https://espace.library.uq.edu.au/view/UQ:371443. Accessed 30 June 2024.

Powathil, G. G., & Parthsarathy, N. B. (2017). Psycho social aspects of tribal unwed mothers. *International Journal of Medicine & Public Health, 7*(2). https://doi.org/10.5530/ijmedph.2017.2.21

Richardson, R., Nandi, A., Jaswal, S., & Harper, S. (2020). The effect of intimate partner violence on women's mental distress: A prospective cohort study of 3010 rural Indian women. *Social Psychiatry and Psychiatric Epidemiology, 55*(1), 71–79. https://doi.org/10.1007/s00127-019-01735-5

Rogg, M. C., & Pezzia, C. (2024). Victimization and distress in indigenous Maya women: A qualitative investigation of gender-based violence and mental health outcomes in rural Guatemala. *Journal of Family Violence, 39*, 193–207. https://doi.org/10.1007/s10896-023-00500-2

Rose-Clarke, K., Pradhan, H., Rath, S., Rath, S., Samal, S., Gagrai, S., … Prost, A. (2019). Adolescent girls' health, nutrition and wellbeing in rural eastern India: A descriptive, cross-sectional community-based study. *BMC Public Health, 19*(1), 1–11. https://doi.org/10.1186/s12889-019-7053-1

Siddiqui, S. (2023). Kalasha people in Pakistan: A mountain indigenous tribe's struggles to protect identity, culture, ancestral lands, and survival. In B. Sengar & A. M. E. Adjoumani (Eds.), *Indigenous societies in the post-colonial world*. Springer. https://doi.org/10.1007/978-981-19-8722-9_16

Singh, P. K., Singh, R. K., Biswas, A., & Rao, V. R. (2013). High rate of suicide attempt and associated psychological traits in an isolated tribal population of North-East India. *Journal of Affective Disorders, 151*(2), 673–678. https://doi.org/10.1016/j.jad.2013.07.018

Singh, P. K., & Rao, V. R. (2018). Explaining suicide attempt with personality traits of aggression and impulsivity in a high risk tribal population of India. *PLoS ONE, 13*(2), Article e0192969. https://doi.org/10.1371/journal.pone.0192969

Tauli-Corpuz, V. (2015). *Report of the special rapporteur on the rights of indigenous people*. Human Rights Council. Special Rapporteur on Rights of Indigenous Peoples. https://digitallibrary.un.org/record/848738?v=pdf#files. Accessed 23 July 2024.

Thornberry, P. (2002). Who is indigenous?: Concept, definition, process. In *Indigenous peoples and human rights* (pp. 33–60). Manchester University Press. http://www.jstor.org/stable/j.ctt155jg1p.7

Thresia, C. U., Srinivas, P. N., Mohindra, K. S., & Jagadeesan, C. K. (2022). The health of indigenous populations in South Asia: A critical review in a critical time. *International Journal of Health Services, 52*(1), 61–72. https://doi.org/10.1177/0020731420946588

United Nations. (2015). *State of the world's Indigenous peoples: Indigenous peoples' access to health services*. United Nations Department of Economic and Social Affairs, Secretariat of the Permanent Forum on Indigenous Issues.

United Nations. (n.d.). *Who are Indigenous peoples*? https://www.un.org/esa/socdev/unpfii/documents/5session_factsheet1.pdf. Accessed 30 June 2024.

United Nations. (2014). *Outcome document of the high-level plenary meeting of the General Assembly known as the World Conference on Indigenous Peoples*. https://documents.un.org/doc/undoc/gen/n14/468/28/pdf/n1446828.pdf?token=RYhCof2ebPMvngtmZ1&fe=true. Accessed 15 July 2024.

Wagha, W. (2012). *Country technical notes on indigenous peoples' issues*. Islamic Republic of Pakistan. https://www.ifad.org/documents/38714170/40224860/pakistan_ctn.pdf/e61c7750-b616-423d-a7b3-cf2f886b47ae?t=1651742302778. Accessed 5 July 2024.

# Chapter 15
# Listening to the Mind-Psychiatric Epidemiology and Mental Health in Breast Cancer Care—Global Perspectives and Insights from India

**Amartya Krishnaditya and Dhananjay D. Mankar**

**Abstract** The present chapter contextualizes the psychiatric epidemiology of breast cancer survivors in India. The prevalence of psychiatric morbidity and its impacts, along with the methodological challenges of measuring such morbidity, are highlighted in this chapter. Employing the Quality of Life in Adult Cancer Survivors (QLACS) measure scale and multiple statistics, the present chapter quantified the chapter's outcomes. The chapter's key findings highlight that the adjusted variation in psychological well-being score was 30.8% (F-statistic = 2.780, *p*-value = 0.0430), which significantly varied based on demography, social support, and financial problems among the sampled women. The correlation between financial problems and psychological well-being was positive (Coeff: 0.6575). The present chapter concludes that although psychological well-being among breast cancer survivors varies based on their demography and socioeconomic background, there is a need to focus on affordable breast cancer services and the promotion of physiological well-being support services for such survivors in India.

**Keywords** Mental health · Psychiatric epidemiology · Breast cancer care · India

## 15.1 Introduction

As aptly stated by Coggon, Rose, and Barker, epidemiology serves as the bedrock of public- health initiatives (Plana-Ripoll et al., 2021). Understanding the determinants of diseases across diverse populations and regions is important to develop

---

A. Krishnaditya (✉)
MIT School of Bioengineering Sciences and Research, Rajbaug Campus, Loni Kalbhor, Maharashtra, India
e-mail: amartyakrishnaditya@gmail.com

D. D. Mankar
School of Health Systems Studies, Tata Institute of Social Sciences, Mumbai, India
e-mail: dhananjay.mankar@tiss.edu

 
P. Chouhan et al. (eds.), *Women's Health Dynamics in South Asia*, Asian Perspectives on Public Health, https://doi.org/10.1007/978-981-95-2321-4_15

preventive measures, evaluate existing healthcare interventions, and target specific policy interventions (Plana-Ripoll et al., 2021). In the public health research domain, psychiatric epidemiology is a well-developed sub-discipline of epidemiology which delves into the intricate world of mental disorders across populations. Concurrently, the subfield also explores the origins of psychiatric conditions, the complex web of factors, causes, and spatial distribution of mental disorders and linked impacts. The key objective of psychiatric epidemiology is to expand the realm of this research in terms of developing a robust framework for population-based scale by strategic interventions to improve the lives of people with mental health issues. In the current era of modern technology, technological advancements have propelled the research work enabling scholars to investigate and understand the nuances of mental health through a different lens apart from the conventional academic viewpoint. This has paved the way for a holistic understanding of the intricate dance between the mind and the environment (Plana-Ripoll et al., 2021).

### *15.1.1 Background of Psychiatric Epidemiology*

The early seeds of psychiatric epidemiology were shown during the Post World War II, when the World Health Organization (WHO) played an instrumental role in shaping international psychiatric epidemiology (Plana-Ripoll et al., 2021). The WHO constitution redefined "health", with the inclusion of mental health underscoring the significance of mental well-being within the holistic concept and conventional aspects of well-being in 1946 (Lovell, 2014). Despite this foundational contribution, the WHO has not been acknowledged enough to nurture the concept of psychiatric epidemiology (Plana-Ripoll et al., 2021). The initial years of the WHO's mental health program grappled with a broad definition of mental health, considering a wide spectrum of aspects (Demazeux, 2014; Lovell, 2014). It faced a constant tug-of-war situation between disorder-specific research and pressing requirements for public health. Limited resources, cultural barriers, and societal apathy were added to the woe (Plana-Ripoll et al., 2021). Following upon these barriers WHO developed an extensive framework for mental health research. Its relevance was questioned by advocates of psychiatric epidemiology "contagion argument" (Plana-Ripoll et al., 2021) theory by drawing parallels between mental illness and infectious diseases. This further led to a debate regarding the feasibility and value of this new approach. The evolution of psychiatric treatments and existing methodological bottlenecks underscored the need for rigorous research methods which led to a critical departure from cultural relativism. The alignment of diverse interests within the WHO, led to the launch of international schizophrenia studies (Lovell, 2014). This was a landmark project that served as a powerful demonstration to understand the significance of mental health research on a global scale (Plana-Ripoll et al., 2021). The development of psychiatric epidemiology highlights its late emergence, early pioneers, and the crucial role played by the WHO in its global expansion after the Second War further, marked by the multifaceted challenges, controversies, and transformative shifts that have shaped its journey (Demazeux, 2014; Plana-Ripoll et al., 2021). Further, the 1960s and 1970s marked a pivotal period in the field of psychiatric epidemiology. Several key milestones have marked this institutional recognition (Plana-Ripoll et al., 2021). The American Psychopathological Association (APA) dedicated its annual meeting to mental disorder epidemiology in 1959, signifying a shift toward growing interest in this field. Around the same time, organizations like the Milbank Memorial Fund (MMF) and the National Institute of Mental Health (NIMH) began funding research in this field, providing financial aid (Plana-Ripoll et al., 2021). The journal "Social Psychiatry' was established in 1966 and gave a platform for publishing research in this nascent field. Columbia University instituted the first training program in psychiatric epidemiology (1967), pioneering its academic integration, which was later funded by NIMH in 1972. The 1970s saw momentum, in such funding-based research programs at other universities that fostered the next generation of psychiatric epidemiologists and solidified the field's academic infrastructure (Plana-Ripoll et al., 2021).

### 15.1.2 Psychiatric Epidemiology: Evolving Landscape of Global Mental Health

The historical narratives and current global perspectives signify the mental health considerations in diverse societal landscapes. Mental health is now considered to play a critical role in contemporary global health dialogues, reflecting a notable shift that was primarily (Plana-Ripoll et al., 2021) concentrated on combating infectious diseases to the detriment of psychiatric considerations (Demazeux, 2014). The evolving landscape of global mental health reflects a more nuanced understanding of mental health disorders. This field employs metrics to understand the quantitative aspect of the burden of mental illness, allowing it to be compared with other health conditions equally (Maths et al., 2007). Although substantial progress has been made in understanding mental health globally, there is still a long way to go. The global treatment gap and proper resource allocation need to be addressed for thorough research on prevalence and associated risks (Wang et al., 2020). These contemporary challenges resonate with historical concerns, emphasizing the requirement for sustained interdisciplinary research and strategic resource allocation. The historical marginalization of mental health finds a modern echo in the exclusion of mental health in global policy interventions, such as the United Nations Millennium Development Goals. Evidences shows that the global health landscape is enriched by perspectives and methods of psychiatric epidemiology, which contribute valuable insights into a wide range of issues, from infectious diseases to the complex interplay between conditions such as HIV-AIDS and depression. Similarly, a recent analysis of the Global Burden of Disease highlights the contribution of mental and substance use problems to non-fatal burdens, which signals a pivotal shift in acknowledging the wider impact of mental health on overall health metrics. A recent analysis of the

Global Burden of Disease highlights the contribution of mental and substance use problems to non-fatal burdens, which signals a pivotal shift in acknowledging the wider impact of mental health on overall health metrics.

### *15.1.3 Intersection of Cancer and Mental Wellness: An Integrated Framework*

The diagnosis of cancer poses a critical threat beyond the realm of physical health, prompting a critical assessment of the mental health landscape in oncological settings (Gopalan et al., 2016). This brings psychiatric epidemiology into the picture and is expected to exhibit a crucial role in oncology by providing a vital understanding of the mental health landscape in this population. In the last three decades, there has been a two-fold increase in the worldwide prevalence of cancer, propelling it to be one of the leading causes of death globally. The redefined form of disease brings a set of profound psychosocial challenges for patients, families, and society, including significant workforce losses. Cancer diagnosis triggers a psychological crisis, shattering the patient's emotional equilibrium and often being perceived as a catastrophic event, which ignites intense emotional responses, encompassing fear, hopelessness, guilt, desperation, and feelings of abandonment (Demazeux, 2014; Wang et al., 2020). While behavioral factors can contribute to cancer development, the psychological turmoil experienced by patients can further manifest as psychiatric complications with distinct neurophysiological and perceptual characteristics. Biological complications coupled with psychological challenges hinder patients' ability to adjust, diminish their quality of life, and negatively influence disease progression and treatment response. Compared to the general population, up to one-third of cancer patients suffer from anxiety and depression (Niedzwiedz et al., 2019; Wang et al., 2020). Depression manifests at a prevalence rate of 20%, while anxiety affects approximately 10% and persists regardless of treatment stage or disease severity (Niedzwiedz et al., 2019; Wang et al., 2020). Neglecting these mental health challenges can lead to serious consequences. If left untreated, these can significantly compromise cancer treatment efficacy, potentially leading to decreased survival rates, increased healthcare expenditure, and a profoundly diminished quality of life (Niedzwiedz et al., 2019). This is a wake-up call that emphasizes the effective implementation of targeted psychological interventions specifically tailored to the requirements of cancer patients (Fernando et al., 2023). The type, stage, and prognosis of cancer, coupled with specific treatment modalities such as radiation, immunotherapy, and chemotherapy, play a decisive role in mental health outcomes (Niedzwiedz et al., 2019). This case emphasizes the intricate relationship between cancer treatments and the potential induction of depression through complex biological mechanisms. Mental health challenges in cancer patients represent a critical public health concern due to their high prevalence and multifaceted consequences. This was further amplified by the COVID-19 (Wang et al., 2020) pandemic, adding to the woes and emphasizing the need for enhanced attention to the psychological well-being of this segment of the population (Wang et al., 2020).

### 15.1.4 Epidemiology of Breast Cancer

Breast cancer, the most prevalent among women (Purkayastha et al., 2017), has drawn attention owing to its distinct psychosocial dimensions. Initial reactions to the diagnosis often revolve around anxieties and the surrounding pain, followed by profound emotional responses to the potential loss of a breast, often symbolically linked to femininity, motherhood, and sexuality (Purkayastha et al., 2017). The associated treatment modalities, including surgery, chemotherapy, and radiotherapy, further impact the quality of life, potentially leading to adverse physiological effects (Purkayastha et al., 2017). Over the past three decades, there has been a concerning ascent in breast cancer cases, with its incidence doubling since 1990 to claim the second leading cause of death, globally (Purkayastha et al., 2017). In 2002, 10.9 million new cancer diagnoses and 6.7 million cancer-related deaths were recorded. Breast cancer accounts for 33% of all diagnoses and contributes to 20% of cancer-related deaths in women (Purkayastha et al., 2017). This trend extends to Turkey, where breast cancer accounts for 35% of cancer cases in women. In Europe, breast cancer ranks third in incidence, accounting for 12.8% of the reported cases. Asia accounts for 29.1% of Age-standardized incidence rates -Western Asia with the highest percentage: 42.8%, followed by Southeastern Asia (28.2%) and Eastern Asia (27%) (Lim et al., 2022; Özmen et al., 2019). Psychiatric dimensions of breast cancer highlight that breast cancer is attributed to a high risk of developing psychiatric disorders, significantly affecting patients' quality of life, treatment adherence, and overall prognosis. This diagnosis often triggers a complex emotional response characterized by fear, hopelessness, guilt, and grief, posing challenges to individual acceptance. Studies indicate that the prominence of psychological issues in breast cancer patients ranges from 30% to 47%, with a persistence of 20–45% even one year after surgery (İzci et al., 2016). The emergence of these psychiatric disorders is a multifaceted phenomenon influenced by a range of factors, including age, sex, personality traits, symptom severity, and socioeconomic status (İzci et al., 2016).

### 15.1.5 Breast Cancer and Mental Health

The occurrence of depression among patients spans between 10% and 25%, signifying a 2–3 times higher likelihood compared to the general population (Shankar et al., 2016). Anxiety levels are high in young and middle-aged women undergoing chemotherapy, as cited in previous studies. Patients with breast cancer encounter simultaneous depression and anxiety (İzci et al., 2016; Shankar et al., 2016), reaching a co-morbidity prevalence of 19% in certain studies. The psychological impact of breast cancer persists, as evidenced by sustained depressive symptoms even six years post-surgery (İzci et al., 2016). Patients with breast cancer are susceptible to a high risk of suicide compared to the general population. This risk is further amplified by factors such as co-morbid depression (Shankar et al., 2016), substance abuse, feelings of hopelessness, limited social support, and advanced disease stage. Studies indicate that 8% of patients with cancer experience suicidal ideation, with this risk potentially escalating to actual attempts at the terminal stage (Shankar et al., 2016). Notably, the risk of suicide is particularly pronounced among single breast cancer patients with advanced disease progression and low socioeconomic status. Similarly, insomnia is a commonly observed symptom in cancer patients, with a prevalence rate of 50% and this rate ranges from 38% to 61% in breast cancer. Factors contributing to sleep disorders include psychological distress resulting from the diagnosis, adverse effects of therapeutic interventions, and menopausal symptoms induced by endocrine therapy. The presence of insomnia is linked with symptoms such as depression and anxiety, and interventions addressing these issues may lead to improvements in sleep quality. Furthermore, the use of medications, particularly sleeping aids, was significantly correlated with clinical insomnia. The treatment modalities—chemotherapy, radiotherapy, and hormonal therapy carry a potential risk of central nervous system (CNS) toxicity, manifesting as cognitive dysfunction, commonly referred to as 'chemo-brain' (Cintrón-García et al., 2020).

Advances in breast cancer treatment modality, from radical surgery to minimally invasive techniques, have revolutionized healthcare. However, this progress has highlighted the crucial need for holistic care encompassing quality of life (QoL) assessment and psychosocial support. Understanding these aspects is vital to public health epidemiology. Studies show that nearly 92% experience distress, with 30% requiring professional intervention (Phoosuwan & Lundberg, 2022). Psychotherapy improves survival rates, reduces recurrence fears, and enhances quality of life. Screening for emotional well-being is crucial for effective QoL management (Avis et al., 2005). In addition, the high prevalence of psychological distress in patients and survivors necessitates the integration of psychotherapy throughout treatment and beyond.

The global ascent in the incidence of breast cancer necessitates an extensive investigation into the psychosocial challenges faced by survivors, particularly regarding their mental health and QoL. The statistics indicating that a significant number of breast cancer survivors experience psychological distress present a stark case that requires professional intervention, thus highlighting the critical need to integrate mental health into cancer care. While the association between cancer and mental well-being is widely explored in India, limited studies explored the mental health well-being among breast cancer survivors in the country. Therefore, the present chapter aims to assess the psychiatric dimension of breast cancer survivors by applying the integrated framework of physical and emotional well-being tools (Gopalan et al., 2016). The chapter findings intend to inform policymakers and healthcare providers about the necessity of targeted interventions and optimized resource allocation for the development of effective psychological support systems, ultimately enhancing the quality of life for breast cancer survivors.

## 15.2 Materials and Methods

### 15.2.1 Study Design

The chapter utilized primary cross-sectional survey data. The survey used the Quality of Life in Adult Cancer Survivors (QLACS) questionnaire to fulfil the study objectives.

### 15.2.2 Study Population

The study employed breast cancer survivors taking into consideration the following inclusion criteria (Gopalan et al., 2016). Breast cancer survivors of all ages and cancer stages, newly diagnosed and long-term survivors were considered. Survivors from all treatment modalities (radiation therapy, chemotherapy, hormonal therapy, or Biological Therapy) and Income Groups were included.

### 15.2.3 Data Collection Tools and Techniques

The study employed 25 participants affiliated with the Nag Foundation, a renowned NGO in Pune specializing in cancer support and survivorship assistance. The standardized QLACS is used to assess the psychological well-being of breast cancer survivors. The QLACS served as the primary framework with Ryff's 18-item scale of psychological well-being. Some modifications were employed in the QLACS with a cross-sectional survey design (Gopalan et al., 2016) to analyze the peripheral factors and their impact on cancer-specific aspects of psychological well-being (Avis et al., 2005; Sohl et al., 2015). This survey instrument was then employed for data collection from the breast cancer survivors. Furthermore, correlation analysis was performed to understand the complex interplay between psychological well-being and various facets of QoL among these survivors. A defined metrics are used for the QLACS questionnaire (Table 15.1).

Structured interviews were also conducted with the survivors to gain insights into their psychological perspectives, societal perceptions post-diagnosis and treatment, and awareness regarding health concepts like breast self-examination and breast cancer screening programs. Interviews with primary caregivers delved into support networks and dynamics surrounding survivor's experiences. Each participant was briefed about the study objectives and ethical approval was obtained before data collection, post which survivors completed the questionnaire and were also interviewed. It was compliant with ethical guidelines to ensure the privacy, confidentiality, and well-being of the participants. Informed consent was taken from all the participants.

**Table 15.1** Defined psychological well-being scale of the QLACS questionnaire, cross-sectional survey on breast cancer survivors

| Scale | Indicators |
|---|---|
| 1 | Never |
| 2 | Seldom |
| 3 | Sometimes |
| 4 | About as often as not |
| 5 | Frequently |
| 6 | Very often |
| 7 | Always |

*Source* Authors estimation

### 15.2.4 Statistical Analysis

Following the data collection and structured interviews, Descriptive and inferential statistical analysis was performed to understand and assess the QoL. The data collected were thoroughly analyzed to identify patterns, associations, and correlations related to psychiatric dimensions of cancer survivorship. Machine learning algorithms (regression analysis and Pearson correlation coefficient) were employed to predict the relations and probable outcomes based on demographic factors, preference for counselling, and similar factors shaping the analysis.

## 15.3 Results

### 15.3.1 Sample Background Characteristics

About 76% of the sampled women were between 36 and 50 years of age (Table 15.2). Most of them were married (88%). Similarly, 88% of the participants were either graduates or postgraduates. The majority of the participants (52%) had an income of less than INR 3 lakh per annum (Table 15.2). 76% of them said that they enjoy life. 88% of the participants said that they had a positive outlook on life. 68% of the participants felt content with their life. 16% of the participants felt depressed very often or always. 16% of the participants felt depressed very often or always. 40% of patients said that they suffered from anxiety. 28% of them worried about little things very often or always. 36% of the participants were bothered by mood swings very frequently. 8% of them were anxious very frequently or always (Table 15.2). 28% of the participants had difficulty doing activities that required concentrating. 40% of the participants had a short attention span. 36% of them were unable to remember things. 24% of the participants forgot what they started to do Table 15.2). 16% of the participants avoided social gatherings and 8% of them avoided new friends. 20% of the participants were reluctant to interact with people and 40% of them were

**Table 15.2** Sampled women background characteristics

| Indicators | Percentage |
|---|---|
| Age–Group [Age 36–50] | 76 |
| Marital status [Married] | 88 |
| Qualification [graduates & above] | 88 |
| Income [≤INR 3 Lakh] | 52 |
| Perspective to enjoyed life [Yes] | 76 |
| Positive outlook toward life | 88 |
| Contentment with life [Yes] | 68 |
| Feeling of depression [Yes] | 16 |
| Pre-existing mental health issues [Yes] | 40 |
| Worrying about little things [Yes] | 28 |
| Mood swings [Yes] | 36 |
| Anxiety | 8 |
| Efficiency in performing activities [No] | 28 |
| Short attention span [Yes] | 40 |
| Recalling virtue [Yes] | 36 |
| Bothered by forgetting [Yes] | 24 |
| *Social affiliation* | |
| Avoided social gatherings | 16 |
| Avoided new friends | 8 |
| Reluctant to interact with people | 20 |
| Hesitant to making new relationships | 40 |
| **Insurance coverage issue [Yes]** | 24 |
| **n** | 25 |

*Source* Author

hesitant to start making new relationships. 24% of them had insurance-related issues (Table 15.2).

### 15.3.2 *Descriptive Statistics of Breast Cancer Survivors*

Among the study population, 68% of them were unaware of basic health terms related to breast self-examination and screening (Fig. 15.1).

In 44% of cases, it was diagnosed 2–4 years ago; while in 24% of cases it was diagnosed 1–2 years back, 20% of cases were diagnosed within the last 5 years, and in 12% of cases it was diagnosed 10–15 years back (Fig. 15.2).

About 52% of the participants said that they felt happy. Stage 1 and Stage 2 together accounted for 72% of all the cases. Surgery and chemotherapy accounted

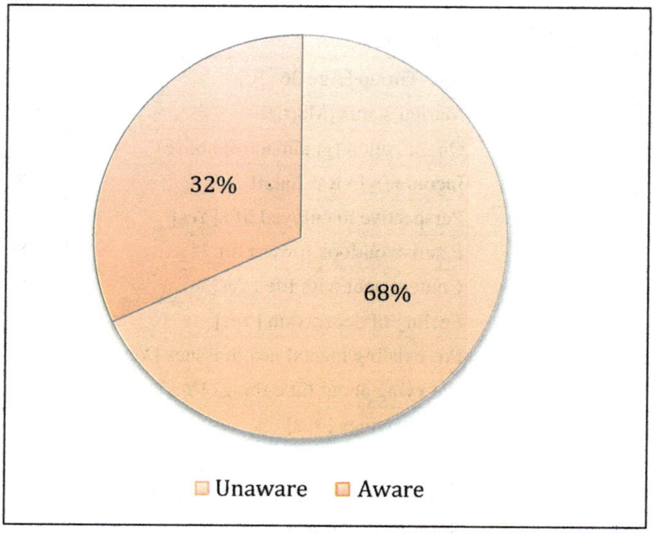


**Fig. 15.1** Awareness about cancer examination and screening among the sampled women

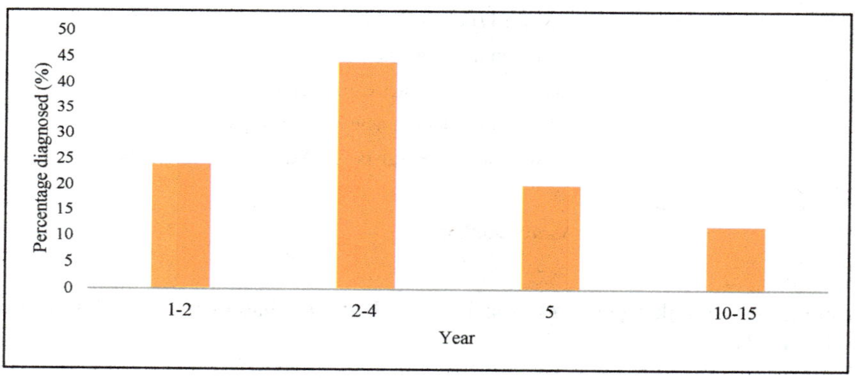


**Fig. 15.2** History of breast cancer diagnosis among the sample women

for the treatment modality in 72% of the cases (Table 15.3). A small percentage of it was accounted for by hormonal therapy, radiation therapy, and a combination of radiation and chemotherapy (Table not shown).

**Table 15.3** Changing perception toward life among sampled women with breast cancer

| Item | Yes | No |
|---|---|---|
| Appreciative toward life | 68% | 32% |
| Help them to cope better with problems | 76% | 24% |
| Worried that family members might get cancer | 24% | 76% |

*Source* Author estimation

### 15.3.3 *Breast Cancer and Financial Problem*

About 28% of them had frequent financial problems owing to cancer treatment 28% of patients said that they had frequent financial problems due to income loss. 36% of participants said that money problems arose because of cancer (Table 15.4).

This ANOVA analysis provides insights into the relationship between financial problems, qualification (education and job category) and various psychological factors in breast cancer survivors (Table 15.5).

Qualification significantly impacts financial problems owing to surgery/treatment ($p$-value = 0.013) and loss of income. This implies that survivors in certain qualification groups faced greater financial hurdles due to cancer (Table 15.5). A cancer diagnosis significantly enhances one's appreciation for life. In this context, it meant that the survivors in certain qualification groups experienced a stronger positive perspective following their cancer journey. The basic minimum qualification of these survivors was graduate, with a few being postgraduates. This qualification category

**Table 15.4** Status of financial constraints among sampled women with breast cancer

| Item | Yes | No |
|---|---|---|
| Due to cancer treatment | 28% | 72% |
| Due to income loss | 28% | 72% |
| Before cancer diagnose | 36% | 64% |

*Source* Authors estimation

**Table 15.5** Result from ANOVA statistical test

| Factors | $p$-value |
|---|---|
| Financial problems owing to surgery/treatment | 0.013 |
| Appreciation for life | 0.013 |
| Coping with problems | 0.006 |
| Sexual functioning | 0.089 |
| Pain and worry | 0.047 |
| Importance of counselling | 0.019 |

*Source* Authors estimation

necessitated further investigation, underscoring a probable association between qualification and appreciation of life post-cancer (Table 15.5). Qualification has a significant influence on perceived benefits in terms of coping with post-cancer challenges ($p$-value = 0.006). It implies that survivors' educational background may have a certain influence on their perception of how their cancer journey has equipped them to handle challenges. This requires further in-depth study to understand the varying opinions across qualification groups, though a common observation infers that survivors with certain minimum qualification levels tend to perceive their cancer experience as enhancing their ability to cope with challenges. This significantly impacts the willingness to go for counselling/psychotherapy ($p$-value = 0.019) with a similar inference that survivors with certain minimum qualification levels tend to understand the importance of psychotherapy (Table 15.5). There is no significant impact on the following aspects (keeping in view that the $p$-value > 0.05 in these factors): positive and negative emotions, social functioning, cancer-related peripheral concerns (worry about recurrence, insurance), treatment-related concerns (feeling unattractive, mood swings), help-seeking behavior, and family concerns (worry about family getting cancer). The income group analysis among breast cancer survivors highlighted a key link between breast cancer survivors and financial hardships. Survivors faced more financial hurdles due to surgery and treatment and lost income ($p$-values = 0.034 and 0.014) (Table 15.5).

### 15.3.4 Findings from Predictive and Correlation Analysis

The main objective is to predict psychological wellness in breast cancer survivors based on factors like financial problems, social support, age, and treatment modality (Table 15.6). The low MSE values imply that the predicted values closely align with the actual psychological well-being scores and the R-squared value illustrates a high proportion of variance in psychological well-being scores based on the selected factors (Table 15.6).

Overall, this linear regression model performs well in the prediction of psychological well-being based on factors including- financial situation, social support network, age, and treatment modality. The linear regression model illustrates its good performance in the prediction of psychological well-being scores (Fig. 15.3).

Figures 15.4 illustrate the density plot of variables of the selected factors: 15.4a—age distribution, 15.4b—social support and 15.4c—financial problem] considered for psychological-well-being prediction. The plots illustrate the need for a large

**Table 15.6** Result from predictive and correlation analysis

| | |
|---|---|
| Mean squared error (MSE) | 0.1974 |
| R-squared | 0.8102 (81%) |

*Source* Authors estimation

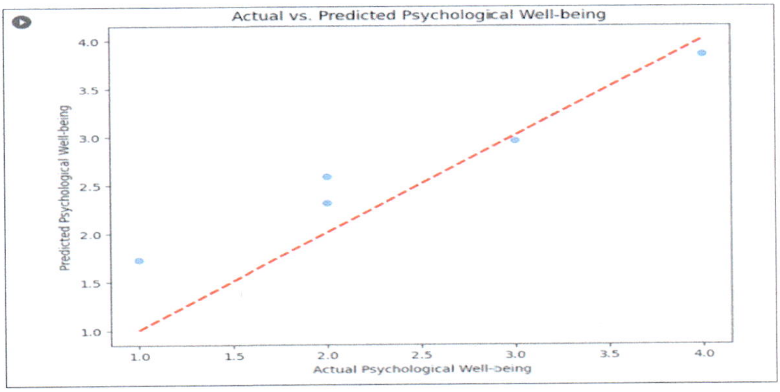


**Fig. 15.3** Graphical presentation of linear regression model showing performance in the prediction of psychological well-being scores

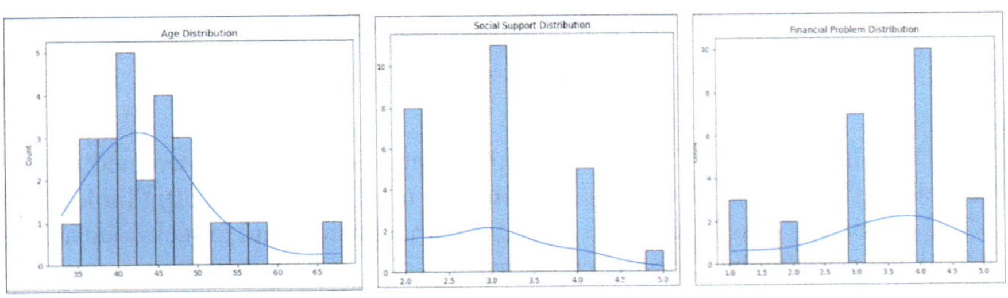


**Fig. 15.4** Density plot of selected variables to explain breast cancer among the sampled women

sample size for deriving definitive conclusions with relatively less even distribution (Fig. 15.4).

### *15.3.5 Likeliness of Breast Cancer Survivors to Seek Counselling*

A random forest classifier algorithm was employed to predict the likelihood of breast cancer survivors seeking counselling and the model was then evaluated. The results show that the precision of the employed predictors of breast cancer was significant (Accuracy: 0.8) and precision varied from 0.50 to 1.00 (Table 15.7).

Based on the accuracy assessment, three classes were considered, which were class 1, class 2, and class 3 (Table 15.8). Class 1: The classifier has good precision (0.50) in identifying those unlikely to seek counselling implying low false positives but, a high recall might be due to a low number of "unlikely" cases in the data

**Table 15.7** Random Forest classifier algorithm showing likeliness of breast cancer survivors to seek counselling

| Classification report | | | | |
|---|---|---|---|---|
| Accuracy: 0.8 | Precision | Recall | fl-score | Support |
| 1 | 0.50 | 1.00 | 0.67 | 1.00 |
| 2 | 1.00 | 0.50 | 0.67 | 2.00 |
| 3 | 1.00 | 1.00 | 1.00 | 2.00 |
| Accuracy | | | 0.80 | 5.00 |
| Macro avg | 0.83 | 0.83 | 0.78 | 5.00 |
| Weighted avg | 0.90 | 0.80 | 0.80 | 5.00 |

*Source* Authors estimation

**Table 15.8** Class categorization of the sampled breast cancer women

| | |
|---|---|
| Class 1 | Survivors unlikely to seek counselling |
| Class 2 | Survivors likely to seek counselling |
| Class 3 | Not applicable (perfectly classified) |

*Source* Authors estimation

(Table 8). The classifier (Class 2) perfectly identifies the group, predicted to seek counselling (Precision: 1.0) but misses half who need it (Recall: 0.50) (Table 15.8).

The classifier (Class 3) identifies a small group with no intent to seek counselling. Overall, the classifier has a decent performance with 80% accuracy but class-specific analysis has some limitations with room for improvement in Class 1 and Class 2. For a more robust prediction in the case of counselling likelihood, pointers like data balancing and alternative algorithms should be considered (Table 15.8).

### 15.3.6 Regression Analysis on Psychological Well-Being

The model explains around 48% of the variance in psychological well-being scores (R-squared = 0.481); Post the variable adjustment the variation reduced to 30.8%. Overall, the model is statistically significant (F-statistic = 2.780, *p*-value = 0.0430), with at least one of the variables having a significant influence on psychological well-being. The normality of the residuals (Omnibus and Jarque–Bera tests), needs improvement though, but its impact is minimal (Table not shown). This analysis provides a starting point for assessing the factors influencing psychological well-being in breast cancer survivors. This necessitates further investigation to explore the significance of individual factors and potential multicollinearity that can redefine the model with a robust framework with more insights. The Pearson correlation coefficient (r) between psychological well-being and financial problems was 0.6575 (Table not shown). This value indicates a moderately strong positive linear relationship implying that as financial problems increase, psychological well-being tends to increase. Although this correlation does not consolidate causation. Robust methodologies with a comprehensive analysis are required, by employing longitudinal studies and experimental survey studies that take into consideration other factors as well—like pre-existing mental health issues, loss of job, or decreased productivity in the work with a cumulative effect on the psychological well-being.

## 15.4 Discussion

The present chapter describes the realm of breast cancer survivorship, delved into their mental health experiences, drawing insights about different demographic and socio-factors that can influence their emotional well-being. Statistical analysis explored the relation of these factors to various psychological aspects, including happiness, anxiety, financial worries, and fear of cancer recurrence, and it was found that differences in socioeconomic factors significantly impacted the Psychiatric landscape of breast cancer patients. For Instance, Income level plays a critical role in shaping experiences with any sort of psychological distress, and financial strain brought on by treatment. Similarly, age groups exhibited distinct patterns in terms of overall life satisfaction, mood fluctuations, and concerns about cancer returning. Social interaction and intimacy also have an important role in the cancer journey. Most of the participants were hesitant to engage in new relationships, owing to fear of social isolation, underscoring the need for social support. Sexual concerns were prevalent on a similar note as most of them struggled with sexual function and avoiding intimacy. While only a third actively sought counselling or therapy (Purkayastha et al., 2017), the majority of them recognized the importance of mental health support alongside mainstream treatment (Shankar et al., 2016). This highlighted the need for an integrated approach that could address both the physical and emotional aspects of the disease (Shankar et al., 2016), highlighting the requirement for tailored programs to the specific requirements of breast cancer patients and survivors across diverse demographic and socioeconomic backgrounds. The Integration of mental health services may incur additional upfront expenditure. This study implies that it could be offset by improved QoL (Purkayastha et al., 2017) for survivors. The QLACS questionnaire, with its inclusion of financial aspects, intends to quantify the potential economic burden associated with mental health interventions. Future research can utilize this data to implement such a program with a cost-effective framework of integrated care that can be used as a reference for increased funding and policy changes. Understanding the specific mental health needs of different cancer survivors and patients is crucial for optimizing care. This study highlights the potential for targeted interventions (Wang et al., 2020) based on demographic factors. By identifying the proportion of the national mental health burden attributable to breast cancer survivors, policymakers can allocate resources more effectively. The present chapter presents a stark picture of elevated anxiety and depression among breast cancer survivors (Shankar et al., 2016), highlighting the profound psychological burden associated with the disease. This finding reinforces the need to move beyond a purely biomedical model of cancer care and embrace a holistic perspective that acknowledges the interconnectedness of cancer care and a comprehensive approach (Demazeux, 2014; Shankar et al., 2016; Purkayastha et al., 2017), with tailored interventions that address the full spectrum of psychological needs encountered in this population.

## 15.5 Conclusion

In conclusion, the journey through cancer extends far beyond conventional diagnosis and treatment, revealing the intricate interplay between physical and emotional well-being. Elevated levels of anxiety and depression among breast cancer survivors underscore the profound psychological burden associated with the disease. Embracing a holistic perspective is crucial, one that acknowledges the interconnectedness of physical and psychological health. A comprehensive approach to cancer care must include tailored interventions that address the full spectrum of psychological needs encountered by survivors. By doing so, we can ensure that cancer care is not only about treating the disease but also about supporting the overall well-being of those affected. This holistic approach is essential for improving the quality of life and long-term outcomes for breast cancer survivors.

## References

Avis, N. E., Smith, K. W., McGraw, S., Smith, R. G., Petronis, V. M., & Carver, C. S. (2005). Assessing quality of life in adult cancer survivors (QLACS). *Quality of Life Research, 14*(5), 1007–1023.

Cintrón-García, J., & Guddati, A. K. (2020). Management of CNS toxicity of chemotherapy and targeted agents: 2020. *American Journal of Cancer Research, 10*(8), 2617–2620. PMID: 32905442; PMCID: PMC7471356.

Demazeux, S. (2014). Psychiatric epidemiology, or the story of a divided discipline. *International Journal of Epidemiology, 43*(suppl_1), i53–i66.

Fernando, A., Tokell, M., Ishak, Y., Love, J., Klammer, M., & Koh, M. (2023). *Mental health needs in cancer: A call for change.* Advance online publication.

Gopalan, M. R., Karunakaran, V., Prabhakaran, A., & Jayakumar, K. L. (2016). Prevalence of psychiatric morbidity among cancer patients—Hospital-based, cross-sectional survey. *Indian Journal of Psychiatry, 58*(3), 275–280.

Hardman, A., Maguire, P., & Crowther, D. (1989). The recognition of psychiatric morbidity on a medical oncology ward. *Journal of Psychosomatic Research, 33*(2), 235–239. https://doi.org/10.1016/0022-3999(89)90051-2. PMID: 2724199.

İzci, F., İlgün, A. S., Fındıklı, E., & Özmen, V. (2016). Psychiatric symptoms and psychosocial problems in patients with breast cancer. *Journal of Breast Health, 12*(3), 94–101.

Karakoyun-Celik, O., Gorken, I., Sahin, S., et al. (2010). Depression and anxiety levels in woman under follow-up for breast cancer: Relationship to coping with cancer and quality of life. *Medical Oncology, 27*, 108–113.

Lim, Y. X., Lim, Z. L., Ho, P. J., & Li, J. (2022). Breast cancer in Asia: Incidence, mortality, early detection, mammography programs, and risk-based screening initiatives. *Cancers (Basel), 14*(17), 4218.

Lovell, A. M. (2014). The World Health Organization and the contested beginnings of psychiatric epidemiology as an international discipline: One rope, many strands. *International Journal of Epidemiology, 43*(Suppl 1), i6-18. https://doi.org/10.1093/ije/dyu125. Epub 2014 Jul 16 PMID: 25031048.

Lovell, A. M. (2014). The World Health Organization and the contested beginnings of psychiatric epidemiology as an international discipline: one rope, many strands. *International Journal of Epidemiology, 43*(suppl_1), i6-i18.

Maths, S. B., Chandrashekar, C. R., & Bhugra, D. (2007). Psychiatric epidemiology in India. *Indian Journal of Medical Research, 126*(3), 183–192.

Montazeri, A. (2008). Health-related quality of life in breast cancer patients: a bibliographic review of the literature from 1974 to 2007. *Health and Quality of Life Outcomes, 6*, 27.

Niedzwiedz, C. L., Knifton, L., Robb, K. A., Katikireddi, S. V., & Smith, D. J. (2019). Title of the article. *BMC Cancer, 19*(943).

Özmen, V., Özmen, T., & Doğru, V. (2019). Breast cancer in Turkey; an analysis of 20,000 patients with breast cancer. *European Journal of Breast Health, 15*(3), 141–146.

Phoosuwan, N., & Lundberg, P. C. (2022). Psychological distress and health-related quality of life among women with breast cancer: A descriptive cross-sectional study. *Supportive Care in Cancer, 30*, 3177–3186.

Plana-Ripoll, O., Lasgaard, M., Mneimneh, Z. N., & McGrath, J. J. (2021). The evolution of psychiatric epidemiology: Where to next? *The Canadian Journal of Psychiatry, 66*(9), 774–777.

Plana-Ripoll, O., Lasgaard, M., Mneimneh, Z. N., & McGrath, J. J. (2021). The evolution @@of psychiatric epidemiology: Where to next? *The Canadian Journal of Psychiatry, 66*(9), 774–777.

Purkayastha, D., Venkateswaran, C., Nayar, K., & Unnikrishnan, U. G. (2017). Prevalence of depression in breast cancer patients and its association with their quality of life: A cross-sectional observational study. *Indian Journal of Palliative Care, 23*(3), 268–273.

Shankar, A., Dracham, C., Ghoshal, S., & Grover, S. (2016). Prevalence of depression and anxiety disorder in cancer patients: An institutional experience. *Indian Journal of Cancer, 53*(3), 432–434.

Sohl, S. J., Levine, B., & Avis, N. E. (2015). Evaluation of the Quality of Life in Adult Cancer Survivors (QLACS) scale for early post-treatment breast cancer survivors. *Quality of Life Research, 24*, 205–212. https://doi.org/10.1007/s11136-014-0749-x

Wang, Y., Duan, Z., Ma, Z., Mao, Y., Li, X., Wilson, A., Qin, H., Ou, J., Peng, K., Zhou, F., Li, C., Liu, Z., & Chen, R. (2020a). Epidemiology of mental health problems among patients with cancer during COVID-19 pandemic. *Translational Psychiatry, 10*(1), 263. https://doi.org/10.1038/s41398-020-00950-y

Wang, Y. H., Li, J. Q., Shi, J. F., Que, J. Y., Liu, J. J., Lappin, J. M., …, Bao, Y. P. (2020b). Depression and anxiety in relation to cancer incidence and mortality: A systematic review and meta-analysis of cohort studies. *Molecular Psychiatry, 25*(7), 1487–1499.

Wang, Y., Duan, Z., Ma, Z., Mao, Y., Li, X., Wilson, A., …, Chen, R. (2020c). Epidemiology of mental health problems among patients with cancer during COVID-19 pandemic. *Translational Psychiatry, 10*(1), 263.

# Chapter 16
# Emotional Health of Women in IT: Comparing Work-From-Home and Hybrid Models Post-COVID-19

**Haritha Guduru and Neha Singh**

**Abstract** The chapter explores how the COVID-19 pandemic affected the emotional health of women working in the IT sector in India and among Non-Resident Indians (NRIs). The chapter highlights the need to understand the unique challenges these women faced during and after the pandemic, in work-from-home (WFH) and hybrid work settings. The available literature focused on a single set of IT employees of a specific region and looked from a general health perspective. The study used a comparative study with qualitative methods, such as semi-structured interviews and focus group discussions (FGDs). Women from different IT roles and organizations in Hyderabad and abroad were selected through snowball sampling that resulted in six case studies. Six psychologists and counsellors participated in FGDs, which used the theory of positive psychology for the recommendations. The findings, based on thematic analysis of positive psychology, revealed significant emotional distress among women that included struggles with work-life balance and financial concerns during the pandemic. Remote work led to feelings of isolation and stress, particularly for those without proper home workspaces and those juggling household responsibilities. The shift to hybrid work brought mixed results; while some women benefited from flexibility, others faced longer work hours and job insecurity. The study provided structured recommendations for both individuals and organizations, stressing the importance of promoting positive emotions, engagement, relationships, meaning, and achievement. Wellness programs, engaging online platforms, and family-friendly policies are suggested to support women's mental health and work-life balance.

**Keywords** Emotional health · Women IT employees · COVID-19 pandemic · Work-from-home and hybrid work · Positive psychology

---

H. Guduru (✉)
Icfai Business School (IBS), IFHE, Hyderabad, India
e-mail: g.haritha@ibsindia.org

N. Singh
Jaipuria Institute of Management, Jaipur, India
e-mail: neha.singh@jaipuria.ac.in



P. Chouhan et al. (eds.), *Women's Health Dynamics in South Asia*, Asian Perspectives on Public Health, https://doi.org/10.1007/978-981-95-2321-4_16

## 16.1 Introduction

COVID-19 began in December 2019 in Wuhan, China, as a respiratory illness. By March 2020, the World Health Organization (WHO) declared it a global pandemic, which prompted worldwide isolation, quarantine, and social distancing measures due to the lack of specific treatments. Organizations globally adopted remote work policies to protect employees. Although some restrictions were eased out in some areas, remote work and social distancing remain prevalent. In India, a nationwide lockdown was imposed on March 25, 2020, and extended as COVID-19 cases rose, leading many businesses to suspend or reduce office operations. This shift decreased travel and increased remote work. While some employees adapted well, many women struggled to balance work-from-home with other responsibilities. As the virus subsided, remote work gradually transitioned to hybrid work, offering some relief but also presenting new challenges.

Indian tech firms gained global prominence in the 1980s and 1990s, particularly after economic liberalization in 1991 (Kumar & Srinivasan, 2023). Many women entered the IT sector due to safety and job opportunities, leading to increased enrolment in technical education programs (Rao & Duggirala, 2022). In 2017–2018, women constituted approximately 34% of the IT-ITES workforce in India. The shift from WFH to hybrid work aimed to enhance work-life balance but often resulted in a continuous work cycle, blurring office and home boundaries. Men generally adapted better than women, who faced significant physical, mental, and emotional health challenges (Kumar & Srinivasan, 2023; NASSCOM, 2023).

Contemporary research extensively covered women's physical health across various sectors during COVID-19, with significant studies focusing on the IT sector in India across different regions (Del Boca et al, 2022; Kottasová, 2020). The research gap is identified in the impact of COVID-19 on women's mental health, particularly emotional well-being, during the transition from WFH to hybrid work modes in the IT sector. This study aims to compare the emotional health of women in the IT sectors of India and women NRIs during the COVID-19 pandemic and post-pandemic transition, focusing on their experiences with WFH and hybrid work modes. The study included semi-structured interviews and focus group discussions (FGDs) to explore these issues. Inputs from FGDs were targeted for interventions designed to improve emotional health, and the effectiveness was evaluated after 45 days. Participants included three women from reputed IT firms of Hyderabad region and three NRI women working in multinational IT firms abroad. They were selected through snowball sampling to ensure diverse representation in roles, experience levels, and responsibilities. The outcome will help identify specific ways to improve emotional well-being for women at the individual level and can aid at developing new organizational policies for women in the IT sector amidst changing work scenarios.

The COVID-19 pandemic significantly altered working conditions, through the adoption of remote work, impacting the emotional health of women in the IT sector (Bertoni and et al. (2023). Remote work, while offering some benefits, also presents challenges to women's mental and physical well-being (Moorthy, 2020).

Social isolation, stalled career growth, and an "always-on" culture often led to increased emotional exhaustion in women (Kottasová, 2020). The blurred boundaries between work and personal life aggravate these issues, causing various health problems, including musculoskeletal issues. Women with children faced additional pressures due to the closure of schools and daycare centres, along with the necessity to manage household chores, creating a demanding environment (Bradbury et al., 2020). Surveys revealed that employees working from home struggled to detach from work and follow out of the schedule routines, with working mothers sacrificing sleep to meet professional responsibilities, leading to health problems (Corsi & Ilkkaracan, 2023).

The lack of dedicated workspaces and privacy compounded these issues, as many women shared their work areas with children attending online classes and other family members working remotely (Del Boca et al., 2022). This constant movement within the home blurred the lines between work and life, making it difficult to detach from job responsibilities (Dingel & Neiman, 2020). Remote work also increases social isolation and depression, especially for those living alone, which affects overall well-being. Continuous home confinement led to increased anxiety and stress, negatively impacting mental and physical health (Hupkau & Petrongolo, 2020). Feelings of irritability and negative emotions, driven by social isolation and anxiety, influenced productivity, work-life balance, and overall well-being (Feng & Savani, 2020). Sedentary lifestyles, fast food consumption, and uncomfortable work environments worsened these issues (Karácsony, 2021). Reduced communication with colleagues and social interactions were major predictors of negative impacts on health (Kaur & Sharma, 2020). Unequal distribution of household chores during the pandemic led to relationship conflicts, reduced satisfaction, and a decline in professional performance (Makridis & Schloetzer, 2022). Studies indicated that women, even when employed, assume a larger share of household responsibilities, leading to higher stress levels and fragmented work and leisure time (Niebuhr et al., 2022). This unequal allocation of chores is associated with reduced working hours and a higher likelihood of women leaving employment (Oakman et al., 2020). Women often expressed dissatisfaction with the division of household chores (Rai & Rai, 2020).

In Indian society, traditional roles expect women to be homemakers and caregivers, a norm that continued even during the lockdown. The shift to remote work forced many women to juggle professional responsibilities and household duties without domestic help. Surveys indicate that the lockdown disproportionately affected women, who bore the brunt of caregiving responsibilities (Feminism India, 2020). This additional burden was not always recognized by employers, which led to increased stress and anxiety among working mothers. The pandemic interrupted household activities, with women taking on more responsibilities for cooking, cleaning, and caring for family members along with work. This situation was further complicated by school closures and the increased need for family care, which unduly increased women's workloads. Balancing these demands with professional work proved challenging, with many women unable to take paid leave despite working from home.

The additional workload and stress during the pandemic regressed progress towards gender equality in the workplace. Women working from home often perform a "double shift," that became suggestive of traditional gender roles. This setback pushed many back into traditional domestic roles. Surveys during the pandemic highlighted significant stress and anxiety faced by women due to new WFH norms (Guy & Arthur, 2020). A Pink Ladder survey revealed many women experienced stress and anxiety, with some managers not respecting work hours. LinkedIn's Workforce Confidence Index showed a higher percentage of working mothers providing full-time childcare compared to working fathers (Cui et al., 2021). Many mothers worked late into the night, negatively impacting their concentration and mental well-being (News 18, 2020).

The pandemic highlighted the distinct mental health challenges faced by men and women. Women are more prone to depression, anxiety, and stress, influenced by industry and job roles (Wade, 2021). Healthcare workers, for instance, experienced higher stress levels due to long hours and uncertain conditions. Women in heteronormative households faced greater stress levels compared to men. The pandemic has brought hybrid working models into focus, offering flexible working options, especially for women. Hybrid models allow greater autonomy over time management compared to in-person work settings (Menon & Sharma, 2020). These models have potential advantages, such as improved work-life balance, cost reductions, and increased productivity (Lee & Tipoe, 2021). The effects of hybrid work are often gendered, with women facing unique challenges in balancing professional and personal responsibilities (Mooi-Reci & Risman, 2021).

The shift to remote work during the COVID-19 pandemic had mixed effects on women's emotional health in the IT sector (Perry-Jenkins & Gerstel, 2020). While offering flexibility and potential for better work-life balance, remote work also exacerbated challenges such as social isolation, blurred work-life boundaries, and increased stress levels. The additional burden of household chores and caregiving responsibilities further impacted women's mental and physical health, leading to reduced professional satisfaction and performance (Sriharan et al., 2020). Addressing these challenges requires a nuanced understanding of gender-specific needs and the development of supportive workplace policies that promote mental well-being and equitable distribution of household responsibilities.

A Deloitte report from 2023 to 2024 noted a reduction in women reporting burnout, decreasing to just under 30% compared to 46% last year. Respondents rated their overall mental well-being as slightly improved. However, over a third (35%) rated their mental well-being as poor or very poor. About half reported higher stress levels than the previous year. Few women received adequate mental health support from their employers, and workplace mental health stigma persisted. The number of women comfortable discussing mental health at work decreased from 43% in 2022 to 25% in 2023. Similarly, the percentage of women disclosing mental health challenges as the reason for taking time off work dropped from 39% in 2022 to 25% in 2023. The pressure to be constantly available worsened, with only 37% of women reporting they could switch off from work, compared to 45% in 2022. Mental health remains a top concern for more than half of women respondents.

The pandemic and lockdowns posed significant challenges for governments, employers, and employees worldwide, impacting business continuity and employee well-being. Working from home (WFH) became essential, establishing a new work pattern that reshaped work dynamics by merging domestic and professional spaces (Karácsony, 2021). This shift disproportionately impacted women professionals, intensifying work-life conflicts and demanding family support. In India, where women typically shoulder domestic duties, balancing work and home responsibilities added extra burdens, affecting their work output (Gueguen & Senik, 2023). Scholars noted that during lockdowns, women faced increased burdens managing childcare, eldercare, and household tasks without usual support services, influencing their work performance.

The term 'hybrid' commonly refers to the integration of technology into daily life, impacting various lifestyle systems like family, education, and work (Delventhal & Parkhomenko, 2021). The growing trend of hybrid workplaces, driven by the COVID-19 pandemic, emphasized the need for flexible work arrangements (Angelici & Profeta, 2023) The study shows the importance of clear communication, defined policies, and proper technology to enhance productivity and work-life balance in hybrid models. The Hybrid Work Model enhances comfort and productivity (Sokolic, 2022) when organizations develop a model that helps holistic working space. Promoting the model for mental health benefits and providing training for effective implementation. Hybrid work offers flexibility, work-life balance, and positive work culture.

WFH, also known as telecommuting, uses Information and Communication Technologies for remote work away from traditional office settings. While some employees appreciate WFH for enhancing work-life balance, employers express concerns over potential productivity declines (Vasconcelos et al., 2015). The widespread job losses and salary cuts, Indian tech firms normalized WFH, to cut down on costs and provided employees with home desktop setups to ensure security and compliance. Companies overlooked the impact of blending professional work with home life on women, who manage unpaid caregiving duties in Indian households. This new work model was made compulsory to bring back the usage of office resources to a minimum. The model comforted some and also brought in challenges related to it. The research addressed a gap by examining women's mental health separately in India and abroad, comparing the experiences of Indian women with NRIs in IT roles to understand how cultural and workplace factors influence emotional health outcomes. The insights from FGDs contributed to both theoretical understanding and practical strategies for supporting women's mental health in globalized work settings.

## 16.2 Materials and Methods

The study aimed to compare the impact of the COVID-19 pandemic on the emotional health of women in the IT sector in India and among Non-Resident Indians (NRIs), focusing on their experiences during COVID-19 and in hybrid work environments post-pandemic. Using qualitative methods, the study conducted semi-structured interviews and focus group discussions (FGDs) with participants selected through snowball sampling. The sample included women from various roles, experience levels, and company sizes in Hyderabad's IT industry and abroad, resulting in six case studies. A group of six psychologists and counsellors participated in FGDs. The findings aligned with the positive psychology theory, specifically the PERMA model, to understand the challenges faced by these women and to provide intervention recommendations aimed at improving their emotional well-being. Follow-up assessments were conducted the effectiveness of these interventions.

The semi-structured interview questionnaire gathered detailed insights into IT professionals' experiences during and after the COVID-19 pandemic, focusing on their emotional well-being in remote and hybrid work setups. Questions included personal details such as age, specific IT roles, and years of industry experience. Participants reflected on their emotional states during the pandemic while working from home, highlighting positive and negative emotions and methods to maintain productivity and well-being. The transition to a hybrid work model was also explored, comparing emotional well-being and satisfaction levels with the previous work-from-home period. The questionnaire addressed challenges during the transition, strategies to overcome them, and suggestions for enhancing work-life balance and emotional health in current and future work scenarios. The interview findings are presented as case studies.

### *16.2.1* Case 1-Saumya: *Senior Consultant Engineer*

During the initial phase of the pandemic, Saumya, who is from Hyderabad city found comfort in spending quality time with her family during maternity leave, enjoying moments with her child and parents. As time passed, she faced increasing challenges. She switched to remote work while managing household chores and caring for elderly parents, which became overwhelming. The inadequate home workspace led to physical health issues, which worsened her mental well-being with the pandemic uncertainties. Learning that many colleagues contracted the virus added to her emotional distress. A ray of light is where companies offered financial benefits that included wellness allowances, and child care allowance which was kind of a relief. The transition from fixed office hours to continuous remote work with higher demands tested Saumya's emotional strength. Concerns about job security during widespread layoffs increased her stress which left her feeling undervalued despite her dedication. The move to a hybrid work model brought new hurdles, such as balancing office and home duties without clear work hour guidelines. Presently, Saumya juggles extended workdays and work hours which often last from 14 to 16-h with household and childcare responsibilities, and travelling to the office three times a week. Although Nitya is able to now connect with social circles, the expectations from the company to work for indefinite hours pose a challenge to maintaining emotional balance and the structured routine she enjoyed before the pandemic.

### 16.2.2 Case 2-Anitha: *Senior Quality Engineer*

An interview with Anitha from Hyderabad a Quality Engineering professional from Accenture, Hyderabad, revealed her journey during the pandemic. At the onset of the lockdown, Anitha was in the fourth week of pregnancy, with health concerns. The emotional turmoil of protecting her unborn child during such uncertain times led to depression and anxiety. At first, her job provided comfort, with the company understanding her need for reduced hours. Later with the layoffs increased worldwide, productivity expectations intensified, that added to her emotional burden. To balance the care of her first child, managing household chores without domestic help, and maintaining her own health became daunting tasks for her each day. Every cough or sneeze filled her with worry about the safety of her pregnancy. This fear persisted throughout her pregnancy, when she struggled to find balance. Despite the relief of a healthy delivery, the lack of maternity leave from the company's understaffing added to her challenges. During the peak of COVID-19, the demand for testing and releasing new apps brought financial incentives which comforted her financially.

Anitha faced new postpartum health challenges that included weight gain and physical ailments like spine and neck issues. Sleepless nights spent to balance childcare and work, coupled with extended workdays of 14 to 15 h, took a toll on her well-being. With the ease of restrictions, support from her parents in childcare brought some relief. The transition to a hybrid work model did not significantly reduce her workload, the schedule of 15 to 16-h days continued with travel and errands of school, and household responsibilities. Anitha expressed frustration over stagnant salaries for the past two years and feeling taken for granted by her employer, with expectations of extended work hours. With the recession news around, looking for a change in career is a risky thing. With all these challenges, she emphasized the necessity of having a job to sustain through post-COVID economic uncertainties.

### 16.2.3 Case 3-Priya: *Scrum Master*

Priya, a Scrum Master at Cognizant Technologies in Hyderabad, shared her experience of working from home during the COVID-19 pandemic, which she believed disrupted the world. Living alone, she faced severe mental, physical, and emotional strain due to isolation. She felt imprisoned and often neglected eating, cooking, or relaxing. Work became her constant companion, and her company, assuming she had more time, assigned abundant tasks. This continuous cycle of work led to severe emotional distress and burnout. She lost interest in social interactions, preferring isolation over gatherings. The solitude and constant work pressure made her accustomed to being alone, that diminished her desire for social contact which was a great blow to her mental well-being. Even after the pandemic, with the shift to a hybrid work model, she struggled to adjust. She became reluctant to go to the office, felt disconnected and lack the motivation to interact with others. Her life now revolves around work that worsened her physical and mental health. Although she was asked to be in the office for ten days a month, she manages only an hour each day, as found it challenging to adapt to the pre-pandemic routine.

### *16.2.4* Case 4-Maya: *Senior Analyst Engineer*

Maya, a Senior Analyst Engineer at Microsoft in Houston, USA, found working from home during the pandemic to be a blessing, despite missing social interactions with colleagues. Her mornings began calmly with her two children, aged 5 and 7. After taking care of their needs, she would start her work, taking breaks as necessary, with her husband assisting with chores and childcare. By evening, they would finish work around 5 or 6 PM and spend time together as a family, engaging in activities like gardening and enjoying happy hours. The absence of a commute saved time and money, reducing stress and improving her overall well-being. Maya continued to collaborate with US clients, and maintained consistent working hours. This flexibility allowed her to feel more balanced at home, as previously there was no one to look after her children when she was at work. She revived traditional Indian games with her children, read them stories, danced to regional songs, and watched movies with her husband.

After the pandemic, as the world transitioned to a hybrid work model, Microsoft, in the USA did not enforce strict office attendance, allowing employees to decide for themselves. This flexibility enabled Mayato to reconnect with her social life on weekends. Weekends were now filled with planned get-togethers, long drives, and meet-ups, enhancing her emotional and social well-being. Despite the initial anxiety and stress during the pandemic, Maya managed to turn it into a positive experience. She found balance and joy in the new routine, demonstrating that with the right mindset and support, challenging times can become periods of growth and happiness.

### *16.2.5* Case 5- Vindhya: *SeniorDeveloper*

Vindhya moved to the UK in 2019, just before the COVID-19 pandemic caused widespread shutdowns. Her husband, a scriptwriter, needed a calm space to work, so she supported him at home. In the beginning, working from home was manageable, and she enjoyed being close to her family. Over a period of time, balancing her husband's creative needs with her own work became difficult. The blurred lines between home and work stressed her, led to feelings of isolation and uncertainty about the future, which impacted her emotional well-being during the pandemic. When the work model shifted to a hybrid system post-pandemic, Vindhya felt some relief. She appreciated the structured routine and the part-time return to the office, which helped her manage both her work and supporting her husband better. Although juggling everything remained challenging, she found ways to maintain emotional balance and felt more satisfied with the compromise between work and home life.

### *16.2.6* Case 6-Manya: *Analyst Engineer*

In early 2020, Manya, an analyst engineer, relocated alone to Australia. Her new beginning was challenging due to the pandemic lockdown. Moving to online work posed significant problems, as she had to navigate everything independently without in-person support, which impacted her focus and job performance. During the pandemic, Manya faced difficulties, struggling to prove herself in a new job, working remotely. Concerns about job security and warnings regarding her work quality added to her stress. She prioritized her job over personal matters, dedicating substantial time to learning and improving her skills through online resources.

When the work environment shifted to a hybrid model post-pandemic, Manya benefited from the opportunity to work in the office. This direct interaction with colleagues and supervisors increased her confidence and competence. It also helped her achieve a better work-life balance. Despite the challenges, Manya's primary concern was job security, mental peace rather than financial issues and personal life.

## 16.3 Thematic Analysis of Cases

The case information collected was put to a thorough understanding using thematic analysis. Various themes emerge out of the case studies that align with the study and case context. The thematic analysis uses qualitative data and is generally applied to texts such as interviews and transcripts. The case text was closely examined for common themes that had a recurring pattern. The analysed cases and themes are as follows in Table 16.1

Saumya and Manya found remote work hard due to poor home setups and lack of support. This situation made them feel isolated and stressed, that harmed their emotional well-being. Vindhya and Manya also had trouble balancing work and personal life during remote work. The lack of clear boundaries between work and home life made it hard for them to keep a healthy balance. Anitha relied on family support and designed regular routines. This helped her to manage stress despite tough work conditions. Saumya and Anitha faced anxiety and stress due to job insecurity and financial worries during the pandemic. These concerns affected their emotional well-being.

Responses to hybrid work models are different. Maya benefited from the flexibility and improved work-life balance, while Anitha struggled with long hours and stagnant salaries. Priya found it hard to readjust to office routines after a long period of isolation. Maya relied on strong family support, which played a crucial role in keeping her emotional well-being during the pandemic. Priya faced challenges due

**Table 16.1** Thematic analysis of the cases

| | Theme | Cases included | Summary of findings |
|---|---|---|---|
| 1 | Emotional Well-being | Saumya, Manya | Both Saumya and Manya struggled with remote work due to home setup challenges and lack of support. Remote work intensified feelings of isolation and stress which negatively affected their emotional well-being |
| 2 | Work-Life Balance | Vindhya, Manya | Vindhya and Manya found it difficult to balance work and personal life during remote work. Blurred boundaries between work and home life made maintaining a mental balance challenging |
| 3 | Coping Mechanisms | Maya, Vindhya | Maya and Vindhya showed flexibility as they maintained routines. Their inclusion with the family and strategies adopted helped them manage stress and maintain emotional well-being amidst tough work conditions |
| 4 | Financial Concerns | Saumya, Anitha | Saumya and Anitha faced anxiety and stress due to job insecurity and financial worries during the pandemic. These factors affected their emotional well-being |
| 5 | Hybrid Work Models | Maya, Anitha, Priya | Maya and Anitha had different responses to hybrid work models. Maya benefited from flexibility and better work-life balance, while Anitha struggled with long work hours and stagnant salaries. Priya found it challenging to readjust to office routines after prolonged isolation |

to a lack of social interactions and increased work pressure, showing the importance of a supportive environment for managing emotional health. The themes show the complex relationship between work models adopted in different countries that reflect on individuals' personal life, and emotional well-being during times of crisis. The thematic analysis stresses the need for effective support systems, irrespective of the country they live in and policies to help employees cope with the challenges of the changing work environment.

### *16.3.1 Focus Discussion Groups (FGDs)*

The thematic analysis was taken to experts for focused discussion groups (FGDs), the areas of concern and potential interventions were identified and focus group discussions were initiated in association with six psychologists and counsellors who specialized in workplace mental health. Experts received summaries of the cases and themes identified, and then engaged in structured discussions to draw out insights and recommendations. These discussions yielded recommendations at two levels: individual and organizational. The recommendations were based on positive psychology, particularly the PERMA theory. Positive psychology focuses on the strengths and virtues that enable individuals and communities to thrive. Developed by Martin Seligman (2022), positive psychology emphasizes the importance of positive experiences, traits, and institutions. The PERMA theory, a cornerstone of positive psychology, identifies five elements essential to well-being: Positive Emotion, Engagement, Relationships, Meaning, and Accomplishment.

The recommendations at the individual level are tabulated and presented post FGDs (Table 16.2) are as follows:

The recommendations from the focus group discussions, to enhance emotional well-being through the PERMA model recommends that for the emotional well-being, individuals should engage in joyful activities, find motivating work aspects, maintain virtual connections, reflect on their work's purpose, and set achievable goals. To improve work-life balance, practicing gratitude, dedicating time to work and personal life, and aligning activities with personal values are essential. Effective coping mechanisms involve enjoying activities, maintaining routines, and leveraging social support. Addressing financial concerns requires mindfulness, skill development, and open discussions about financial worries. Adapting to hybrid work models involves embracing flexibility, engaging deeply at work, and nurturing colleague relationships. Cultivating gratitude, staying engaged in supportive activities, and recognizing resilience are key to maintaining emotional well-being.

The recommendations for the organizations drawn from the focus-grouped discussed were tabulated in Table 16.3 as follows:

The FGDs suggestion to support employee well-being was based on the PERMA model. The organizations that offer remote work, should offer wellness programs and also provide engaging online tools which facilitate virtual team-building activities and highlight the purpose of employees' work, and celebrate achievements. For the improvement of work-life balance, organizations should support personal achievements, promote productivity, introduce family-friendly policies, align goals with personal values, and recognize balanced accomplishments. In addressing coping mechanisms, organizations should provide mental health resources, encourage routine maintenance, facilitate peer support programs, communicate resilience importance, and acknowledge efforts in managing work-life balance. For financial concerns, offering financial wellness programs, career development opportunities, open communication about job security, and recognizing efforts towards financial stability are recommended. In hybrid work models, promoting flexibility benefits, supporting engagement during office days, facilitating social interactions, communicating the value of hybrid models, and recognizing balanced performance is essential. Lastly, fostering a supportive work environment, encouraging engagement in support networks, promoting strong workplace relationships, emphasizing support's importance, and celebrating resilience and support among employees is crucial for building a resilient and positive workplace.

**Table 16.2** Recommendations for the individuals through FGDs

| | Theme | Cases included | Recommendations for individuals (PERMA) |
|---|---|---|---|
| 1 | Emotional Well-being | Saumya, Manya | **Positive Emotions**: Engage in activities that bring joy and relaxation<br>**Engagement**: Find aspects of work that are engaging and focus on them<br>**Relationships**: Maintain regular virtual interactions with family and friends<br>**Meaning**: Reflect on the purpose and impact of your work<br>**Accomplishment**: Set small, achievable goals to build a sense of accomplishment |
| 2 | Work-Life Balance | Vindhya, Manya | **Positive Emotions**: Practice gratitude for small wins in balancing work and life<br>**Engagement**: Dedicate focused time to work and personal activities<br>**Relationships**: Spend quality time with family and friends<br>**Meaning**: Ensure that both work and personal activities align with personal values<br>**Accomplishment**: Track progress in both professional and personal goals |
| 3 | Coping Mechanisms | Maya, Anitha | **Positive Emotions**: Engage in relaxing and enjoyable activities<br>**Engagement**: Keep a routine that includes engaging tasks<br>**Relationships**: Rely on and strengthen family and social support<br>**Meaning**: Find meaning in daily routines and family interactions<br>**Accomplishment**: Celebrate small successes and progress in managing stress |
| 4 | Financial Concerns | Saumya, Anitha | **Positive Emotions**: Practice mindfulness to manage anxiety<br>**Engagement**: Focus on learning new skills for job security<br>**Relationships**: Discuss financial concerns with supportive people<br>**Meaning**: Reflect on the purpose behind financial stability<br>**Accomplishment**: Set and achieve small financial goals |
| 5 | Hybrid Work Models | Maya, Anitha, Priya | **Positive Emotions**: Focus on the positives of hybrid work flexibility<br>**Engagement**: Engage deeply in work during office days<br>**Relationships**: Foster relationships with colleagues during in-office days<br>**Meaning**: Find meaning in the balance hybrid work offers<br>**Accomplishment**: Achieve balance in work and personal life |

### *16.3.2 The Intervention*

In the experiment, each member followed the recommendations from the focus group discussions (FGDs) based on the PERMA model of positive psychology for about 45 days. The initial data before FGDs before the intervention of emotional well-being

**Table 16.3** Recommendations for the organizations through FGDs

| | Theme | Cases included | Recommendations for Organizations (PERMA) |
|---|---|---|---|
| 1 | Emotional Well-being | Saumya, Manya | **Positive Emotions:** Offer wellness programs to boost employee morale<br>**Engagement:** Provide engaging online work platforms and tools<br>**Relationships:** Facilitate regular virtual team-building activities<br>**Meaning:** Highlight the purpose and impact of employees' work<br>**Accomplishment:** Recognize and celebrate employees' achievements |
| 2 | Work-Life Balance | Vindhya, Manya | **Positive Emotions:** Encourage and support employees' personal achievements<br>**Engagement:** Promote focus and productivity during work hours<br>**Relationships:** Support family-friendly policies and practices<br>**Meaning:** Align organizational goals with employees' personal values<br>**Accomplishment:** Recognize and reward balanced work and personal achievements |
| 3 | Coping Mechanisms | Maya, Anitha | **Positive Emotions:** Provide access to mental health resources<br>**Engagement:** Encourage employees to maintain routines<br>**Relationships:** Facilitate peer support programs<br>**Meaning:** Communicate the significance of resilience in the workplace<br>**Accomplishment:** Recognize employees' efforts in managing work-life balance |
| 4 | Financial Concerns | Saumya, Anitha | **Positive Emotions:** Offer financial wellness programs<br>**Engagement:** Provide opportunities for career development<br>**Relationships:** Foster open communication about job security<br>**Meaning:** Emphasize the importance of financial stability<br>**Accomplishment:** Recognize efforts towards financial security and stability |
| 5 | Hybrid Work Models | Maya, Anitha, Priya | **Positive Emotions:** Promote the benefits of hybrid work flexibility<br>**Engagement:** Support employees' engagement during office days<br>**Relationships:** Facilitate social interactions in hybrid settings<br>**Meaning:** Communicate the value of hybrid work models<br>**Accomplishment:** Recognize balanced work performance in hybrid models |

was procured and tabulated then the intervention with recommendations lasted for 45 days. Saumya and Manya addressed their remote work challenges by engaging in enjoyable activities, focusing on interesting work tasks, and maintaining regular virtual interactions with family and friends. They also reflected on their work's purpose and set small, achievable goals. Vindhya and Manya worked on their work-life balance by practicing gratitude for small successes, dedicating focused time to work and personal activities, and ensuring their activities matched their personal values. They tracked their progress in both professional and personal areas. Maya and Anitha used coping strategies by maintaining consistent routines, engaging in relaxing activities, and relying on family and social support. They found meaning in their routines and celebrated small achievements in managing stress. Anitha and Saumya addressed financial concerns by practicing mindfulness to handle anxiety, focusing on skill development for job security, and discussing financial worries with supportive individuals. Maya, Anitha, and Priya adapted to hybrid work models by focusing on the benefits of flexibility, engaging deeply during office days, building relationships with colleagues, and finding meaning in the balance between work settings. They also celebrated their achievements in managing both work and personal life. These efforts led to various improvements in their mood, stress levels, and overall well-being. The post-intervention interviews were conducted to note the changes. The following Table 16.4 consolidates the pre and post-intervention emotional well-being of individuals:

## 16.4 Discussion

The study aimed to improve emotional health through interventions based on the PERMA model of positive psychology, which focuses on Positive Emotions, Engagement, Relationships, Meaning, and Accomplishment. The impact of these interventions was measured at three points: 30 days, 45 days, and 60 days, showing a gradual improvement in participants' emotional well-being, work engagement, and work-life balance. The regular monitoring allowed researchers to understand the effectiveness of the interventions and make necessary adjustments to ensure continued support.

Saumya showed a small reduction in stress by 30 days, mainly due to improvements in her workspace and starting to engage in small tasks at work. By 45 days, her stress levels were lower as she became more involved in her work and started interacting with colleagues occasionally. At 60 days, she was more emotionally stable, better managing her work-life balance, and staying engaged in her work. This progress aligns with Bertoni et al. (2023), who found that remote work can increase job satisfaction, though Saumya's early isolation was also a challenge, as discussed by Kottasová (2020). Manya showed mild improvement in her mood after 30 days, having set up simple daily routines and started talking to colleagues for support. By 45 days, her emotional state had improved further, and her relationships at work were stronger. By 60 days, Manya had found a better balance between work and her personal life, highlighting the importance of consistent routines and support during

**Table 16.4** Pre and post-intervention observations on individual's emotional well-being

| Case name | Before intervention | 30 days of post-intervention | 45 days of post-intervention | 60 days of post-intervention |
|---|---|---|---|---|
| Saumya | High stress, feelings of isolation, inadequate home setup | Stress slightly reduced. Began focusing on work tasks and setting up a proper workspace | Stress continued to decrease. Workspace improvements helped her manage tasks more effectively | Stress significantly reduced. Managed work-life balance better and felt emotionally stable |
| Manya | High stress, struggle with remote work setup, lack of support | Slight improvement in mood. Started following a daily routine and reaching out to colleagues | Mood improved further. Regular work patterns and communication with peers increased | Emotional state became stable. Work and personal life were better balanced |
| Vindhya | Difficulty balancing work and personal life, frequent stress | Made small changes to time management. Felt less stress during quieter work periods | Balance improved. More focus on separating work and home responsibilities. Stress reduced | Work-life balance was steady. Personal and work tasks were managed with confidence |
| Maya | Less consistent routines | Started following a routine. Took breaks to spend time with family | Routines improved further. Participated more in family activities | Maintained consistent routines. Felt emotionally stronger due to support from family |
| Anitha | High anxiety about financial stability and stress balancing work-life | Anxiety started reducing with mindfulness activities. Began tracking finances | Anxiety decreased more. Financial planning and workload balance improved | Anxiety was under control. Financial planning and work-life balance were well managed |
| Priya | Difficulty adapting to hybrid work, weak office relationships | Began attending office regularly but avoided extended interactions | Felt more comfortable in the office. Started talking more with colleagues | Fully adjusted to the office schedule. Built strong workplace relationships |

transitions, as noted by Farré et al. (2021). Vindhya made small changes to balance her work and home life in the first 30 days, including practicing gratitude. By 45 days, she had improved her time management and felt less stressed. At 60 days, Vindhya had a steady balance between her responsibilities and continued her gratitude practices, which supports the findings of Feng and Savani (2020). Her early struggles reflect the systemic challenges discussed by Oakman et al. (2020).

Maya began following a structured routine for 30 days, spending more time with her family and taking breaks to reduce stress. By 45 days, her emotional state improved due to more active engagement with her family and friends. At 60 days, Maya had settled into stable routines and experienced significant emotional well-being, demonstrating the importance of strong relationships during difficult times.

Anitha showed a slight reduction in anxiety by 30 days, using mindfulness practices and starting to track her finances. By 45 days, she managed her financial concerns better, and her anxiety continued to decrease. By 60 days, Anitha had gained confidence in handling her finances and balancing work-life responsibilities. These changes reflect the value of mindfulness in reducing stress, as highlighted by Moorthy (2020), and her financial concerns are similar to the challenges discussed by Corsi and Ilkkaracan (2023). Priya had difficulty adjusting to hybrid work at first, but by 30 days, she started attending the office more regularly, even though her interactions were limited. By 45 days, she adapted to the hybrid model and began building connections with colleagues. At 60 days, Priya had fully adjusted to the hybrid work environment and built strong professional relationships, addressing the challenges of hybrid work identified by Makridis and Schloetzer (2022).

A key take away from the study is the importance of regular wellness sessions. These sessions, which include mindfulness and stress management techniques, were effective in reducing anxiety and helping participants manage the challenges of hybrid work. Over time, they created a supportive environment where employees could share experiences, build connections, and improve their emotional well-being. These sessions also helped participants set boundaries, prioritize tasks, and manage responsibilities, especially for women balancing multiple roles. Regular check-ins, such as those that identified Saumya's workspace adjustments, Manya's need for routines, and Priya's challenges with hybrid work, enabled timely support and adjustments, as seen in the study by Farré et al. (2021). Organizations should prioritize such programs to create a positive, supportive workplace that fosters emotional and professional growth for employees.

### *16.4.1 Future Scope and Limitations*

Future research can be conducted by exploring the emotional health of women in the IT sector across different regions of India and among NRIs in various countries. It can look into how cultural, economic, and workplace factors affect their well-being. A larger and more diverse sample, as well as the use of a mixed-method approach, will be helpful to offer a broader understanding. Helping women to track their progress over time could show the long-term effects of the COVID-19 pandemic, particularly as hybrid work modes continue to develop. This study has some limitations, which include its focus on specific regions and a small sample size, which might not fully represent the broader population. The use of snowball sampling also has introduced some bias, limiting how widely the findings can be applied. The qualitative approach, while providing detailed insights, may not capture how widespread these issues are, and the cross-sectional design does not show changes in emotional health over time. Checking on these limitations in future, research would improve understanding of how specific company policies and practices impact women's emotional health during and after the pandemic.

## 16.5 Conclusion

The shift from remote work to hybrid work models during the COVID-19 pandemic brought mixed outcomes for women in the IT sector in India. The remote work offered flexibility, but it also caused stress due to inadequate home office setups, feelings of isolation, and challenges in managing both work and home duties. Hybrid work, which combined remote and in-office work, provided a more balanced approach but still left women facing long hours and stagnant salaries. Though this model was intended to improve work-life balance by allowing for in-person collaboration and better separation between work and home life, it hasn't fully resolved the issues. To better support women, the study suggests that individuals should focus on the PERMA approach to boost emotional well-being gradually and follow it regularly for over a period of time. This involves engaging in activities that bring them joy, finding meaning in work, strong relationships with people, living with purpose, and setting small goals that lead to a sense of achievement. For organizations, there is a need to refine hybrid work policies. The organizations can bring in inclusiveness by integrating wellness programs to support mental health, creating engaging work environments, and implementing family-friendly policies. Organizations should also try to focus on career development opportunities and provide support networks to help women manage their professional and personal responsibilities. These steps are essential to improve the effectiveness of hybrid work arrangements, to help women achieve a better work-life balance, and to increase job satisfaction with positive emotional health.

## References

Angelici, M., & Profeta, P. (2023). Smart-working: Work flexibility without constraints. *Management Science*. https://doi.org/10.1287/mnsc.2023.4767

Bertoni, M., Cavapozzi, D., Pasini, G., & Pavese, C. (2023). Remote working and mental health during the first wave of COVID-19 pandemic. *IZA DP*, 14773.

Bradbury, A. (2020). Mental health stigma: The impact of age and gender on attitudes. *Community Mental Health Journal, 56*(5), 933–938. https://doi.org/10.1007/s10597-020-00559

Choudhury, P., Khanna, T., Makridis, C. A., & Schirmann, K. (2022). *Is hybrid work the best of both worlds? Evidence from a field experiment* (Working Paper, 22-063).

Corsi, M., & Ilkkaracan, I. (2023). COVID-19, gender, and labor. In K. F. Zimmermann (Ed.), *Handbook of labor, human resources and population economics*. Springer. https://doi.org/10.1007/978-3-319-57365-6_323-1

Covid-19: Why are women more vulnerable to mental health issues? (2020, May 5). https://feminisminindia.com/2020/05/05/covid-19-women-vulnerable-mental-health-issues/

Cui, R., Ding, H., & Zhu, F. (2021). Gender inequality in research productivity during the COVID-19 pandemic. *Manufacturing & Service Operations Management, 24*(2).

Del Boca, D., Oggero, N., Profeta, P., & Rossi, M. C. (2022). The impact of COVID-19 on the gender division of housework and childcare: Evidence from two waves of the pandemic in Italy. *IZA Journal of Labor Economics, 11*(1).

Deloitte. (2023). *Women at work: India 2023.* Deloitte. Retrieved July 18, 2024, from https://www2.deloitte.com/content/dam/Deloitte/in/Documents/about-deloitte/in-ad-2023Deloitte_Women-at-Work_India.pdf

Deloitte. (2024). *Women at work: A global outlook 2024.* Deloitte. Retrieved July 18, 2024, from https://www.deloitte.com/content/dam/assets-shared/docs/collections/2024/deloitte-women-at-work-2024-a-global-outlook.pdf?dl=1

Delventhal, M. J., & Parkhomenko, A. (2021). *Spatial implications of telecommuting* (Working Paper). https://papers.ssrn.com/sol3/papers.cfm?abstract_id=3746555

Dingel, J. I., & Neiman, B. (2020). How many jobs can be done at home? *National Bureau of Economic Research.* https://doi.org/10.3386/w26948

Envoy. (n.d.). *What is a hybrid work model?* Envoy. Retrieved July18, 2024, from https://envoy.com/blog/what-is-a-hybrid-work-model/

Feng, Z., & Savani, K. (2020). Covid-19 created a gender gap in perceived work productivity and job satisfaction: Implications for dual-career parents working from home. *Gender in Management: An International Journal, 35*(7/8), 719–736.

Financial Express. (2021). Work from home should be assimilated as routine part of our work-life; Here's why. https://www.financialexpress.com/jobs/work-from-home-should-be-assimilated-as-routine-part-of-our-work-life-heres-why/2268802/. Accessed 3 July 2021.

Gallup. (2023). *The future of hybrid work: Key questions answered with data.* Gallup. Retrieved July 18, 2024, from https://www.gallup.com/workplace/390632/future-hybrid-work-key-questions-answered-data.aspx

Gueguen, G., & Senik, C. (2023). Adopting telework: The causal impact of working from home on subjective well-being. *British Journal of Industrial Relations, 61*, 832–868.

Guy, B., & Arthur, B. (2020). Academic motherhood during COVID-19: Navigating our dual roles as educators and mothers. *Gender, Work & Organization, 27*(5), 887–899.

HiBob. (n.d.). *Hybrid working model.* HiBob. Retrieved July 18, 2024, from https://www.hibob.com/hr-glossary/hybrid-working-model/

Hindustan Times. (2021). Women spent more time doing household chores than men during COVID-19 study. https://www.hindustantimes.com/lifestyle/relationships/women-spent-more-time-ng-household-chores-than-men-during-covid-19-study-101615687274563.html. Accessed 14 March 2021.

Hupkau, C., & Petrongolo, B. (2020). Work, care and gender during the COVID-19 crisis. *Covid Economics, 54*, 1–28.

Karácsony, P. (2021). Impact of teleworking on job satisfaction among Slovakian employees in the era of COVID-19. *Problems and Perspectives in Management, 19*(3), 1–9.

Kasarla, H. (2020, May 2). India's lockdown is blind to the woes of its women. https://thewire.in/women/indias-lockdown-is-blind-to-the-woes-of-its-women

Kaur, T., & Sharma, P. (2020). A study on working women and work from home amid coronavirus pandemic. *Journal of Xi'an University of Architecture & Technology, XII*, 1400–1408.

Kottasová, I. (2020, May 24). Coronavirus is killing more men. But the lockdown is disastrous for women and their rights. *CNN World.* https://www.cnn.com/2020/05/24/world/women-rights-coronavirus-intl/index.html. Accessed 9 July 2020.

Kumar, K. B. (2020, June 12). Is work from home feasible in the long run? https://www.thehindu.com/opinion/op-ed/is-work-from-home-feasible-in-the-long-run/article31807666.ece

Kumar, R., & Srinivasan, S. (2023). The future of work in the era of AI: The case of India's IT industry. *Journal of Future Studies, 27*(2), 123–150.

Lee, I., & Tipoe, E. (2021). Changes in the quantity and quality of time use during the COVID-19 lockdowns in the UK: Who is the most affected? *PLoS ONE, 16*(11), Article e0258917. https://doi.org/10.1371/journal.pone.0258917

Makridis, C., & Schloetzer, J. (2022). Does working from home increase job satisfaction and retention? Evidence from the COVID-19 pandemic. *Georgetown McDonough School of Business Research Paper*, no. 4016657. Washington DC: McDonough School of Business, Georgetown University.

Mantri, G. (2020, August 14). The pandemic has set back women's progress in the workplace. Retrieved on July 5, 2024 from https://www.thenewsminute.com/article/pandemic-has-set-back-women-s-progress-workplace-130731

Mathur, N. (2020, September 10). Nearly 50% of India's working women more stressed due to pandemic: LinkedIn. Retrieved on July 1, 2024 from https://www.livemint.com/companies/news/nearly-50-of-india-s-working-women-more-stressed-due-to-pandemic-linkedin-11599722943378.html

Menon, S., & Sharma, S. (2020). A study on the status of women's empowerment in urban Bangalore, India. *Journal of International Women's Studies, 21*(5), 54–64.

Mooi-Reci, I., & Risman, B. J. (2021). The gendered impacts of COVID-19: Lessons and reflections. *Gender & Society, 35*(2), 161–167. https://doi.org/10.1177/08912432211001305

Moorthy, S. (2020, April 1). Working from home, IT employees battle job pressures and mental health issues. *Money Control*. https://www.moneycontrol.com/news/business/coronavirus-working-from-home-it-employees-battle-job-pressures-mental-health-issues-5096171.html. Accessed 22 August 2020.

NASSCOM. (2023). *IT-BPM sector in India: Strategic review 2023*. National Association of Software and Service Companies.

News 18. (2020, August 26). WFH is destroying work-life balance and affecting mental health amid pandemic. Retrieved on16 July from https://www.news18.com/news/buzz/wfh-is-destroying-work-life-balance-and-affecting-mental-health-amid-pandemic-2821601.html

Niebuhr, F., Borle, P., Börner-Zobel, F., & Voelter-Mahlknecht, S. (2022). Healthy and happy working from home? Effects of working from home on employee health and job satisfaction. *International Journal of Environmental Research and Public Health, 19*(3), 1122.

Oakman, J., Kinsman, N., Stuckey, R., Graham, M., & Weale, V. (2020). A rapid review of mental and physical health effects of working at home: How do we optimise health? *BMC Public Health, 20*, 1825.

Vasconcelos, P., Furtado, E., & Pinheiro, P. (2015). A hybrid approach for modeling alternatives of flexible working. *Procedia Computer Science*. https://doi.org/10.1016/j.procs.2015.07.162

Perry-Jenkins, M., & Gerstel, N. (2020). Work and family in the second decade of the 21st century. *Journal of Marriage and Family, 82*(1), 420–453.

Rai, S., & Rai, S. (2020). A study on impact of COVID-19 on women workers in India. *The Indian Journal of Labour Economics, 63*, 901–921.

Rao, M. S., & Duggirala, M. (2022). The future of work in the digital era: Evidence from the Indian IT industry. *Information Systems Frontiers, 24*, 279–298. https://doi.org/10.1007/s10796-021-10078-7

Roy, R. (2021). Working from home: Women in the Indian tech-industry through the pandemic. *Journal of Comparative Literature and Aesthetics, 44*(1, Spring), 108–119.

Satpathy, I., & Patel, P. (2022). An empirical study on employees working from home and their mental wellbeing: With reference to IT professionals in Mumbai. *International Journal of Research and Analytical Reviews, 9*(4), 738–747.

Savić, D. (2020). COVID-19 and work from home: Digital transformation of the workforce. *Grey Journal (TGJ), 16*(2), 101–104.

Selvaratnam, T. (2020, April 7). The shadow pandemic: How the COVID-19 crisis is exacerbating gender inequality. https://www.msnbc.com/know-your-value/the-shadow-pandemic-how-covid-19-crisis-exacerbating-gender-inequality-n1190611

Sharma, K., & Mishra, M. (2020). Mental health during COVID-19: An Indian perspective. *International Journal of Social Psychiatry, 66*(7), 627–629.

Shrivastava, S. (2020, October 29). Work-from-home phenomenon may erode urban working women's rights: Study. https://www.business-standard.com/article/current-affairs/work-from-home-phenomenon-may-erode-urban-working-women-s-rights-study-120102900086_1.html

Singh, D., & Nayak, S. (2021). Women's work and employment during COVID-19 lockdown. *Social Change, 51*(4), 503–518.

Singh, S. (2020, May 26). Impact of COVID-19 on women and children. *The Times of India*. https://timesofindia.indiatimes.com/blogs/voices/impact-of-covid-19-on-women-and-children/

Sokolic, D. (2022). Remote work and hybrid work organizations. Conference. *Economic and Social Development*, Aveiro.

Sriharan, A., Ratnapalan, S., Tricco, A. C., Lupea, D., Ayala, A. P., Pang, H., & Lee, D. D. (2020). Occupational stress, burnout, and depression in women in healthcare during COVID-19 pandemic: Rapid scoping review. *Frontiers in Global Women's Health, 1*, Article 596690. https://doi.org/10.3389/fgwh.2020.596690

Taylor, S. (2020). What is work-life balance and how does it impact your mental health? *Psych Central*. https://psychcentral.com/lib/what-is-work-life-balance-and-how-does-it-impact-your-mental-health/

Wade, M., (2021). The disparate impact of COVID-19 on the mental health of female and male caregivers. *Social Science & Medicine, 275,* 113801. https://doi.org/10.1016/j.socscimed.2021.113801

# Chapter 17
# Moderating Role of Social Support in Association of Well-Being and Psychological Problems Among Pakistani Pregnant Women

**Najma Iqbal Malik, Mohsin Atta, Ambar Zahra, Quratulain, Jam Bilal Ahmad, and Farooq Ahmed**

**Abstract** This chapter elucidates the empirical endeavour to investigate the relationship between psychological distress, body image dissatisfaction, and mental health in working and non-working women in the course of pregnancy, in addition to the moderating role of social support. This chapter covered the cross-sectional study and was conducted on a purposive sample of 213 pregnant women. Findings revealed that women's negative observations about their body image also dissatisfaction with their body are positively correlated to psychological distress but negatively correlated to mental well-being and non-significant correlation with social support. Psychological distress is negatively correlated to mental well-being and social support, and its constructs are negatively allied to mental distress. The outcomes of the Hierarchical Regression analysis showed that body image dissatisfaction significantly negatively, social support positively, and psychological distress did not significantly predict mental well-being. Marriage duration of 16 years or above was positively predicted, and the age range of 31 to 40 years was significantly strongly and positively predicted, but higher secondary education negatively predicted mental well-being. Moreover, high-level social support was revealed to be a significant moderator in the association of dissatisfaction with body image as well as mental well-being. Results revealed that working women suffered from mental health problems and perceived more social support compared to non-working females. This chapter may help families, especially

N. I. Malik · M. Atta · Quratulain
Department of Psychology, University of Sargodha, Sargodha, Punjab, Pakistan

A. Zahra
Counseling Centre, University of Sargodha, Sargodha, Punjab, Pakistan

J. B. Ahmad
Taxila Institute of Asian Studies, Quaid-I-Azam University Islamabad, Islamabad, Pakistan

F. Ahmed (✉)
Department of Anthropology, The Islamia University of Bahawalpur, Bahawalpur, Punjab, Pakistan
e-mail: farooq.ahmed@iub.edu.pk

 
P. Chouhan et al. (eds.), *Women's Health Dynamics in South Asia*, Asian Perspectives on Public Health, https://doi.org/10.1007/978-981-95-2321-4_17

spouses to understand their partner's well-being-related problems during pregnancy, as well as the importance of social support. It also helps human resource management to facilitate pregnant females by establishing a comfortable environment to get maximum output from them at work.

**Keywords** Psychological distress · Body image dissatisfaction · Mental well-being · Social support · Pakistan

## 17.1 Introduction

In different stages of pregnancy, females suffer from increased body weight and physical changes, which results in generating negative thoughts about their body image, self-control, body dissatisfaction, and risk of distress for example anxiety, stress, depression, also low self-esteem (Watson-Singleton, 2017). According to Arvidsdotter et al. (2016), psychological distress (PD) is a condition of emotional distress allied with multiple stressors (events, situations or persons that are triggering stress) plus demands that are tough to deal with in a daily lifetime. Pregnancy is an irreplaceable mother experience with deep mental, emotional, physical, as well as biochemical consequences on women. Mental well-being is a most important global well-being concern plus a key determinant in social mobility and efficacy. Pregnant females are susceptible because of body variations that they undergo during the phases of pregnancy that may perhaps disturb the mental well-being of mothers.

During the prenatal and post-partum periods, about one-fifth of pregnant women have mental health problems including anxiety, depression, psychosis, substance misapplication, and eating disorders, which might last up to a year (Alipour et al., 2018). Body image is a multifaceted concept where various opinions, beliefs, feelings, and plusbehaviours play a vigorous part in an individual's personal assessment regarding their bodily look and overall attitude towards their body (Cash, 2017). The importance of body image for psychophysical development is frequently discussed in psychological research (Izydorczyk et al., 2020) in addition to medical past research works (Bai et al., 2019).

The bulk of current scientific investigations concerning physique image dissatisfaction in women emphasizes measuring the image of the body in the view of their physique image after giving birth (Zielinski et al., 2017), sexual life quality (Thomas et al., 2019), well-being after and before childbirth (Tutkuviene et al., 2018), body regulation and social inclusion (Keshwani et al., 2021). Research also indicates significant relationships between body image dissatisfaction and mental well-being during pregnancy, as evidenced by various longitudinal and causal studies. These studies highlight how changes in body image can influence psychological health, particularly in new mothers. For instance Han et al. (2016) a study tracked 39,315 women in the Norwegian Mother and Child Cohort find out that body image concerns mediate the relationship between depressive symptoms and weight gain, particularly in women with higher pre-pregnancy BMI. A more recent study examining the 136 pregnant women demonstrate that body image dissatisfaction varies during pregnancy and post-partum, with higher dissatisfaction levels in overweight women (Linde et al., 2024).

The care and assistance people believe others are providing are social support (Xiao et al., 2020). Social support tends to be the safeguard against body image issues and mental problems associated with pregnancy (Izydorczyk et al., 2021). Furthermore, it can improve self-efficacy and subjective well-being in dealing with anxiety plus stress (Ginja et al., 2018). Pregnancy situations, the sensation of maternity, also the presence of people always there for the pregnant female may perhaps cause her to have fewer desire for environmental mastery in the course of her pregnancy (Fahami et al., 2018).

The majority of explorations has shown a connection between motherly mental well-being social webs, with the best mental health outcomes being experienced by mothers who are well-supported. For example, mothers who received little or inadequate help following the delivery of their baby are five times more expected to have post-partum depression symptoms than women who gained enough support (Ginjaet al., 2018). Kok et al. (2020) suggested that societal support functions as a protective factor by buffering maternal education and psychological distress, thus enhancing the well-being of both working and non-working pregnant women. Body image is a big concern during this period. These issues affect the mental health plus well-being of the female.

There is a dearth of multivariate longitudinal studies on pregnancy-related psychological issues. In order to have more in-depth insights longitudinal studies, (indicating that body image dissatisfaction is linked to mental well-being, particularly through factors like self-esteem, pregnancy-specific worries, and social support) require further investigation to establish a strong causal relationship. Linde et al. (2022) in prospective longitudinal design with a quantitative approach also emphasized the need for further longitudinal investigations in this particular domain.

Pregnancy affects both working and non-working women at some time. In the context of the stress-buffering postulate, support from society is particularly beneficial during high stress. This hypothesis provides a theoretical base to explain the negative influence of physique image dissatisfaction on mental well-being and the beneficial part of social support that helps individuals maintain their well-being and adapt more effectively to challenging circumstances. Certain studies concentrated on both working and non-working women in a Western cultural context, e.g., Milgrom et al. (2021) examined psychological factors and depressive symptoms in Australia, and Reichenheim et al. (2018) found social support as a protector in contrast to the adverse impacts of spouse violence on psychological well-being among Brazilian pregnant women. No research was carried out in Pakistan with this combination of study variables and population of interest, i.e., pregnant working and non-working pregnant women. In Pakistan, more than 50% of the population comprises females, and there is a growing trend for women to leave their homes for work. Childbearing and motherhood are their obligations, whether they work or not. In the process of motherhood, women go through different phases which affect their mental and physical health. So, research in this area will be useful for Pakistani females and other

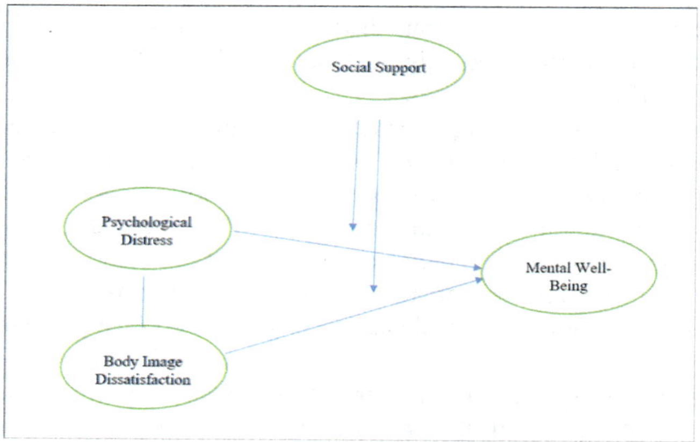


**Fig. 17.1** Conceptual structure of the chapter

South Asian women because they share nearly the same culture. In low-income counties, e.g., Pakistan, there are certain mental healthcare system challenges, such as an inadequacy of mental health professionals and scarce funding. These issues prevent pregnant women's access to necessary mental health services.

Keeping in view the aforementioned discourse and exploration of existing literature, the following investigation questions are under consideration in the current chapter: (1) Is there a relationship between study variables in working and non-working pregnant women? (2) Would psychological distress, body image dissatisfaction, and social support be significant predictors of mental well-being? (3) Would demographic variables be significant predictors of mental well-being? (4) Would perceived Social Support be a significant moderator in the link between body image and mental well-being? (5) Would there be significant differences between working and non-working women concerning psychological distress, body image, social support, and mental well-being? (Fig. 17.1)

## 17.2 Materials and Methods

### *17.2.1 Design and Participants*

This chapter is designed to investigate the link between psychological distress, physique image dissatisfaction, plus mental well-being in working and non-working women during pregnancy, and also to discover the moderating role of support from society. The sample of this study was extracted by means of a purposive sampling method from different hospitals in Punjab, which included 213working pregnant ($n$ = 111) and non-working pregnant women ($n$ = 101) from both public and private hospitals during February 2021 to August 2021.

### 17.2.2 Inclusion and Exclusion Criteria for Data Collection

Women with an age range of 20–50 years who attended antenatal check-ups at any time of their pregnancy were included in this study. Only those females were selected who had a marriage duration of at least one year. Mothers who did not go to regular antenatal check-ups were excluded from this study. Those who were unmarried, widows, separated, and divorced from their partners were also excluded.

### 17.2.3 Instruments

#### 17.2.3.1 Kessler Psychological Distress Scale

This scale was constructed by Kessler and Mroczekin 1994 with Cronbach's alpha 0.91. This scale was a five-point Likert scale, and the alpha reliability of this scale in the present study was 0.93.

#### 17.2.3.2 Body Shape Questionnaire 16-A

This questionnaire developed by Cooper et al. in 1987, and the current study used this to examine concerns regarding the shape and weight of the body undergone by those individuals who have eating-related disorders or physique image and dissatisfaction-related problems (Cooper et al., 1987). This scale reliability in the literature was 0.0.89. However, alpha reliability in the present study was 0.94.

#### 17.2.3.3 Warwick–Edinburg Mental Well-Being Scale (WEMWBS)

This scale was constructed by Stewart-Brown et al. in 2009. WEMWBS is a measure of mental well-being based on 14 item scale with 5 points Likert scale. This scale reliability in the literature was 0.91 and 0.92. However, the alpha reliability of this scale in the present study was 0.95.

#### 17.2.3.4 Multi-Dimensional Scale for Perceived Social Support (MSPSS)

This inventory was constructed by Zimet et al. in 1988. In the literature, the original reliability of the whole scale was 0.88, for significant others 0.91, for households 0.87 and for associates 0.85. However, the alpha reliabilities for the social support scale, in the present study, were 0.96 with subscales as significant others 0.89, the family was 0.90, and friends 0.92.

### 17.2.4 Procedure and Ethical Consideration

The Institutional Research Committee, Department of Psychology, University of Sargodha, Pakistan, reviewed and approved this study (SU/PSY/793-b). The sample was approached after obtaining permission from the concerned hospital authorities. As the participants of this investigation were literate as well as illiterate, the researcher applied different protocols for both types of samples. Both types of sample was debriefed regarding the study's goal in a different way. Significant ethical principles such as informed consent (verbal and written) for voluntary participation and confidentiality were the essential protocols equally provided to both literate and illiterate women. Although the interview method was used for collecting data from illiterate ladies. In this method, the researcher asked each illiterate participant about her demographics, and after getting demographic information, the researcher, statement by statement, asked about the rest of the questionnaire of the illiterate women.

### 17.2.5 Data Analysis

IBM SPSS (statistical packages for social sciences) 22 version software was used to test the study hypothesis. Descriptive statistics were evaluated for mean, standard deviation, and frequency. Alpha reliability, Pearson correlation, multiple linear regression, hierarchal regression analysis, and independent-sample *t*-test accounted for analysing the data.

## 17.3 Results

The results of this chapter were analysed by the use of SPSS. Before testing the present study hypothesis, reliabilities and descriptive statistics of the data were calculated after that, Pearson Correlation, Hierarchical Regression, Moderation through Process Macro, and Independent sample *t*-test were applied.

Table 17.1 illustrates the frequency and percentages of the demographic attributes of the two samples of the study concerning working and non-working pregnant women.

Table 17.2 shows the alpha reliability of measurements ranging from 0.89 to 0.96, which indicates satisfactory internal consistency. Results point out that psychological distress has a significant positive association with body image dissatisfaction ($r = 0.23$, $^{**}p < 0.01$) but a negative association with mental well-being ($r = -0.14$, $^{**}p < 0.01$), also with social support ($r = -0.40$, $^{**}p < 0.01$), along its subscales (significant others, family and friends). Furthermore, results indicate that Body image dissatisfaction has a significant negative association with mental well-being ($r = -$

**Table 17.1** Demographic characteristics of working and non-working women

| | Working | | Non-working | | Total | |
|---|---|---|---|---|---|---|
| Variables | *n* | (%) | *n* | (%) | *n* | (%) |
| *Age* | | | | | | |
| 20–30 years | 54 | (48.6) | 62 | (60.8) | 119 | (55.9) |
| 31–40 years | 56 | (50.5) | 38 | (39.3) | 91 | (42.7) |
| 41–45 years | 01 | (.9) | 2 | (2.0) | 3 | (1.4) |
| *Education* | | | | | | |
| No Formal Education | 6 | (5.4) | 1 | (1.0) | 7 | (3.3) |
| Primary | 1 | (0.9) | 8 | (7.0) | 9 | (4.2) |
| Elementary | 3 | (2.7) | 7 | (6.9) | 10 | (4.7) |
| Secondary | 2 | (1.8) | 33 | (32.4) | 35 | (16.4) |
| Higher Secondary | 1 | (0.9) | 24 | (23.5) | 25 | (11.7) |
| Graduation | 14 | (12.6) | 16 | (15.7) | 30 | (14.1) |
| Post-graduation | 84 | (75.7) | 13 | (12.7) | 97 | (45.5) |
| *Marriage duration* | | | | | | |
| 1–5 years | 73 | (65.8) | 55 | (53.9) | 128 | (60.1) |
| 6–10 years | 34 | (30.6) | 29 | (28.4) | 63 | (29.6) |
| 11–15 years | 3 | (2.7) | 8 | (7.8) | 11 | (5.2) |
| 16 and above | 1 | (0.9) | 10 | (9.8) | 11 | (5.2) |
| *Relation with husband* | | | | | | |
| Cousin | 46 | (36.9) | 49 | (48) | 95 | (44.6) |
| Out of family | 65 | (58.6.) | 53 | (52) | 118 | (55.4) |
| *No of children* | | | | | | |
| No children | 41 | (36.9) | 29 | (28.4) | 70 | (32.9) |
| 1–2 | 50 | (47.7) | 49 | (48) | 102 | (47.9) |
| 3–4 | 16 | (14.4) | 18 | (17.6) | 34 | (16.0) |
| 5–6 | 1 | (0.9) | 6 | (5.9) | 7 | (3.3) |
| *Pregnancy duration* | | | | | | |
| 1st trimester | 27 | (24.5) | 20 | (19.6) | 47 | (22.1) |
| 2nd trimester | 29 | (26.1) | 37 | (36.3) | 66 | (31.0) |
| 3rd trimester | 55 | (49.5) | 45 | (44.1) | 100 | (46.9) |
| *Miscarriages* | | | | | | |
| No miscarriages | 86 | (77.5) | 84 | (82.4) | 170 | (79.8) |
| 1 miscarriage | 16 | (14.4) | 9 | (8.8) | 25 | (11.7) |
| 2 miscarriages | 7 | (6.3) | 8 | (7.8) | 15 | (7.0) |
| 3 or above miscarriages | 2 | (1.8) | 1 | (1.0) | 3 | (1.4) |

(continued)

**Table 17.1** (continued)

| | Working | | Non-working | | Total | |
|---|---|---|---|---|---|---|
| Variables | *n* | (%) | *n* | (%) | *n* | (%) |
| *Monthly income* | | | | | | |
| 10–30 thousand | 14 | (12.6) | 51 | (50) | 65 | (35.5) |
| 31–50 thousand | 58 | (52.3) | 28 | (27.5) | 86 | (40.4) |
| 51–1 lac | 17 | (15.3) | 19 | (18.6) | 36 | (16.9) |
| 1 lac and above | 22 | (19.8) | 4 | (3.9) | 26 | (12.2) |
| *Family system* | | | | | | |
| Nuclear | 46 | (41.4) | 38 | (37.3) | 84 | (39.4) |
| Joint | 65 | (58.6) | 64 | (62.7) | 129 | (60.6) |
| *Residence* | | | | | | |
| Rural | 24 | (21.6) | 44 | (43.1) | 68 | (31.9) |
| Urban | 87 | (78.4) | 58 | (56.9) | 145 | (68.1) |

Authors' estimation references

0.19, $^{**}p < 0.01$), and a non-significant relationship with other study variables. Moreover, results indicate that mental well-being has a significant positive relationship with social support ($r = 0.25$, $^{**}p < 0.01$) also its subscales.

Table 17.3 displays the effect of psychological distress, body image dissatisfaction also social support on mental well-being in working and non-working pregnant Pakistani women. In model 1, the $R^2$ value of 0.03 showed that body image described a 3% change in mental well-being with $F$ (1, 211) = 7.69, $p < 0.01$. The outcome shown that body image significantly and negatively predicted mental well-being ($\beta = -0.18$, $p < 0.01$). In model 2, the $R^2$ value of 0.07 shown that body image plus psychological distress described 7% change in the mental well-being with $F$ (2, 210)

**Table 17.2** Mean, standard deviation, alpha reliability, and and Correlation analysis for psychological distress, body image dissatisfaction, mental well-being, and social support

| Scales | *M* | *SD* | *α* | 1 | 2 | 3 | 4 | 5 | 6 | 7 |
|---|---|---|---|---|---|---|---|---|---|---|
| KPDS | 24.72 | 9.97 | 0.93 | 1 | 0.23** | −0.14** | −0.40** | −0.36** | −0.37** | −0.39** |
| BSQ | 42.61 | 18.98 | 0.94 | | 1 | −0.19** | −0.04 | −0.03 | −0.05 | −0.03 |
| WEMWBS | 52.76 | 12.92 | 0.95 | | | 1 | 0.25** | 0.21** | 0.23** | 0.26** |
| MSPSS | 59.11 | 17.33 | 0.96 | | | | 1 | 0.92** | 0.95** | 0.92** |
| Others | 19.81 | 6.21 | 0.89 | | | | | 1 | 0.84** | 0.74** |
| Family | 19.82 | 6.12 | 0.90 | | | | | | 1 | 0.81** |
| Friends | 19.48 | 6.31 | 0.92 | | | | | | | 1 |

Authors' estimation references: KPDS = XXXlucida psychological distress scale; BSQ = body shape questionnaire; WEMWEBS = warwick–edinburg mental well-being scale; MSPSS = multidimensional scale for perceived social support
$^{**}p < 0.01$

$= 8.09$, $p < 0.001$. The outcomes showed that body image dissatisfaction ($\beta = -0.23$, $p < 0.01$) plus psychological distress ($\beta = -0.19$, $p < 0.01$) negatively and significantly predicted mental well-being. The $\Delta R^2$ value of 0.04 discovered a 4% variation in the variance of model 1 and model 2 with $\Delta F\ (1, 210) = 8.22$, $p < 0.01$.

In model 3, the $R^2$ value of 0.11 showed that body image dissatisfaction plus social support elucidated 11% change in mental well-being with $F\ (3, 209) = 8.76$, $p < 0.001$. The outcomes revealed that body image dissatisfaction ($\beta = -0.22$, $p < 0.01$) negatively, but social support ($\beta = 0.21$, $p < 0.01$) positively and significantly predicted mental well-being. However, in model 3, in the presence of social support, psychological distress did not significantly predict mental well-being. The $\Delta R^2$ value of 0.04 discovered 4% change in the variance of model 2 and model 3 with $\Delta F$ (1, 209) $= 9.46$, $p < 0.01$.

Table 17.4 displays the effect of 16 years and above marriage duration, 31 to 40 years of age, and higher secondary education on mental well-being in working and non-working pregnant Pakistani women. The $R^2$ value of 0.13 shows that the predictors XXXlucidated 13% change in the outcome variable with $F\ (3, 209) = 10.68$, $p < 0.001$. The findings revealed that 16 years and above marriage duration significantly positively predicted mental well-being ($\beta = 0.13$, $p < 0.05$), 31 to 40 years of age strongly positively and significantly predicted mental well-being ($\beta = 0.26$, $p < 0.001$) and higher secondary education significantly negatively predicted mental well-being ($\beta = -0.15$, $p < 0.05$).

Table 17.5 showed that the model presented an interaction of body image and social support predicting mental well-being and was significant with $\{R^2 = 0.15$, $\Delta F\ (3, 209) = 12.90$, $p < 0.001\}$ and product of body image and social support

**Table 17.3** Hierarchical regression results for mental well-being

| Variable | *B* | 95% CI | | *SE B* | *β* | $R^2$ | $\Delta R^2$ |
|---|---|---|---|---|---|---|---|
| | | *LL* | *UL* | | | | |
| **Model 1** | | | | | | 0.03 | 0.03** |
| Constant | 47.32*** | 43.09 | 51.55 | 2.14 | | | |
| Body Image Dissatisfaction | −0.12** | −0.03 | −0.21 | 0.04 | −0.18** | | |
| **Model 2** | | | | | | 0.07 | 0.04** |
| Constant | 52.30*** | 46.91 | 57.69 | 2.73 | | | |
| Body Image Dissatisfaction | −0.15** | −0.06 | −0.24 | 0.04 | −0.23** | | |
| Psychological Distress | −0.25** | −0.42 | −0.07 | 0.08 | −0.19** | | |
| **Model 3** | | | | | | 0.11 | 0.04** |
| Constant | 40.06*** | 30.59 | 49.52 | 4.79 | | | |
| Body Image Dissatisfaction | −0.15** | −0.06 | −0.24 | 0.04 | −0.22** | | |
| Psychological Distress | −0.13 | −0.32 | 0.05 | 0.09 | −0.10 | | |
| Social Support | 0.16** | 0.05 | 0.26 | 0.05 | 0.21** | | |

Authors' estimation references: *Note* CI = confidence interval, *LL* = lower limit, *UL* = upper limit
***$p < 0.001$, **$p < 0.01$

**Table 17.4** Multiple regression coefficients of age, marriage duration, and education on mental well-being

| Variables | *B* | *SE* | *t* | *p* | 95%CI |
|---|---|---|---|---|---|
| Constant | 50.17 | 1.18 | 42.25 | 0.000 | [47.83, 52.51] |
| Marriage Duration (16 years or above) | 7.87 | 3.77 | 2.08 | 0.03 | [0.42, 15.31] |
| Age (31 to 40 years) | 6.78 | 1.70 | 3.97 | 0.000 | [3.41, 10.15] |
| Education (higher secondary) | −6.09 | 2.62 | −2.32 | 0.02 | [−11.26, −0.92] |

Authors' estimation references: *Note* CI = confidence interval
$^{***}p < 0.001$, $^{*}p < 0.05$

significantly and negatively predicted the mental well-being with (B = −0.008, $t = -3.63$, $p < 0.001$). This shows that social support negatively moderated the association between body image plus the mental well-being of pregnant working and non-working Pakistani females. The availability of higher social support weakens the negative association between body image and mental well-being. By receiving social support, pregnant women perceive their body shape, weight, and physical changes as less negative, increasing their psychological well-being.

The interaction plot perceives social support as the moderator in the relationship between body image and mental well-being (Fig. 17.2). The steep line in the above graph demonstrates that the high level of social support negatively moderated the link between body image dissatisfaction and mental well-being. This relationship is weakened because of the high level of social support.

Table 17.6 exhibited that the model presented an interaction of psychological distress and social support predicting mental well-being, which was significant ($B = 0.01$, $t = -1.76$, $p =$ n.s.). This revealed that social support did not moderate the link between psychological distress and the mental well-being of pregnant working and non-working Pakistani women.

Table 17.7 shows a significant mean difference between working and non-working pregnant women regarding psychological distress, body image dissatisfaction, and social support. Mean scores indicate that non-working women ($M = 26.32$, $t\,(211) =$

**Table 17.5** Summary of the results for moderating role of social support in the association of body image and mental well-being

| Predictors | B | SE | *p* |
|---|---|---|---|
| Constant | 15.27 | 6.58 | 0.02 |
| Body image Dissatisfaction | −0.67 | 0.15 | 0.000 |
| Social support | 0.52 | 0.10 | 0.000 |
| Body image dissatisfaction x Social Support | −0.008 | 0.00 | 0.000 |
| $R^2$ | 0.15 | | |

Authors' estimation references: $^{***}p < 0.001$, $^{*}p < 0.05$

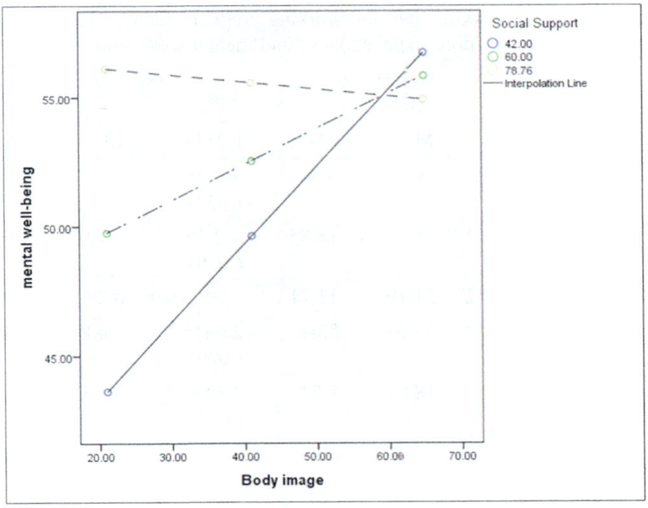


**Fig. 17.2** Moderation graph of social support in the relationship of body image dissatisfaction and mental well-being. *Source* Authors' Illustrations

**Table 17.6** Summary of the results for moderating role of social support in the association of psychological distress and mental well-being

| Predictors | B | SE | *p* |
|---|---|---|---|
| Constant | 55.46 | 7.46 | 0.00 |
| Psychological Distress | −0.48 | 0.26 | 0.06 |
| Social support | −0.02 | .12 | 0.89 |
| Social support x Psychological Distress | 0.01 | 0.00 | 0.08 |
| $R^2$ | 0.08 | | |

Authors' estimation references: $^{***}p < 0.001$, $^{*}p < 0.05$.

−2.26, $p < 0.05$) are in more psychological distress as compared to working women. Results also indicate that non-working women ($M = 45.78$, $t$ (211) = −2.35, $p <$ 0.05) are more concerned with their body image as compared to working women. Furthermore, the result indicates that working women ($M = 62.07$, $t$ (211) = 2.24, $p < 0.01$) perceived more social support as compared to no working women".

## 17.4 Discussion

Current research focused on examining the link between psychological distress, body image dissatisfaction, and mental well-being in working and non-working women during pregnancy and the role of social support. The finding indicates that psychological distress has a significant positive link with body image dissatisfaction and

**Table 17.7** Differences in working and non-working pregnant females regarding psychological distress, body image dissatisfaction, social support, and mental well-being

| | Working (111) | | Non-working (102) | | | 95% CI | | Cohen's *d* |
|---|---|---|---|---|---|---|---|---|
| Scales | M | SD | M | SD | t(211) | LL | UL | |
| KPDS | 23.25 | 10.13 | 26.32 | 9.58 | −2.26* (.024) | −5.74 | 0.69 | .003 |
| BSQ | 39.71 | 18.71 | 45.78 | 18.85 | −2.35* (.019) | −7.93 | 2.55 | .941 |
| WEMWBS | 54.20 | 12.52 | 51.19 | 13.21 | 1.71 (.089) | 0.28 | 7.36 | .238 |
| MSPSS | 62.07 | 18.64 | 55.89 | 5.64 | 2.64** (.009) | −4.88 | 4.71 | .339 |
| Sig. to others | 20.83 | 6.55 | 18.69 | 5.54 | 2.54* (.012) | −1.82 | 1.61 | .532 |
| Family | 20.71 | 6.51 | 18.64 | 5.79 | 2.24* (.026) | −2.04 | 1.34 | .347 |
| Friends | 20.52 | 6.60 | 18.35 | 15.22 | 2.54* (.012) | −1.38 | 2.10 | .399 |

Authors' estimation references: *Note.* KPDS = Kessler psychological distress scale; BSQ = body shape questionnaire; WEMWEBS = Warwick–Edinburg mental well-being scale; MSPSS = multi-dimensional scale for perceived social support
$p^* < 0.05, p^{**} < 0.01$

a negative relationship with mental well-being and social support along with its subscales (significant others, family, and friends). Furthermore, the finding indicates that body image dissatisfaction has a significant negative link with mental well-being plus a non-significant relationship with other study variables. Moreover, findings indicate that mental well-being has a significant positive link with social support and its sub-factors. Findings are supported by previous literature. Previous studies found a negative significant link between body image dissatisfaction and psychological well-being among women (Dotse & Asumeng, 2015). In Italy, research has been led by researchers Ruini et al. (2003) to understand the link between psychological distress and psychological well-being. According to the researcher, the degrees of psychological distress may necessarily cause Italian females to have lesser mental well-being scores.

This study also indicates that body image dissatisfaction and psychological distress are significant negative predictors, but social support significantly and positively predicted mental well-being. Existing literature also makes evident that the plateful role of social support among both working and non-working pregnant women has been explored more in a Western context, e.g., Milgrom et al. (2021) in Australia and Reichenheim et al. (2018) in Brazilian pertinent samples found the protective and benefiting part of social support concerning mental health. Khadija et al. (2021) found social support and its construct, i.e., tangible, emotional, informational, and social network support, as positive predictors of mental well-being in Pakistani pregnant women; Shahid et al. (2021) explored that social support enhances mental well-being by reducing psychological stressors in pregnant women, but there is a dearth of literature in Asian culture. So, for the present study, it was deemed appropriate to examine both working and non-working pregnant women to have an empirical insight into the phenomenon being studied.

Some researchers have established that pregnant females who are extra self-conscious and concerned about their body shape have more depression symptoms. It is possible that those ladies were extra concerned regarding their physique image and size because they expected to have more trouble dealing with it after giving birth (Silveira et al., 2015). Conditions of pregnancy, the emotion of parenthood, and the presence of others who constantly assist the mother may cause her to have far less need for a better environment throughout pregnancy (Fahami et al., 2018). Pregnancy is frequently viewed as a strength to improve body image satisfaction by reinforcing a sense of femininity and self-acceptance.

A study determined that body shape changes during pregnancy, the pregnant is happy regardless of the changes in body image, and education contributes to improving body shape by changing the behaviours reflecting the body image. Mean scores indicate that pregnant women have only mild concern with body shape. Thus, it might not negatively affect the mental well-being of pregnant females (Ardahan & Bayik, 2014). The levels weakened all throughout the pregnancy, and self-esteem was higher in the first trimester than in the advanced trimesters of pregnancy (Sema et al., 2015).

Besides this, the present study made a significant contribution by revealing that their mental well-being is strongly and significantly positively impacted in women aged between 31 and 40. However, in the sample women having a marriage duration of 16 years or above, their mental well-being is significantly positively impacted. However, women have higher secondary education, and their mental well-being is significantly negatively impacted. It means that the age range of 31 to 40 years is a strong and higher predictor of mental well-being in working and non-working Pakistani pregnant women than other under-study variables. This research was unique in revealing three significant demographic predictors of mental well-being in an underrepresented population in psychological science research. The stress-buffering postulate proposes that social support tends to eliminate or at least buffer the negative relationship between perceived stressors and their outcomes, which is vividly visible in the present study findings (Cohen & McKay, 2020).

Moderation test displays that social support has a moderating role in the link between body image dissatisfaction and mental well-being. According to a study, high levels of perceived social support are linked to healthier physical plus psychological well-being results. Particular mental health issues may perhaps be linked to a lack of social support, resulting in conflicting proof about the moderating role of stress in the link between social support plus psychological health results (Ioannou et al., 2019).

Social support, as a significant environmental resource in an individual's social life, influences an individual's physical plus psychological health and conceptual patterns. It is linked with the onset, growth, regulation, and also prevention of depression (Wang et al., 2014). A good social support system is able to protect a stressed person and has a mutually helpful function in preserving a positive emotional experience. Social support can facilitate adaptive behavioural responses to severe or long-lasting stressors by providing informational, emotional, and/or material resources. The stress-buffering model conceptualizes this interaction (Quinlan-Davidson et al., 2021). The strong and weak tie theory distinguished that in times of stress and depression, close friends, and family members are usually tied strongly to provide all kinds of support (Griffiths et al., 2011).

On the other hand, sometimes visible social support is perceived as weaker than invisible support. Especially in Pakistani society, people tend to trust and rely more on God than family members and friends; thus, the stress-buffering hypothesis may not be supported. Present findings did not accept the postulate that social support moderates between psychological distress plus mental well-being in pregnant women (Table 17.6). Hence, the stress-buffering postulate recommends that social support can buffer the negative influences of stress on well-being. Yet, it is worth mentioning that not all studies support this hypothesis. There are also some contrary results (Lakey & Lutz, 2016). A plausible explanation may be that the relationship is much more complex and depends upon numerous factors like religious beliefs, social and familial bonds, perception in terms of type, and the power of support by the pregnant women. There is also some evidence in support of the present finding, e.g., Krause (2015) found that religious involvement overwhelms and turns social support into a non-significant predictor of well-being, and Brown et al. (2021) established that social support does not universally perform as a buffer between distress and mental health. They, in pregnant women, look that social support did not attenuate the relationship between stress and mental health problems, including anxiety plus depression. Social ties could provide only supportive information, but all these have been found to generate negative thoughts and spread rumours with negative emotions during the pandemic COVID 19, which can further cause more preoccupation among pregnant women (Liu et al., 2021).

This study also discovered that there were considerable differences in psychological distress, body image dissatisfaction, and social support between working and non-working pregnant females. Findings specify that non-working females were extra psychologically distressed as compared to working females. Moreover, non-working females were extra concerned with their body image dissatisfaction as compared to working women. Furthermore, the result indicates that working females perceived extra social support than non-working women. Present findings should be seen in the social and familial context of the collectivist culture within which the study was conducted. Hence, working women experience more confidence due to financial autonomy, exposure to the work environment, and multi-tasking, which divert their minds positively, and they find less time to be worried about body shape dissatisfaction and psychological distress. Moreover, at home, they are surmised to receive more social support from family because their family members assume that a working woman is already burdened with job-related work, so she is treated more congenially than a non-working woman when pregnant. In Pakistani society, the role of a housewife is considered to be strongly associated with a woman who is responsible for all domestic matters. These domestic matters exert pressure on non-working women and incline them to be more worried about body shape dissatisfaction and cause them to experience high psychological distress. This situation leads pregnant non-working women to experience lesser social support from family.

Lack of support for pregnant women has been stated to cause caregiving and financial strain, leading to anxiety plus psychological distress in the female (Lancaster et al., 2010). The link between psychological distress, pregnancy outcome, plus social support is quite complicated. According to the findings, striking psychological resources, mainly social stability and social participation, which give instrumental and emotional support, are protective and secure the impact of life stress on a mother's emotional well-being (Glazier et al., 2004). Their findings matched the present study. Housewives emerged to be at the greatest risk of prenatal depression because of their frequent exposure to important elements like stressful life events, low education, dearth of social support, low income, immigrant status, and marital stress, all of which were independently related to prenatal depressive symptoms Matsuzaki et al., 2011).

This research chapter has some identifiable limitations, such as the low generalizability of findings due to the limited sample size, which consisted of 102 pregnant non-working and 111 working pregnant women. Including a larger sample size would improve the trustworthiness and generalizability of the findings. Some respondents were illiterate and had difficulty responding to and understanding the questions. It is suggested that in the future, only literate females will be included for more reliable results. Females from different trimesters were considered for the study. Most females were from the first and second trimesters. Body image dissatisfaction issues worsen in the third trimester in pregnant females. It is suggested that in upcoming investigations, only females from the third trimester be included for more reliable and new findings.

## 17.5 Conclusion

This chapter was aimed at determining the relationship between psychological distress, body image dissatisfaction, and mental well-being in pregnant working and non-working Pakistani women besides examining the moderating role of social support. The present study concluded that social support and 16 years or above marriage duration are positive predictors. Still, body image/shape and higher secondary education are significant negative key determinants of mental health during pregnancy. However, psychological distress does not significantly predict mental well-being. However, it is also concluded that 31 to 40 years is the age group, which is a strong and positive key determinant of mental health during pregnancy in working and non-working women. As a result, it is suggested that this concern be taken into account when providing pregnancy care and mental health planning for pregnant women. Furthermore, data on physical fluctuations throughout pregnancy and after childbirth must be provided to women to assist them better, consider variations in their bodies, and avoid the development of impractical expectations throughout pregnancy and after childbirth. According to the findings, social support has a high moderating influence on body image dissatisfaction and mental health. Other people's social support throughout pregnancy can benefit the pregnant mothers' mental health.

**Acknowledgements** A special thanks to hospital administrations for permitting this research and to all the patients who contributed in this research.

**Funding** This research received no external funding.

**Conflict of Interest** The authors declare no conflict of interest.

## References

Alipour, Z., Kheirabadi, G. R., Eslami, A. A., & Kazemi, A. (2018). Psychological profiles of risk for antenatal depression and anxiety in Iranian sociocultural context. *Journal of Education and Health Promotion, 7*(1), 160. https://doi.org/10.4103/jehp.jehp_201_17

Ardahan, M., & Bayik, A. B. (2014). Body image perception and the effectiveness of a body image education in pregnant housewives. *The Journal of Nursing Care, 3*(03), 2167–1168. https://doi.org/10.4172/2167-1168.1000163

Arvidsdotter, T., Marklund, B., Kylén, S., Taft, C., & Ekman, I. (2016). Understanding persons with psychological distress in primary health care. *Scandinavian Journal of Caring Sciences, 30*(4), 687–694. https://doi.org/10.1111/scs.12289

Bai, L., Arver, B., Johansson, H., Sandelin, K., Wickman, M., & Brandberg, Y. (2019). Body image problems in women with and without breast cancer 6–20 years after bilateral risk-reducing surgery—A prospective follow-up study. *The Breast, 44*, 120–127. https://doi.org/10.1016/j.breast.2019.01.013

Brown, H. K., Qazimi, E., Griffith, E., Wood, A. M., & Sheeran, P. (2021). The stress-buffering effect of social support on maternal mental health during the COVID-19 pandemic. *Psychological Medicine, 51*(2), 277–287.

Cash, T. F. (2017). Multidimensional body–self relations questionnaire (MBSRQ). In *Encyclopedia of feeding and eating disorders* (pp. 551–555). https://doi.org/10.1007/978-981-287-104-6_3

Cohen, S., & McKay, G. (2020) Social support, stress and the buffering hypothesis: A theoretical analysis. In *Handbook of psychology and health* (Vol. 4, pp. 253–267). Routledge.

Cooper, P. J., Taylor, M. J., Cooper, Z., & Fairbum, C. G. (1987). The development and validation of the Body Shape Questionnaire. *International Journal of Eating Disorders, 6*(4), 485–494. https://doi.org/10.1002/1098-108X(198707)6:4%3C485::AID-EAT2260060405%3E3.0.CO;2-O

Dotse, J. E., & Asumeng, M. (2015). Relationship between body image satisfaction and psychological well-being: The impact of Africentric values. *Journal of Social Science Studies, 2*(1), 320–342. https://doi.org/10.5296/jsss.v2i1.6843

Fahami, F., Amini-Abchuyeh, M., & Aghaei, A. (2018). The relationship between psychological well-being and body image in pregnant women. *Iranian Journal of Nursing and Midwifery Research, 23*(3), 167–171. https://doi.org/10.4103/ijnmr.IJNMR_178_16

Ginja, S., Coad, J., Bailey, E., Kendall, S., Goodenough, T., Nightingale, S., & Lingam, R. (2018). Associations between social support, mental well-being, self-efficacy and technology use in first-time antenatal women: Data from the BaBBLeS cohort study. *BMC Pregnancy and Childbirth, 18*(1), 1–11. https://doi.org/10.1186/s12884-018-2049-x

Glazier, R. H., Elgar, F. J., Goel, V., & Holzapfel, S. (2004). Stress, social support, and emotional distress in a community sample of pregnant women. *Journal of Psychosomatic Obstetrics & Gynecology, 25*(3–4), 247–255. https://doi.org/10.1080/01674820400024406

Griffiths, K. M., Crisp, D. A., Barney, L., & Reid, R. (2011). Seeking help for depression from family and friends: A qualitative analysis of perceived advantages and disadvantages. *BMC Psychiatry, 11*, 1–12.

Han, S., Brewis, A. A.,& Wutich, A. (2016). Body image mediates the depressive effects of weight gain in new mothers, particularly for women already obese: Evidence from the Norwegian Mother and Child Cohort Study. *BMC Public Health, 16*, 664. https://doi.org/10.1186/s12889-016-3363-8

Ioannou, M., Kassianos, A. P., & Symeou, M. (2019). Coping with depressive symptoms in young adults: Perceived social support protects against depressive symptoms only under moderate levels of stress. *Frontiers in Psychology, 9*, 2780. https://doi.org/10.3389/fpsyg.2018.02780

Izydorczyk, B., Truong Thi Khanh, H., Lizińczyk, S., Sitnik-Warchulska, K., Lipowska, M., & Gulbicka, A. (2020). Body dissatisfaction, restrictive, and bulimic behaviours among young women: A Polish-Japanese comparison. *Nutrients, 12*(3), 666. https://doi.org/10.3390/nu1203 0666

Izydorczyk, B., Walenista, W., Kamionka, A., Lizińczyk, S., & Ptak, M. (2021). Connections between perceived social support and the body image in the group of women with diastasis recti abdominis. *Frontiers in Psychology, 12*, Article 707775. https://doi.org/10.3389/fpsyg. 2021.707775

Keshwani, N., Mathur, S., & McLean, L. (2021). The impact of exercise therapy and abdominal binding in the management of diastasis recti abdominis in the early post-partum period: A pilot randomised controlled trial. *Physiotherapy Theory and Practice, 37*(9), 1018–1033.

Kessler, R. C., & Mroczek, D. (1994). *Final versions of our non-specific psychological distress scale*. University of Michigan. Survey Research Center of the Institute for Social Research.

Khadija, A., Atta, M., & Malik, N. I. (2021). Impact of social support on mental well-beingin pregnant women. *Pakistan Journal of Psychology, 52*(2), 41–53.

Kok, R., Avendano, M., & Mackenbach, J. (2020). The buffering effects of social support on the association between maternal education and psychological distress in pregnant women. *PLoS ONE, 15*(12), Article e0243711.

Krause, N. (2015). Trust in God and psychological distress: Exploring variations by religious affiliation. *Mental Health, Religion & Culture, 18*, 235–245.

Lakey, B., & Lutz, C. J. (2016). Social support and preventive and therapeutic interventions to promote mental health. In I. H. Gotlib & C. L. Hammen (Eds.), *Handbook of depression* (3rd ed., pp. 386–401). The Guilford Press.

Lancaster, C. A., Gold, K. J., Flynn, H. A., Yoo, H., Marcus, S. M., & Davis, M. M. (2010). Risk factors for depressive symptoms during pregnancy: A systematic review. *American Journal of Obstetrics and Gynecology, 202*, 5–14. https://doi.org/10.1016/j.ajog.2009.09.007

Linde, K., Lehnig, F., Nagl, M., Stepan, H., & Kerstingal, K. (2022). Course and prediction of body image dissatisfaction during pregnancy: A prospective study. *BMC Pregnancy and Childbirth, 22*, 719.https://doi.org/10.1186/s12884-022-05050-x

Linde, K., Lehnig, F., Treml, J., Nagl, M., Stepan, H., & Kersting, A. (2024). The trajectory of body image dissatisfaction during pregnancy and postpartum and its relationship to Body-Mass-Index. *PLoS ONE, E19*(8), e0309396. https://doi.org/10.1371/journal.pone.0309396

Liu, C., Huang, N., Fu, M., Zhang, H., Feng, X. L., & Guo, J. (2021). Relationship between risk perception, social support, and mental health among general Chinese population during the CoViD-19 pandemic. *Risk Management and Healthcare Policy, 14*, 1843–1853. https://doi.org/ 10.2147/RMHP.S302521

Matsuzaki, M., Haruna, M., Ota, E., Murayama, R., & Murashima, S. (2011). Factors related to the continuation of employment during pregnancy among Japanese women. *Japan Journal of Nursing Science, 8*(2), 153–162. https://doi.org/10.1111/j.1742-7924.2010.00169.x

Milgrom, J., Holt, C. J., Gemmill, A. W., Ericksen, J., Leigh, B., & Buist, A. E. (2021). Psychosocial factors associated with depressive symptoms during pregnancy in Australian women. *Journal of Affective Disorders, 284*, 94–101.

Quinlan-Davidson, M., Kiss, L., Devakumar, D., Cortina-Borja, M., Eisner, M., Tourinho Peres, M. F. (2021). The role of social support in reducing the impact of violence on adolescents' mental health in São Paulo, Brazil. *PLoS ONE, 16*(10), e0258036. https://doi.org/10.1371/journal.pone.0258036

Reichenheim, M. E., Moraes, C. L., Lopes, C. S., & Lobato, G. (2018). Social support protects against the negative effects of partner violence on mental health among Brazilian pregnant women. *PLoS ONE, 13*(12), Article e0209462.

Ruini, C., Ottolini, F., Rafanelli, C., Tossani, E., Ryff, C. D., Fava, G. A. (2003). The relationship of psychological well-being to distress and personality. *Psychotherapy and Psychosomatics, 72*(5), 268–275. https://doi.org/10.1159/000071898

Sema, I., Bulent, K., Mehmet, N., Askin, A. (2015). Body image perception and self-esteem during pregnancy. *International Journal of Women Health and Reproductive Sciences, 3*(4), 196–200. https://doi.org/10.15296/ijwhr.2015.41

Shahid, A., Malik, N. I., Shahid, F., Ullah, I., & Abbass, Z. (2021). Psychosocial predictors of mental health among pregnant women. *Perspectives in Psychiatric Care, 58*(3), 1071–1076. https://doi.org/10.1111/ppc.12900

Silveira, M. L., Ertel, K. A., Dole, N., & Chasan-Taber, L. (2015). The role of body image in prenatal and post-partum depression: A critical review of the literature. *Archives of Women's Mental Health, 18*(3), 409–421. https://doi.org/10.1007/s00737-015-0525-0

Stewart-Brown, S., Tennant, A., Tennant, R., Platt, S., Parkinson, J., & Weich, S. (2009). Internal construct validity of the Warwick-Edinburgh mental well-being scale (WEMWBS): A Rasch analysis using data from the Scottish health education population survey. *Health and Quality of Life Outcomes, 7*(1), 1–8. https://doi.org/10.1186/1477-7525-7-15

Thomas, H. N., Hamm, M., Borrero, S., Hess, R., & Thurston, R. C. (2019). Body image, attractiveness, and sexual satisfaction among midlife women: A qualitative study. *Journal of Women's Health, 28*(1), 100–106. https://doi.org/10.1089/jwh.2018.7107

Tutkuviene, J., Juskaite, A., Katinaite, J., Silove, S., Drasutis, J., Sargautyte, R., & Drasutiene, G. (2018). Body image issues in Lithuanian females before and during pregnancy. *Anthropologischer Anzeiger; Bericht Uber die Biologisch-Anthropologische Literatur, 75*(1), 9–17. https://doi.org/10.1127/anthranz/2018/0779

Wang, X., Cai, L., Qian, J., & Peng, J. (2014). Social support moderates stress effects on depression. *International Journal of Mental Health Systems, 8*(1), 1–5. https://doi.org/10.1186/1752-4458-8-41

Watson-Singleton, N. N. (2017). Strong Black woman schema and psychological distress: The mediating role of perceived emotional support. *Journal of Black Psychology, 43*(8), 778–788. https://doi.org/10.1177/0095798417732414

Xiao, H., Zhang, Y., Kong, D., Li, S., & Yang, N. (2020) The effects of social support on sleep quality of medical staff treating patients with coronavirus disease 2019 (COVID-19) in January and February 2020 in China. *Medical Science Monitor: International Medical Journal of Experimental and Clinical Research, 26*, e9235491–e9235498. https://doi.org/10.12659/MSM.923549

Zielinski, R., Low, L. K., Smith, A. R., & Miller, J. M. (2017). Body after baby: A pilot survey of genital body image and sexual esteem following vaginal birth. *International Journal of Women's Health, 9*, 189–198. https://doi.org/10.2147/IJWH.S123051

Zimet, G. D., Dahlem, N. W., Zimet, S. G., & Farley, G. K. (1988). The multi-dimensional scale of perceived social support. *Journal of Personality Assessment, 52*(1), 30–41. https://doi.org/10.1207/s15327752jpa5201_2

9789819523207